Immunology
of the
Bacterial Cell Envelope

Immunology of the Bacterial Cell Envelope

Edited by
D. E. S. Stewart-Tull
Department of Microbiology
University of Glasgow
and
M. Davies
Department of Pathology
University of Bristol

A Wiley-Interscience Publication

JOHN WILEY & SONS
Chichester · New York · Brisbane · Toronto · Singapore

Library of Congress Cataloging in Publication Data
Main entry under title:

Immunology of the bacterial cell envelope.

'A Wiley – Interscience publication.'
Includes index.
1. Bacterial cell walls.   2. Immunology.
I. Stewart-Tull, D. E. S.(Duncan E. S.)
II. Davies, M. (Martin), 1932 –
[DNLM: 1. Bacterial—cytology.   2. Bacteria—immunology. QW 4 133]
QR77.3.146   1985   616'.014   84-20993

ISBN 0 471 90552 6

British Library Cataloguing in Publication Data:
Immunology of the bacterial cell envelope.
1. Bacteria   2. Cell membranes
3. Immunology
I. Stewart-Tull, D. E. S.   II. Davies, M.
589.9'0875   QR77

ISBN 0 471 90552 6

Phototypeset by Dobbie Typesetting Service, Plymouth, Devon
Printed by BAS Printers Ltd, Over Wallop, Hampshire

Contents

v

Preface

Originally, the publishers suggested that the review on the *Immunology of Peptidoglycans* in Annual Reviews of Microbiology could be extended. However, in view of the rapid advances in immunology, especially in immunochemistry, immunosuppression and immunopotentiation, it seemed timely to gather together available information on the immunological activities of bacterial cell surface components. The aim was to complement existing volumes dealing with the chemistry of surface structures, but sufficient chemical data has been provided to acquaint the non-chemist with the subject.

Within the limits of pagination, it was necessary to be selective on the choice of topics. Some readers may consider that bacterial flagella and immunochemistry of lipopolysaccharides are major omissions, whereas others may agree these have been covered adequately in existing textbooks.

The task for an individual to write a comprehensive encyclopaedic volume would be immense and it seemed obvious to call on research workers with particular knowledge. Their contributions fall into one of two categories; those dealing with (1) the innate antigenicity of the component and (2) the effect on the mammalian immune response. A small degree of overlap between chapters has been allowed to provide continuity and expression of individual viewpoints.

The capacity of a bacterial organism to produce disease is conditioned by entry into the host, multiplication *in vivo*, interference with host defence and immune mechanisms and damage to the host. Some surface components are important in adherence of organisms to host surfaces (e.g. *Escherichia coli* pili, *Streptococcus pyogenes* lipoteichoic acid), interference with host defences (e.g. *Escherichia coli* and *Neisseria gonorrhoeae* outer membrane proteins), toxicity (e.g. Gram-negative lipopolysaccharides) and long-term persistence in tissues (e.g. streptococcal peptidoglycan in arthritis). On the other hand, bacterial surface components are antigens in whole cell vaccines and with the new development of sub-cellular vaccines, it is important to know their effect on the host immune system.

Elegant studies on the immunochemistry of cell envelope constituents followed the classical work of Michael Heidelberger and his colleagues on capsular antigens of *Streptococcus pneumoniae*. In student days he mixed horse anti-pneumococcal polysaccharide antiserum and polysaccharide to form a visible precipitate, as a demonstration during a lecture. The vivid memory remains and it was a great pleasure to receive the contribution from this pioneer immunologist some twenty-eight years after his retirement.

Our thanks are due to Dr Stephen Thornton for his great enthusiasm in the initial planning of the book, to all the contributors and to our families for their patience.

D. E. Stewart-Tull

M. Davies

Contributors

Frank W. Chorpenning *Department of Microbiology, The Ohio State University, 484 West 12th Avenue, Columbus, OH 43210, USA*

Martin Davies *Reproductive Immunology Research Group, Department of Pathology, The Medical School, University of Bristol, Bristol, BS8 1TD, UK*

James P. Duguid *Bacteriology Department, University of Dundee Medical School, Ninewells Hospital, Dundee, UK*

Robert A. Eisenberg *Department of Medicine, School of Medicine, University of North Carolina at Chapel Hill, Chapel Hill, NC 27514, USA*

Ronald E. Esser *Departments of Microbiology and Immunology, School of Medicine, University of North Carolina at Chapel Hill, Chapel Hill, NC 27514, USA*

John H. Freer *Department of Microbiology, Alexander Stone Building, University of Glasgow, Garscube Estate, Bearsden, Glasgow G61 1QH, UK*

Michael Heidelberger *New York University Medical Center School of Medicine, 550 First Avenue, New York, NY 10016, USA*

Berno Heymer *Universität Ulm, Abteilung für Pathologie, 7900 Ulm/Donau, Oberer Eselsberg, FRG*

Timo K. Korhonen *Department of General Microbiology, University of Helsinki, Mannerheimintie 172, SF-00280, Helsinki 28, Finland*

Shozo Kotani *Department of Microbiology and Oral Microbiology, Osaka University Dental School, 1-8 Yamadaoka, Suita, Osaka 565, Japan*

Christine McCartney   *Department of Bacteriology and Immunology, The Royal Infirmary, Glasgow, G4 0SF, UK*

Auli Pere   *Department of Microbiology, University of Helsinki, Mannerheimintie 172, SF-00280, Helsinki 28, Finland*

Mikael Rhen   *Department of Microbiology, University of Helsinki, Mannerheimintie 172, SF-00280, Helsinki 28, Finland*

Karl H. Schleifer   *Lehrstuhl für Mikrobiologie, Technische Universität München, Arcisstrasse 21, 8000 Munich 2, FRG*

John H. Schwab   *Departments of Microbiology and Immunology, School of Medicine, University of North Carolina at Chapel Hill, Chapel Hill, NC 27514, USA*

Peter H. Seidl   *Lehrstuhl für Mikrobiologie, Technische Universität München, Arcisstrasse 21, 8000 Munich 2, FRG*

Cyril J. Smyth   *Department of Microbiology, Moyne Institute, Trinity College, Dublin 2, Ireland*

Duncan E. S. Stewart-Tull   *Department of Microbiology, Alexander Stone Building, University of Glasgow, Garscube Estate, Bearsden, Glasgow, G61 1QH, UK*

Haruhiko Takada   *Department of Microbiology and Oral Microbiology, Osaka University Dental School, 1-8 Yamadaoka, Suita, Osaka 565, Japan*

Vuokko Väisänen-Rhen   *Department of General Microbiology, University of Helsinki, Mannerheimintie 172, SF-00280, Helsinki 28, Finland*

Alastair C. Wardlaw   *Department of Microbiology, University of Glasgow, Glasgow G12 8QQ, UK*

Immunology of the Bacterial Cell Envelope
Edited by D. E. S. Stewart-Tull and M. Davies
© 1985 John Wiley & Sons Ltd.

CHAPTER 1

Historical Immunochemical Survey of Pneumococcal Polysaccharides

Michael Heidelberger
*New York University Medical Center, School of Medicine,
550 First Avenue, New York, NY 10016, USA*

It was Pasteur, in 1861, who first reported the formation of a gum from microorganisms, 'petites globules réunis en chapelet', growing in solutions of sucrose. Another instance was added by Buchanan (1909), and in 1921 Toenniessen described polysaccharide material from an encapsulated pathogenic Friedländer's bacillus (*Klebsiella* K2), as did also Kramár in 1922. None of these microbiologists appears to have looked for serological activity, and so the significance of these findings remained obscure.

After a serological study had led Dochez and Gillespie (1913) to the concept of three 'fixed types' of pneumococcus, types PnI, PnII and PnIII, each with its individual specificity, Dochez and Avery (1917) discovered a heat-stable 'soluble specific substance' (SSS) in fluid cultures of each of these types: a substance which precipitated specifically only in anti-Pn sera raised in animals injected with pneumococcus of the homologous type. SSS was also found in the blood of patients with type I, II, or III pneumococcal septicaemia. Owing to this solubility and diffusibility it was anticipated that SSS would also appear in the urine of septicaemic cases. Accordingly, Dochez and Avery requested that a sample from a suitable case of type II pneumonia be sent from the ward to their laboratory. Type II antiserum was added and no precipitation occurred. The two brilliant investigators sat looking glumly at the clear fluid and wondering in what way their intuition had failed them. Finally, one of them got up and read the name on the sample bottle. It was from the wrong patient! The proper specimen was soon obtained and, as had been hoped, showed rapid precipitation.

Dochez had gone on to the College of Physicians and Surgeons of Columbia University when Avery and I started to characterize the soluble specific substance (SSS). We began with PnII because Avery said PnI had capsules which were too small. Although type III had the largest, it was considered a streptococcus, not pneumococcus, by some workers. We concentrated large volumes of autolysed meat-infusion broth cultures of PnII on a huge water-bath under a hood. The concentrate from about 300 litres was precipitated with sufficient alcohol to give a three-layer separation when centrifuged. Most of the SSS was in the middle gray, gummy layer and the other layers were discarded. As a meticulous microbiologist, Avery was horrified at some of my techniques: the simplest and cheapest way to free the suspension of the middle layer from large amounts of glycogen (mainly from the meat-infusion broth) was to spit liberally into it, stir well, and let the mixture stand for a while. Also, for location of serologically active fractions I chose a bottle of old anti-PnII that was half full of mould but still had enough antibody left to give immediate precipitin reactions. He was also dubious about centrifuging slow and weakly turbid precipitates but I convinced him of its utility by adding control tubes.

We were soon astonished to find less and less nitrogen in our most active fractions, since up to that time serological activity was considered to be a property solely of proteins. Avery said: 'Could it be a carbohydrate?' So I boiled a small portion with acid and got a strong test for a reducing sugar which turned out to be glucose. We also noted an acidic component (Heidelberger and Avery, 1923, 1924) which was later shown to be D-glucuronic acid, and L-rhamnose was entirely missed (Stacey, 1947; Butler and Stacey, 1955). Our own work was with small quantities of material, before the days of paper or column chromatography, when the only way to identify a sugar was actual isolation in crystalline form or as a known derivative. Only recently has the structure of SSS-II been shown rigorously to be (Kenne *et al.*, 1975):

$$
\left[
\begin{array}{l}
\rightarrow 3)\alpha\text{L-Rham}(1\rightarrow3)\alpha\text{L-Rham}(1\rightarrow3)\beta\text{L-Rham}(1\rightarrow4)\beta\text{D-Glc}(1\rightarrow \\
\qquad\qquad\qquad\qquad (2) \\
\qquad\qquad\qquad\qquad \uparrow \\
\alpha\text{D-GlcA}(1\rightarrow6)\alpha\text{D-Glc}(1)
\end{array}
\right]_n
$$

While the study of SSS-II, and of SSS-III which followed it, was proceeding we were also alert to the functions of SSS and other constituents of pneumococci. SSS was recognized as the capsular polysaccharide of pneumococci and by others also as the principal antigen giving rise to the protective action of type-specific antisera (Avery and Heidelberger, 1923, 1925; Zozaya *et al.*, 1930; Heidelberger *et al.*, 1930).

The soluble specific substance type III rapidly revealed differences from SSS-II. When SSS-III was precipitated from aqueous solution with alcohol, it separated as dense fibres; SSS-II deviated the plane of polarized light to the right but SSS-III was laevorotatory and yielded an insoluble free acid. At this point we were joined by Walther F. Goebel who, like me, had been a 'post-doc' for a year with Richard Willstätter. We soon identified glucose again as a component of SSS-III, as well as a derivative of glucuronic acid (Heidelberger *et al.*, 1925) which turned out to be a new type of sugar acid which we called an aldobionic acid (Heidelberger and Goebel, 1926, 1927) now termed aldobiouronic acid. Such acid disaccharides were later recognized as major components of hemicelluloses: existing around the world in enormous megatonnage, but first discovered in a few grams of SSS-III. The aldobiouronic acid of SSS-III is cellobiouronic acid (Hotchkiss and Goebel, 1937) and SSS-III is a polymeric salt of this acid in which the repeating units are joined through $\beta(1\rightarrow3)$ linkages: (Reeves and Goebel, 1941):

$$\text{$\dashv$3)βD-GlcA(1$\rightarrow$4)βD-Glc(1$\vdash_{\overline{n}}$}$$

SSS-I turned out to be very different from the nitrogen-free SSS-II and SSS-III. A strong acid and a weak base, SSS-I had about 5% of nitrogen, one-half of which was eliminated by HNO_2 with the simultaneous appearance of reducing sugars and disappearance of precipitation in anti-PnI. Hydrolysis with aqueous acids led to unmanageable purple tars, but galacturonic acid was recognized as the acidic component (Heidelberger *et al.*, 1925). After some puzzling data on the part of others, an 'A substance' (Pappenheimer and Enders, 1933) was isolated from PnI without the use of alkali: 'A substance' precipitated anti-PnI rabbit sera more completely than did SSS-I as originally prepared. Simultaneously, Avery and Goebel (1933) showed that 'native' SSS-I contained a labile *O*-acetyl group easily removed by alkali, so that SSS-I as first isolated was actually a deacetylated derivative. (For quantitative data on the effect of this on specific precipitation, see Heidelberger *et al.*, 1936, 1950). A structure,

$$\text{$\dashv$3)-2,4,6-trideoxy-4-amino$-\alpha$D-GalNHAc(1$\rightarrow$4)αD-GalA(1$\rightarrow$3)αD-GalA(1$\vdash_{\overline{n}}$}$$

has been proposed for SSS-I (Lindberg *et al.*, 1980), but it does not give the location of the immunologically important *O*-acetyl group (see also Guy *et al.*, 1967).

Since SSS-I, -II, and -III are chemically different, this provided a sound basis for the understanding of serological type-specificity among pneumococci. Similar findings with other families of microorganisms followed in other laboratories and more carbohydrate chemists, microbiologists, and immunologists became interested in this field of study. (For a recent review see Kenne and Lindberg, 1983). But polysaccharides are not the '*whole* secret of bacterial specificity' (see Heidelberger, 1977) as Rebecca Lancefield (1928) convincingly showed with the type-specific 'M proteins' of *Streptococcus haemolyticus*, group A, although it has a group-specific polysaccharide analogous to that of pneumococcus.

Early in the study of pneumococci Avery (1915) had found atypical PnII strains that were 'weakly and incompletely' agglutinated by anti-PnII sera. Many cases of pneumonia were caused by strains which he designated IIA and IIB; these were later given type numbers V and VI. I wondered what made SSS-V and SSS-VI different from SSS-II, and, also, what similarities they showed as members of type II. Accordingly, when I 'retired' to Selman A. Waksman's Institute of Microbiology at Rutgers University in 1955, I sent supplies of SSS-II and SSS-V to my friend Maurice Stacey in Birmingham, reserving SSS-VI for Paul A. Rebers and myself. The immunochemistry of SSS-II, -V and -VI developed rapidly and unexpectedly: only the principal findings are touched upon here. SSS-II has already been discussed. Stacey had assigned SSS-V to a brilliant young member of his department, S. A. Barker, who found that it contained two amino sugars new to natural products (Barker *et al.*, 1966). One, 2-amino-2,6-dideoxy–L-talopyranose, they called 'pneumosamine' and the other was 2-amino-2,6-dideoxy–L-galactopyranose. Both were probably present in SSS-V as *N*-acetyl derivatives. I had also noted that substances which cross-reacted strongly with anti-PnII, because of their lateral non-reducing end-groups of D-glucuronic acid, usually precipitated anti-PnV less strongly. This suggested that SSS-V might have fewer such end-groups of GlcA than SSS-II, or that in SSS-V the GlcA might be linked 1,2-(Heidelberger, 1962). The latter alternative was the actual one and it explained what we needed to know. A tentative structure has been proposed for SSS-V (cited in Kenne and Lindberg, 1983). SSS-VI not only showed an unexpected relationship to the teichoic acids (Baddiley, 1970) but became the first polysaccharide in which the phosphorus-free repeating unit could be isolated practically quantitatively and in crystalline form (Rebers and Heidelberger, 1961). Its rather weak relationship to SSS-II is mediated by its content of $\alpha(1,3)$-linked L-rhamnose.

In these days of radioimmunological assays, which measure nanograms and picograms of antibodies with reasonable accuracy, it is difficult to imagine the crudity of what were called 'quantitative' methods in immunology up to the early 1930s. With the available relative dilution methods, often carried out all the way down the line with the same pipette, it was possible to estimate that one antiserum might be roughly twice as strong as another, but there was no indication of their actual antibody content. Fundamental questions such as were antibodies actually globulins or merely associated with globulins, or was complement a substance or a colloidal state of fresh serum, were impossible to answer.

Strangely enough microanalytical chemical methods had never been effectively used. Rigorous application of these, with the help of Forrest E. Kendall, became a priority after my appointment at Columbia's College of Physicians and Surgeons as the first full-time chemist in a department of medicine. For the first time nitrogen-free antigens, pneumococcal SSS-II and SSS-III were available, also antibodies partially purified by Felton's (1925) simple method. Complete details will be found in Heidelberger and Kendall, 1929, 1935a,b). This unforeseen use of bacterial capsular polysaccharides made it possible to measure precipitins in units of weight, to extend the method to anti-protein sera, and eventually to isolate analytically pure antibody, proving that antibodies were actually globulins (Heidelberger and Kabat, 1938), and providing a firm basis for the development of immunology. (Additional details and references in Heidelberger, 1979.)

Although mice and rabbits could be immunized with killed pneumococci against infection by pneumococcus, the whole cells proved too toxic for effective use in man. Therefore the use of purified capsular polysaccharides, the immunodominant antigens of type specificity, were tried since these had been found to be immunogenic in mice and man. Ekwurzel *et al.* (1938) conducted a massive experiment with the Civilian Conservation Corps that went 'agley'. The young people's outdoor activities were so healthful that the vaccinated and unvaccinated camps failed to show great differences. Another opportunity came when the Surgeon General of the US Army asked me to see what could be done about a well-studied epidemic that had been going on for several years at an aviation camp during World War II. Although the fatalities were low there was inconvenience in teaching how to kill. As a preliminary we immunized volunteer medical students in order to find the optimal dosage, and we measured the formation of antibodies (Heidelberger *et al.*, 1946). Helped by a paper of Wood (1941) which showed that rats could be cured of an already established infection of PnI by about three times the blood concentration of a rabbit anti-PnI as the average antibody formed by the volunteers, I recommended that prevention be tried with the next incoming population. About 8000 trainees were injected subcutaneously with about 70 μg each of Pn SSS-I, -II, -V, and -VII, these being the polysaccharides of the types that had been responsible for roughly 60% of the infections up to that time. A parallel line of entrants was injected with saline alone. Within two weeks there were no more cases of the types injected among the immunized group. It seemed puzzling at first that the non-immunized group showed about a 50% reduction in pneumonias due to these four types but it was found that the immunized trainees had ceased to be carriers of these types and so the unimmunized half was exposed to one-half as many contacts with them. Also, the number of cases due to pneumococcal types not immunized against was nearly equal in both groups (MacLeod *et al.* 1945). Thanks to the fine field work of Colin M. MacLeod and his associates, this was one of the best conducted epidemiological studies in medical history. It showed that once the infecting types of pneumococci are known, an epidemic of pneumococcal pneumonia can be stopped in a closed population within two weeks. Vaccines are now commercially available with 14–15 type-specific pneumococcal polysaccharides (Austrian *et al.*, 1976) and a second generation with 23 types is expected to be released in July 1983 (Robbins *et al.*, 1983). With these there appear to be no complications caused by the 'competition of antigens' that worried the early immunologists who were using proteins.

The study of cross-reactions of polysaccharides among and between types and families of microorganisms has been a fruitful source of information relating chemical structures to immunological specificity (see, for example, Heidelberger and Nimmich, 1976, and subsequent papers). Another instance: while I was at the College of Physicians and Surgeons I happened to read two papers in the *Journal of the American Chemical Society* by Kenyon and his colleagues on oxidized cotton (Unruh and Kenyon, 1942; Yackel and Kenyon, 1942). In great excitement I asked for samples, realizing that Kenyon's group by, oxidizing some of the 6-CH_2OH positions to -COOH, had converted cotton into an immunologically active polysaccharide which should precipitate anti-PnIII and -VIII sera. The structure of SSS-VIII is (Jones and Perry, 1957):

$$\rightarrow 4)\beta\text{D-GlcA}(1\rightarrow4)\beta\text{D-Glc}(1\rightarrow4)\alpha\text{D-Glc}(1\rightarrow4)\alpha\text{D-Gal}(1\rightarrow_{\overline{n}}$$

Tests on the dissolved and neutralized samples verified the prediction (Heidelberger and Hobby, 1942). At luncheon one day in the faculty dining room I recounted this story and found that the surgeons were using small, sterile, oxidized cotton pads as a haemostat and packing that could be left in a wound because it would be slowly neutralized and solubilized by the body fluids and washed away. Analogy with the solubility and elimination of SSS-II observed by Dochez and Avery 25 years before prompted an offer to tell the surgeons just how long it would take patients to dispose of the pads. This was entertainingly done by precipitating anti-PnIII or -VIII serum with a few drops of the subject's serum or neutralized urine, so that one could tell almost to the hour when the last traces of oxidized cotton were gone. An accidentally discovered cross-reaction was thus almost immediately put to practical use.

In the foregoing pages I have tried to show the increased knowledge of microbiology gained by the discovery of the specific soluble substances of pneumococcus and the theoretical and practical results that followed. I hope that I have succeeded.

REFERENCES

Austrian, R., Douglas, R. M., Schiffman, G., Coetzee, A. M., Koornhof, H. J., Hayden-Smith, S., and Reid, R. D. W. (1976). Prevention of pneumococcal pneumonia by vaccination. *Trans. Assoc. Am. Physicians*, **89**, 184–194.

Avery, O. T. (1915). A further study on the biologic classification of pneumococci. *J. Exp. Med.*, **22**, 804–819.

Avery, O. T., and Goebel, W. F. (1933). Isolation and properties of the acetyl polysaccharide of Pneumococcus type I. *J. Exp. Med.*, **58**, 731–754.

Avery, O. T., and Heidelberger, M. (1923). Immunological relationships of cell constituents of pneumococcus. *J. Exp. Med.*, **38**, 81–85.

Avery, O. T., and Heidelberger, M. (1925). Immunological relationships of cell constituents of pneumococcus. II. *J. Exp. Med.*, **42**, 367–376.

Baddiley, J. (1970). Structure, biosynthesis and function of teichoic acids. *Acc. Chem. Res.*, **3**, 98–105.

Barker, S. A., Bick, S. M., Brimacombe, J. S., How, M. J., and Stacey, M. (1966). Structural studies on the capsular polysaccharide of pneumococcus type V. *Carbohydr. Res.*, **2**, 224–233.

Buchanan, R. E. (1909). The gum produced by *Bacillus radicicola*. *Zentralbl. Bakteriol.*, *Abt. 2*, **22**, 371–396.

Butler, K., and Stacey, M. Immunopolysaccharides. IV. Structural studies on the type II Pneumococcus polysaccharide. *J. Chem. Soc.*, **1955**, 1537–1541.

Dochez, A. R., and Avery, O. T. (1917). Elaboration of specific soluble substance by pneumococcus during growth. *J. Exp. Med.*, **26**, 477–493.

Dochez, A. R., and Gillespie, L. J. (1913). Biologic classification of pneumococci by means of immunity reactions. *J. Am. Med. Assoc.*, **61**, 727–730.

Ekwurzel, G. M., Simmons, J. S., Dublin, L. I., and Felton, L. D. (1938). Studies on immunizing substances in pneumococci. VIII: Report on field tests to determine the prophylactic value of a pneumococcus antigen. *Public Health Rep. USPHS*, **53**, 1877–1893.

Felton, L. D. (1925). The protective substance in antipneumococcic serum. I. Type I. *J. Infect. Dis.*, **37**, 199–224.

Guy, R. C. E., How, M. J., Heidelberger, M., and Stacey, M. (1967). Capsular polysaccharide of Pneumococcus type 1. *J. Biol. Chem.*, **242**, 5106–5111.

Heidelberger, M. (1962). Immunochemistry of pneumococcal types II, V, and VI. IV. Cross-reactions of type V antipneumococcal sera and their bearing on the relation between types II and V. *Arch. Biochem. Biophys. Suppl.*, **1**, 169–173.

Heidelberger, M. (1977). A 'pure' organic chemist's downward path. Chapter 1. *Annu. Rev. Microbiol.*, **29**, 1–12.

Heidelberger, M. (1979). A 'pure' organic chemist's downward path. Chapter 2. The years at P and S. *Annu. Rev. Biochem.*, **48**, 1–21.

Heidelberger, M., and Avery, O. T. (1923). The soluble specific substance of Pneumococcus. *J. Exp. Med.*, **38**, 73–79.

Heidelberger, M., and Avery, O. T. (1924). The soluble specific substance of Pneumococcus. Second paper. *J. Exp. Med.*, **40**, 301–316.

Heidelberger, M., and Goebel, W. F. (1926). On the nature of the specific polysaccharide of type III Pneumococcus. *J. Biol. Chem.*, **70**, 613–623.

Heidelberger, M., and Goebel, W. F. (1927). On the chemical nature of the aldobionic acid from the specific polysaccharide of type III Pneumococcus. *J. Biol. Chem.*, **74**, 613–618.

Heidelberger, M., and Hobby, G. L. (1942). Oxidized cotton, an immunologically specific polysaccharide. *Proc. Natl. Acad. Sci. USA*, **28**, 516–518.

Heidelberger, M., and Kabat, E. A. (1938). Quantitative studies on antibody purification. II. Dissociation of antibody from pneumococcus specific precipitates and specifically agglutinated pneumococci. *J. Exp. Med.*, **67**, 181–199.

Heidelberger, M., and Kendall, F. E. (1929). Quantitative study of the precipitin reaction between type III pneumococcus polysaccharide and purified homologous antibody. *J. Exp. Med.*, **50**, 809–823.

Heidelberger, M., and Kendall, F. E. (1935a). Precipitation reaction between type III pneumococcal polysaccharide and homologous antibody. II. Conditions for quantitative precipitation of antibody in horse sera. *J. Exp. Med.*, **61**, 559–562.

Heidelberger, M., and Kendall, F. E. (1935b). Precipitation reaction between type III pneumococcal polysaccharide and homologous antibody. III. Quantitative study and theory of the reaction mechanism. *J. Exp. Med.*, **61**, 563–591.

Heidelberger, M., and Nimmich, W. (1976). Immunochemical relationships between bacteria belonging to two separate families: pneumococci and *Klebsiella*. *Immunochemistry*, **13**, 67–80.

Heidelberger, M., Goebel, W. F., and Avery, O. T. (1925). The soluble specific substance of Pneumococcus. Third paper. *J. Exp. Med.*, **42**, 727–745.

Heidelberger, M., Sia, R. H. P., and Kendall, F. E. (1930). Specific precipitation and mouse protection in type I antipneumococcus sera. *J. Exp. Med.*, **52**, 477–483.

Heidelberger, M., Kendall, F. E., and Scherp, H. W. (1936). The specific polysaccharides of types I, II, and III of Pneumococcus. A revision of methods and data. *J. Exp. Med.*, **64**, 559–572.

Heidelberger, M., MacLeod, C. M., Kaiser, S. J., and Robinson, B. (1946). Antibody formation in volunteers following injection of pneumococci or their type-specific polysaccharides. *J. Exp. Med.*, **83**, 303–320.

Heidelberger, M., MacLeod, C. M., Markowitz, H., and Rose, A. S. (1950). Improved methods for the preparation of the specific polysaccharides of Pneumococcus. *J. Exp. Med.*, **91**, 341–349.

Hotchkiss, R. D., and Goebel, W. F. (1937). Chemoimmunological studies on the soluble substance of Pneumococcus. III. Structure of the aldobionic acid from the type III polysaccharide. *J. Biol. Chem.*, **121**, 195–203.

Jones, J. K. N., and Perry, M. B. (1957). Structure of the type VIII pneumococcus specific polysaccharide. *J. Am. Chem. Soc.*, **79**, 2787–2793.

Kenne, L., and Lindberg, B. (1983). Bacterial polysaccharides. In *The Polysaccharides*, Vol. 2 (Ed. G. O. Aspinall), pp.287–409. Academic Press, New York.

Kenne, L., Lindberg, B., and Svensson, S. (1975). Structure of the capsular polysaccharide of Pneumococcus type II. *Carbohydr. Res.*, **40**, 69–75.

Kramár, E. (1922). Chemical properties of bacterial capsules. *Zentralbl. Bakteriol Abt. 1 Orig.*, **88**, 401–406.

Lancefield, R. C. (1928). Antigenic complex of *Streptococcus haemolyticus*. II. Chemical and immunological properties of the protein fractions. *J. Exp. Med.*, **47**, 469–479.

Lindberg, B., Lindkvist, B., Lönngren, J., and Powell, D. A. (1980). Structural studies of the capsular polysaccharide from *Streptococcus pneumoniae* type 1. *Carbohydr. Res.*, **78**, 111–117.

MacLeod, C. M., Hodges, R. G., Heidelberger, M., and Bernhard, W. G. (1945). Prevention of pneumococcal pneumonia by immunization with specific capsular polysaccharides. *J. Exp. Med.*, **82**, 445–465.

Pappenheimer, A. M., Jr., and Enders, J. F. (1933). Specific carbohydrate of type I Pneumococcus. *Proc. Soc. Exp. Biol. Med.*, **31**, 37–39.

Pasteur, L. Sur la fermentation visqueuse et la fermentation butyrique. *Bull. Soc. Chim.*, **1861**, 30–33.

Rebers, P. A., and Heidelberger, M. (1961). The specific polysaccharide of type VI pneumococcus. II. The repeating unit. *J. Am. Chem. Soc.*, **83**, 3056–3059.

Reeves, R. E., and Goebel, W. F. (1941). Chemoimmunological studies on the soluble specific substance of Pneumococcus. V. Structure of the type III polysaccharide. *J. Biol. Chem.*, **139**, 511–519.

Robbins, J. B., Lee, C.-J., Rastogi, P. H., Schiffman, G., Austrian, R., Henrichsen, J., Magela, P. H., and Broome, C. V. (1983). Considerations for formulating the second generation of pneumococcal capsular polysaccharide vaccines with emphasis on the cross-reactive types within groups. *J. Infect. Dis.*, **148**, 1136–1149.

Stacey, M. (1947). Aspects of immunochemistry. *Q. Rev. Chem. Soc.*, **1**, 179–245.

Toenniessen, E. (1921). Untersuchungen über die Kapsel (Gummihülle) der pathogenen Bakterien. II. Die chemische Beschaffenheit der Kapsel und ihr dadurch bedingtes Verhalten gegenüber der Fixierung und Färbung. *Zentralbl. Bakteriol. Abt. 1 Orig.*, **85**, 225–237.

Unruh, C. C., and Kenyon, W. O. (1942). Investigation of the properties of cellulose oxidized by nitrogen dioxide. I. *J. Am. Chem. Soc.*, **64**, 127–131.

Wood, W. B., Jr. (1941). Studies on the mechanism of recovery in pneumococcal pneumonia. I. Action of type specific antibody upon the pulmonary lesion of experimental pneumonia. *J. Exp. Med.*, **73**, 201–222.

Yackel, E. C., and Kenyon, W. O. (1942). Oxidation of cellulose by nitrogen dioxide. *J. Am. Chem. Soc.*, **64**, 121–127.

Zozaya, J., Boyer, J., and Clark, J. (1930). Standardization of antipneumococcic serum types I and II. *J. Exp. Med.*, **26**, 471–476.

Immunology of the Bacterial Cell Envelope
Edited by D. E. S. Stewart-Tull and M. Davies
© 1985 John Wiley & Sons Ltd.

CHAPTER 2

Immunochemistry and Biological Activity of Peptidoglycan

B. Heymer,* P. H. Seidl[†] and K. H. Schleifer[†]
*Universität Ulm, Abteilung für Pathologie,
7900 Ulm/Donau, Oberer Eselsberg, FRG, and [†]Lehrstuhl für Mikrobiologie,
Technische Universität München, Arcisstrasse 21, 8000 Munich 2, FRG

I. INTRODUCTION

There are numerous reviews on the immunochemistry (Schleifer and Krause, 1971a,b; Rogers, 1974; Schleifer, 1975; Schleifer and Seidl, 1977; Beveridge,

1981; Seltmann, 1982) as well as on the biological activity (Rotta, 1975; Heymer, 1975a,b; Heymer and Rietschel, 1977; Rotta *et al.*, 1979, 1981; Kotani *et al.*, 1981; Dziarski, 1981; Stewart-Tull, 1980) of peptidoglycan (PG). Hence, it is not the purpose of the present chapter simply to recapitulate data already extensively described in those presentations. Instead, it would appear to be more worthwhile, in addition to a brief survey of the various aspects of PG, to point out the more recent findings in this field and to discuss critically the relevance of observations made on the biological activity of PG so far. Therefore, emphasis will be put on answers to questions such as: Are the biological properties of PG restricted to or specific for a particular type of PG or are they more or less common to all PGs? Does PG possess a unique core structure representing the biologically active centre? Is there an explanation for the conflicting results published on the biological activity of PG? Which biological effects of PG may be relevant for man?

There are some obvious limitations imposed on the present chapter by the fact that certain aspects of PG are discussed in the contributions of Stewart-Tull, Schwab, and Takada and Kotani. Consequently, topics dealt with in those chapters will be omitted — as far as possible — from the following presentation.

II. CHEMICAL STRUCTURE OF PEPTIDOGLYCAN

All eubacteria, with the exception of Mycoplasmatales, contain peptidoglycan (murein) as an essential cell wall polymer (Kandler, 1982; Schleifer and

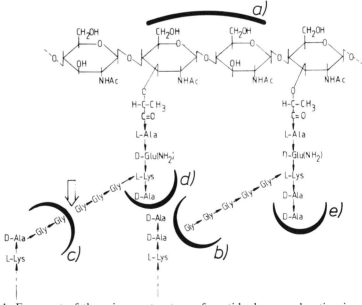

Figure 1. Fragment of the primary structure of peptidoglycan and antigenic epitopes of peptidoglycan

Stackebrandt, 1983). It is a heteropolymer consisting of a polysaccharide backbone (glycan strand) which is cross-linked through oligopeptides (Figure 1). The chemical structure of the glycan strand resembles that of chitin. Like chitin, it consists of $\beta(1\rightarrow4)$-glycosidically linked N-acetylglucosamine residues. However, unlike chitin, each alternate N-acetylglucosamine residue is substituted by a D-lactic acid ether in its C-3 hydroxyl group. This derivative of glucosamine is called muramic acid. The carboxyl group of muramic acid is substituted by an oligopeptide (peptide subunit) which contains alternating L- and D- amino acids. Adjacent peptide subunits are cross-linked either directly or via an interpeptide bridge (Figure 1). This gives rise to a huge macromolecule encompassing the bacterial cell.

Extensive studies on the chemical structure of the PG of various bacteria have revealed the existence of almost 100 different primary structures of PG (peptidoglycan or murein types). A first review on this topic was published by Schleifer and Kandler (1972). More recent data on the chemical structure of PG have been included in various reviews (Schleifer and Kandler, 1983; Schleifer and Seidl, 1984; Schleifer and Stackebrandt, 1983). The main characteristics of the primary structure of PGs can be summarized as follows. The glycan part of the various PGs is rather uniform. Only a few variations, such as acetylation or phosphorylation of the muramyl 6-hydroxyl group or the occasional absence of N-acetyl or peptide substituents, are known. In some mycobacteria and coryneform bacteria the N-acetyl group of muramic acid can be oxidized to N-glycolyl (Uchida and Aida, 1977).

The peptide subunits consist of alternating L- and D-amino acids. However, differences in the amino acid sequence can be found in various PG types (Schleifer and Kandler, 1972; Schleifer and Seidl, 1984). In some bacteria a minor portion of the peptide subunits may consist of pentapeptides revealing C-terminal D-alanyl–D-alanine residues. They represent a remnant of the PG precursor. From three to six chemically different amino acids can be present in a particular PG type. Certain typical amino acids of proteins, such as branched or aromatic amino acids, cysteine, methionine, arginine, histidine or proline, have never been found as constituents of PG.

The peptide subunits of PG can be cross-linked in two different ways (Schleifer and Kandler, 1972). The cross-linkage of group A PGs extends, as depicted in Figure 1, from the distal amino group of the diamino acid in position 3 of one peptide subunit to the carboxyl group of D-alanine in position 4 of an adjacent peptide subunit. It can occur either in a direct way (e.g. most gram-negative bacteria) or via an interpeptide bridge. Group B cross-linkage is rather rare and found only among certain coryneforms and a few anaerobic organisms (Schleifer and Seidl, 1984). It is characterized by a cross-linkage between the α-carboxyl group of glutamic acid in position 2 in one peptide subunit and the C-terminal D-alanine in position 4 of an adjacent peptide subunit (Schleifer and Kandler,

1972). There is always an interpeptide bridge containing a diamino acid necessary to cross-link the two carboxyl groups.

III. IMMUNOCHEMISTRY OF PEPTIDOGLYCAN

Since the first description of antibodies to PG by Abdulla and Schwab (1965), intensive studies have subsequently been performed concerning the immunogenicity of PG (Karakawa and Krause, 1966; Karakawa *et al.*, 1966, 1967, 1968, 1970; Hisatsune *et al.*, 1967; Hughes *et al.*, 1971; Helgeland and Grov, 1971). It is noteworthy that attempts to raise antibodies in rabbits against solubilized PG have been unsuccessful, irrespective of the dose administered, the methods of immunization used, the immunization schedule, and the addition of adjuvant. The coupling of soluble PG to bovine serum albumin by diazotization, in contrast, gave strong precipitating antisera (Goldstein *et al.*, 1973).

Although it was possible to obtain anti-PG sera from rabbits which had been immunized intravenously or intradermally with particulate PG from various bacterial species (Abdulla and Schwab, 1965; Karakawa and Krause, 1966; Karakawa *et al.*, 1966, 1968; Rolicka and Park, 1969; Helgeland and Grov, 1971; Hughes *et al.*, 1971), the antibody response was never as marked as that achieved when rabbits had been immunized intravenously with vaccines prepared from heat-killed whole cells of gram-positive cocci (Abdulla and Schwab, 1965; Karakawa *et al.*, 1966, 1967, 1968). Immunization procedures employing complete Freund's adjuvant (Rolicka and Park, 1969; Karakawa *et al.*, 1970; Hughes *et al.*, 1971; Goldstein *et al.*, 1973) should be avoided since they may also result in antibodies to the PG part of the peptidoglycolipid, wax D (Koga and Pearson, 1973).

However, antisera to group A-variant streptococci were found to be a rich source of antibodies to PG. Detection of cross-reactivity in such sera led to intensive studies on the specificity of antibodies to PG (Krause, 1975; Schleifer and Seidl, 1977).

Up to now, these studies have led to the discovery of at least five independent antigenic epitopes of PG (compare Figure 1): the glycan strand, epitope *a*; N-terminal and C-terminal sequences of the interpeptide bridge, epitopes *b* and *c*; the uncross-linked peptide subunit tetrapeptide Ala–D-Glu (diamino acid–D-Ala), epitope *d*; and the uncross-linked peptide subunit pentapeptide Ala–D-Glu (Lys–D-Ala–D-Ala), epitope *e*.

A. Antigenic Properties of the Glycan Strand

Early studies on the antigenic properties of PG indicated that the peptide moiety and the hexosamine polymer of PG were major antigenic determinants (Karakawa and Krause, 1966; Karakawa *et al.*, 1966, 1967, 1968). Evidence for this assumption stemmed from the fact that both a peptide moiety and a hexosamine-rich moiety, isolated from lytic enzyme digests, inhibited the PG precipitin reaction. From the apparent cross-reactivity between streptococcal A polysaccharide and PG and the capacity of *N*-acetylglucosamine to inhibit the PG precipitin reaction (Karakawa *et al.*, 1967), it was concluded that this amino sugar played an immunodominant role. However, cross-reactivity caused by impurities in the antigen preparations used could not be completely excluded. Rolicka and Park (1969) demonstrated that antibodies against the glycan chain recognized *N*-acetylglucosamine and *not* *N*-acetylmuramic acid as the immunodominant sugar, whereas Wikler (1975) reported that *N*-acetylmuramic acid was the immunodominant sugar. Schleifer and Seidl (1977) were finally able to resolve this controversy. Although the monomer acetylamino sugars were strong inhibitors of the PG precipitin reaction, the antibody-combining site seemed to be complementary to the size of a tetrasaccharide (Rolicka and Park, 1969; Schleifer and Seidl, 1977).

The occurrence of antibodies to the glycan strand of PG led to the question whether the synthetic immunoadjuvant *N*-acetylmuramyl–alanyl–D-isoglutamine (MDP) would bind to such antibodies or not (Audibert *et al.*, 1978). An answer to this question might indicate whether reactivity of MDP with natural PG antibodies could induce clinical hazards, preventing the application of MDP or its derivatives in man. Studies were performed employing the corresponding ^{14}C- or ^{125}I-labelled compounds in Farr-type binding and inhibition assays. No binding of [^{14}C]-MDP could be detected with naturally occurring or experimentally induced PG antibodies. Such lack of reactivity was surprising since MDP represents part of the monomeric subunit of the PG backbone. Although MDP in isolated form did not elicit an immune response (Audibert *et al.*, 1976), it became immunogenic when it was coupled with an appropriate carrier (Reichert *et al.*, 1980; Chedid *et al.*, 1979). Both conjugates, carrying MDP substitutents on the γ-carboxyl group of glutamic acid of MDP or on the anomeric C-1 carbon atom of the *N*-acetylmuramyl portion of MDP, were immunogenic and the antibodies reacted with free synthetic MDP. It was most surprising that carrier-bound *N*-acetylmuramyl–D-Ala–D-Glu-NH$_2$, in contrast to *N*-acetylmuramyl–Ala–D-Glu-NH$_2$, was incapable of inducing an immune response (Chedid *et al.*, 1979).

Recently, employing as an antigen low-molecular-weight glycopeptides from *Bacillus subtilis* PG, a Farr-type hapten binding assay and an enzyme-linked immunoadsorbent assay were developed for the sensitive detection of human antibodies to the glycan moiety of PG (Seidl *et al.*, in preparation). The specificity of the test systems used was examined in detail and it was possible to establish that the antibody population detected in human sera by the glycopeptide did not recognize a single *N*-acetylamino sugar, thus excluding interaction of terminal acetylamino sugars of bacterial polysaccharides. Neither did *N*-acetylglucosamine residues present in human glycoproteins nor MDP bind to these antibodies. By means of adsorption experiments with PGs from numerous bacterial strains including *Escherichia coli, Enterobacter aerogenes, Staphylococcus aureus, Streptococcus pyogenes, B. subtilis,* it was possible to characterize the glycan strand as a kind of common antigen for all eubacteria. Furthermore, the independence of human antibodies directed against the glycan moiety and those directed against the peptide part was clearly demonstrated, thus corroborating the data of Schleifer and Krause (1971b) which were obtained from work with rabbit hyperimmune sera.

The contradictory reports on the specificity of antibodies to the glycan moiety of PG (*N*-acetylglucosamine or *N*-acetylmuramic acid as the determinant sugar, specific antibodies to MDP, or glycan strand specific antibodies which bound neither to *N*-acetylglucosamine, *N*-acetylmuramic acid nor to MDP) only reflect its enormous immunochemical complexity, as already indicated by Grov and Oeding (1971). Ryc *et al.* (1982) as well as Wagner and Wagner (1978) assumed that on whole cells the glycan subunits are not accessible to antibodies. Recently, however, employing specific antibodies, it was possible to make the glycan moiety visible with the indirect ferritin technique (P. H. Seidl, K. H. Schleifer, G. Wanner, unpublished observations).

B. Antigenic Properties of the Interpeptide Bridge

Early studies by Helgeland *et al.* (1973) and Ranu (1975) indicated that the interpeptide bridge of PG contains an independent antigenic site. Proof for this assumption was obtained by applying synthetic peptidyl-protein immunogens carrying as substituents peptides with structural similarity to C-terminal or N-terminal sequences of the interpeptide bridge (Seidl and Schleifer, 1977, 1978a, 1979). All PGs hitherto examined are not completely cross-linked (Schleifer and Kandler, 1972). Thus, at least 10% of the interpeptide bridges show unsubstituted amino groups (Figure 1). Furthermore, glycine peptides with a free amino or carboxyl group in staphylococcal peptidoglycans are the products of endopeptidases splitting Gly–Gly bonds in the interpeptide bridge (Wadström, 1973). These C-terminal and N-terminal sequences in the interpeptide bridge represent two independent antigenic epitopes of PG.

Since the different PG types are a very valuable criterion for the differentiation of gram-positive cocci (Schleifer and Kandler, 1972), highly specific antisera against the particular interpeptide bridges were applied for the serological separation of staphylococci from micrococci (Seidl and Schleifer, 1978b). It is noteworthy that the difference of even one amino acid (alanine or glycine) in the interpeptide bridge of PG could be serologically detected (Seidl and Schleifer, 1979).

Recently, employing interpeptide bridge antisera raised by immunization with (tri-alanyl–ϵ-aminocaproyl)$_{22}$–albumin or with (pentaglycyl–ϵ-aminocaproyl)$_{20}$–albumin, the respective interpeptide bridges were specifically made visible on the cell surface of *Staphylococcus aureus* or *Streptococcus pyogenes*, thus providing corroborative evidence that the interpeptide bridge is an important epitope (P. H. Seidl, K. H. Schleifer, G. Wanner, N. Franken, and P. Zwerenz, unpublished observations).

C. Antigenic properties of the peptide subunit

1. Uncross-linked Pentapeptide Ala–D-Glu(Lys–D-Ala–D-Ala)

Because of the cross-reactivity between streptococcal and staphylococcal PGs, Karakawa *et al.* (1968) suggested that this immunological cross-reactivity might be dependent in part upon the similarity of their tetrapeptides. Studies with synthetic random polypeptides, e.g. $poly(Glu^{42}-Lys^{28}-D-Ala^{30})_n$, indicated the importance of D-alanine in the antigenic specificity of PG (Karakawa *et al.*, 1970). Employing a series of synthetic peptides as inhibitors in the quantitative PG precipitin reaction, Schleifer and Krause (1971a) were able to demonstrate an antibody population in antisera against A-variant streptococci with specificity for the pentapeptide Ala–D-Glu(Lys–D-Ala–D-Ala). These antibodies were directed against the carboxy terminal group of the pentapeptide and did not bind to the tetrapeptide Ala–D-Glu(Lys–D-Ala). D-alanyl–D-alanine was characterized as the immunodominant group, the contribution of the other amino acids to the antigenic site of the pentapeptide being of less importance (Lys, D-Glu) or insignificant (Ala).

These findings were confirmed (Schleifer and Seidl, 1974; Seidl and Schleifer, 1975) by employing peptidyl-protein immunogens carrying as substituents synthetic pentapeptides (e.g. Gly–Ala–Ala–D-Ala–D-Ala; Gly–γD-Glu–Lys–D-Ala–D-Ala) and by Zeiger and Maurer (1973) using the random polypeptide $(Glu^{60}Ala^{40})_n$ substituted by Ala–D-Glu(Lys–D-Ala–D-Ala). The assumption that uncross-linked Ala–D-Glu(Lys–D-Ala–D-Ala) represented an antigenic determinant for animals and humans was corroborated by Farr-type hapten binding and inhibition studies of corresponding animal as well as human sera (Heymer *et al.*, 1975a, 1976; Audibert *et al.*, 1978; Zeiger *et al.*, 1981; Pope *et al.*, 1982). Furthermore, the immunodominant role of the C-terminal D-alanyl–D-alanine in the antibody response to the group-A variant streptococcal vaccine was shown in the direct ferritin technique (Ryc *et al.*, 1982) by employing specific antibodies to the D-alanyl–D-alanine moiety for radioimmunological detection of PG (Eisenberg *et al.*, 1982), and by demonstrating cross-reactivity between (R)-D-Ala–D-Ala and β-lactam antibiotics (Seidl *et al.*, 1983). However, a much more complex specificity was detected in human sera (Seidl *et al.*, 1983.; P. H. Seidl, K. H. Schleifer, G. Wanner, N. Franken, and P. Zwerenz, unpublished observations). As in animal antisera (Schleifer and Krause, 1971a), in some human sera antibodies to Ala–D-Glu(Lys–D-Ala–D-Ala) were exclusively or predominantly directed to C-terminal (R)-D-Ala–D-Ala as the immunodominant group. In contrast, in some human sera lysine and/or

D-glutamic acid seemed to contribute significantly to the antigenic site, the sequence (R)-D-Ala–D-Ala playing a minor role.

2. Uncross-linked Tetrapeptide Ala–D-Glu(diamino acid–D-Ala)

Helgeland *et al.* (1973) have already mentioned that uncross-linked Ala–D-Glu(Lys–D-Ala) might be an antigenic determinant of PG. Studies on the immunochemistry of PGs of gram-negative bacteria characterized the uncross-linked tetrapeptide Ala–D-Glu(meso-A_2pm–D-Ala) as an antigenic epitope (Nguyen-Huy *et al.*, 1976). The C-terminal meso-A_2pm–D-Ala of the peptide was immunodominant; Ala–D-Glu(Lys–D-Ala) or (R)-D-Ala–D-Ala peptides were poor inhibitors of the precipitin reaction. Recently, Ala–D-Glu(Lys–D-Ala) was characterized as an additional antigenic determinant of PG in the human. The antibodies were directed against the C-terminal Lys–D-Ala moiety, and normally no cross-reactivity between Ala–D-Glu(Lys–D-Ala) and Ala–D-Glu(Lys–D-Ala$_2$) was observed (Seidl *et al.*, 1983; P. H. Seidl, K. H. Schleifer, G. Wanner, N. Franken, and P. Zwerenz, unpublished observations). These studies explain the binding of *N*-acetylmuramyl–alanyl–D-isoglutaminyl–lysyl[^{125}I]–D-alanine to some sera (Audibert *et al.*, 1978) probably owing to antibody specificity for Ala–D-Glu(Lys–D-Ala).

Thus, an enormous complexity was found in the specificity of PG antibodies. The five main antigenic epitopes further reveal a great heterogeneity. Monospecific test systems detecting antibodies to distinct chemically defined structures should therefore be useful for further elucidation of the immunochemical properties of PG.

IV. OCCURRENCE OF PEPTIDOGLYCAN ANTIBODIES

A. Methods of Determination

Because of the possible diagnostic role of PG antibodies, many assay systems have been developed for their determination, including immunoprecipitation (Rolicka and Massell, 1973; Schachenmayr *et al.*, 1975), latex agglutination (Heymer *et al.*, 1973a), immunodiffusion (Helgeland and Grov, 1975), enzyme-linked immunosorbent assay (Verbrugh *et al.*, 1981; Wilhelm *et al.*, 1982; Seidl *et al.*, 1983; Johnson *et al.*, 1984; Franken *et al.*, 1984), solid-phase radioimmunoassay (Schopfer *et al.*, 1980; Wheat *et al.*, 1983), Farr-type radioactive hapten-binding assay (Heymer *et al.*, 1975a, 1976; Audibert *et al.*, 1978; Zeiger *et al.*, 1981; Pope *et al.*, 1982). With the exception of Seidl *et al.* (1983), Franken *et al.* (1984), Heymer *et al.* (1975a, 1976), Audibert *et al.* (1978), Zeiger *et al.* (1981) and Pope *et al.* (1982), these authors employed 'purified' PG preparations for antibody determination. However, such preparations are somewhat unsatisfactory since 'purified' PGs may contain other antigenic cell wall components such as proteins, lipoteichoic acids, teichoic acids, polysaccharides or lipopolysaccharides as impurities. Procedures for extraction of PG (Schopfer *et al.*, 1980; Verbrugh *et al.*, 1981; Wheat *et al.*, 1983; Wilhelm *et al.*, 1982) either result in incomplete extraction of PG or cause severe chemical modifications of PG (Schleifer, 1975). In conclusion, all assay systems established on the basis of 'purified' PG may detect not only antibodies to PG but also to other cell wall associated polymers. Proof for specific and exclusive measurement of antibodies to PG was hitherto only furnished by procedures based on chemically well-defined antigens or haptens (Seidl *et al.*, 1983; Franken *et al.*, 1984; Heymer *et al.*, 1975a, 1976; Zeiger *et al.*, 1981).

B. Immunoglobulin Classes

Specific antibodies to PG of the immunoglobulin IgG class (Helgeland and Grov, 1971; Heymer *et al.*, 1973a; Zeiger *et al.*, 1981; Verbrugh *et al.*, 1981; Wilhelm *et al.*, 1982; Wheat *et al.*, 1983; Seidl *et al.*, 1983), of the IgA class (Helgeland and Grov, 1971; Zeiger *et al.*, 1981; Wilhelm *et al.*, 1982; Franken *et al.*, 1984), of the IgM class (Zeiger *et al.*, 1981; Verbrugh *et al.*, 1981; Wilhelm *et al.*, 1982; Wheat *et al.*, 1983; Seidl *et al.*, 1983), and of the IgE class (Schopfer *et al.*, 1980) have been reported. However, only Zeiger *et al.* (1981), Seidl *et al.* (1983) and Franken *et al.* (1984) used chemically well-defined antigens thus clearly proving that the immunoglobulin class identified was directed to a PG sequence. With respect to 'specific IgM to PG', Verbrugh *et al.* (1981), Wilhelm *et al.* (1982) and Wheat *et al.* (1983) probably measured rheumatoid factor and not only specific IgM to PG. Thus, one should be aware of the fact that all indirect immunoassay systems may be severely disturbed by the presence of rheumatoid factor. This holds particularly true for sera exhibiting both specific IgG and IgM to the same antigen. Similarly, the reported occurrence of IgE with specificity for PG (Schopfer *et al.*, 1980) cannot yet be accepted since assays demonstrating the destruction of IgE (56°C, 4 h; or treatment with 0.1 M mercaptoethanol) were not performed. Moreover, the data obtained appear somewhat dubious since binding was found only to wall preparations of *Staphylococcus aureus* and not to those of other bacteria.

C. Biological Role and Diagnostic Significance

Little is known about the biological role and the potential diagnostic significance of PG antibodies. An association between the occurrence of PG antibodies in the sera of patients and certain disease processes was reported for 'rheumatic diseases' (Rolicka and Massell, 1973; Heymer *et al.* 1976; Pope *et al.*, 1982; Wheat *et al.*, 1983; Johnson *et al.*, 1984), for endocarditis (Zeiger *et al.*, 1981; Wheat *et al.*, 1983), for staphylococcal infections of deep tissue sites (Verbrugh *et al.*, 1981), for 'complicated bacteraemia' (Wheat *et al.*, 1983), for pneumonia, streptococcal nephritis, osteomyelitis, lymphadenitis and scarlet fever (Seidl *et al.*, 1983).

As pointed out, the immune response to PG is very complex. Since PG reveals at least five main antigenic determinants there is a great heterogeneity of antibodies to PG. Therefore, assay systems detecting antibodies to one chemically defined structure of PG (Heymer *et al.*, 1975a,b, 1976; Zeiger *et al.*, 1981; Seidl *et al.*, 1983; Franken *et al.*, 1984) are superior to assay systems using complex material as antigen and measuring a 'mixed' antibody response to PG. Moreover, it should be stressed that antibodies of the various immunoglobulin classes and to the various antigenic determinants of PG may occur simultaneously and independently in the same serum. Therefore, it is most likely that only immunoassays permitting the selective determination of antibodies of a particular immunoglobulin class (Seidl *et al.*, 1983; Franken *et al.*, 1984) will enable the precise definition of the biological role and diagnostic significance of PG antibodies.

V. BIOLOGICAL ACTIVITY OF PEPTIDOGLYCAN

After the discussion of the various chemical and immunological features of PG one may now better appreciate the complex biological properties of this unique bacterial component. Taking into account what has been detailed thus far it is not surprising that the spectrum of biological activities (listed in Table 1) is relatively complex and, at a first glance, rather perplexing. Nevertheless, there is a common denominator among several of the properties given; e.g. the immunoadjuvant effect and the polyclonal B-cell activation. Furthermore, it is evident that many of the activities indicated in Table 1 may cooperate to produce the phenomenon mentioned last, namely the induction of inflammation.

Table 1   Biological Activity of Peptidoglycan

1.	Induction of antibody formation (and cellular immunity?)
2.	Immunomodulation (e.g. immunoadjuvanticity)
3.	Endotoxin-like properties (e.g. pyrogenicity, local Shwartzman reaction)
4.	Complement activation (through classical and alternative pathways)
5.	Polyclonal B-cell activation (e.g. mitogenic effect, Ig secretion)
6.	Effects on macrophages (e.g. on phagocytosis, chemotaxis)
7.	Effects on granulocytes (e.g. on phagocytosis, chemotaxis)
8.	Release of mediators (e.g. histamine, prostaglandins)
9.	Complex biological effects (e.g. increase of tumoricidal activity)
10.	Induction of inflammation (in experimental animals and in man)

A. Endotoxin-like Properties

Among the earliest observations on the biological properties of PG were reports indicating certain similarities with endotoxin of gram-negative bacteria. In

Table 2. Endotoxin-like Activity of Peptidoglycan

Test animal	Source of PG	Phenomenon observed	Reference
Limulus polyphemus	Various bacterial species	Gelation of amoebocyte lysate	Wildfeuer *et al.*, 1974
Rabbit	Various bacterial species	Induction of fever	Rotta and Schleifer, 1974
Mouse	*Streptococcus pyogenes*	Stimulation of non-specific resistance to bacterial infection	Rotta, 1975
Rabbit	*S. pyogenes Staphylococcus epidermidis*	Induction of fever	Heymer and Rietschel, 1977
Rabbit	*S. pyogenes*	Lysis of platelets	Rotta *et al.*, 1979
Rabbit/ guinea pig	Various bacterial species	Local Shwartzman reaction	Rotta *et al.*, 1979, 1981

particular Rotta systematically studied streptococcal and other PGs for such activities (Rotta, 1975). Some of the findings are summarized in Table 2. Of the characteristics listed, induction of fever by PG has been investigated most intensively (Rotta *et al.*, 1981). While there is little doubt that sonically solubilized PGs of numerous different gram-positive bacteria possess a characteristic pyrogenic activity distinct from that of endotoxin, the fever-inducing potency of PG as determined in rabbits is $> 10^3$ less intense than that of endotoxin (Heymer and Rietschel, 1977). With few exceptions the same holds true with respect to the other endotoxin-like properties listed in Table 2. The possibility that these activities might simply be due to an endotoxin contamination of the PG preparations employed has been ruled out by a number of experiments. Thus, it was shown that the ability of PG to induce gelation of amoebocyte lysate of *Limulus polyphemus* could be specifically destroyed by pretreatment of preparations with lysozyme (Wildfeuer *et al.*, 1974). It also was demonstrated that rabbits made resistant to lipid A (the active part of endotoxin) still remained sensitive to a pyrogenic challenge with PG (Heymer and Rietschel, 1977). This indicates that the phenomena observed can safely be ascribed to PG. However, the fact that PG and endotoxin in spite of a completely different chemical structure produce similar biological effects could mean that they — at least in some instances — activate the same mediator system.

B. Activation of Complement by Peptidoglycan

The first indication that PG might be able to activate complement came from the observation that fresh plasma was required to induce lysis of platelets by PG (Rotta, 1975). Shortly thereafter Bokisch (1975) demonstrated that streptococcal and in particular staphylococcal PG in fact activate the complement

Table 3   Activation of Complement by Peptidoglycan

Source of serum	Source of PG	Pathway activated	Reference
Man	*Streptococcus pyogenes* *Staphylococcus aureus* *Staph. epidermidis*	Both pathways	Bokisch, 1975
Mouse/ guinea pig	*Staph. aureus*	Alternative	Pryjma *et al.*, 1976
Man	*S. pyogenes* *Staph. epidermidis* *Bordetella pertussis*	Not specified	Heymer and Rietschel, 1977
Man	*S. pyogenes*	Alternative	Greenblatt *et al.*, 1978
Man	*S. pyogenes* *Staph. aureus*	Alternative	Semeraro *et al.*, 1979
Guinea pig	*S. pyogenes*	Alternative	Gallis, 1979
Man	*Staph. aureus*	Alternative	Verbrugh *et al.*, 1980
Man	Various bacterial species	Not specified	Wilkinson *et al.*, 1981
Man	*Neisseria gonorrhoeae*	Classical	Peterson and Rosenthal, 1982

system by both the classical as well as the alternative pathways. Since then—as is evident from Table 3—the interaction of PG with complement has been studied and confirmed by many other investigators. Because the complement system harbours some of the most potent mediators of inflammation (Williams and Jose, 1981; Vogt, 1982; Boyle and Borsos, 1983), this ability of PG is of prime importance. In addition there are three aspects to consider: (1) As can be seen from the data summarized in Table 3, PGs from various bacterial species can activate complement by the alternative pathway, i.e. independently of the presence of PG antibodies. (2) Activation of complement through the classical pathway is also likely to occur in many situations since PG antibodies are present in many animal as well as human sera (Schachenmayr *et al.*, 1975; Johnson *et al.*, 1982; Pope *et al.*, 1982; Zeiger *et al.*, 1981). (3) There are several properties of PG such as the generation of chemotactic activity (Heymer and Rietschel, 1977) or the opsonization of *Staphylococcus aureus* (Peterson *et al.*, 1978) that are known to be totally dependent on complement. In other words, at least some of the biological activities of PG are definitely mediated by the complement system. Whether this also holds true with respect to the inflammatory reactions induced by PG has still to be determined.

C. Polyclonal B-cell Activation

In the course of studies attempting to define the target cell of the immunoadjuvant activity of PG (see chapters by Stewart-Tull and Takada and Kotani), it was found that PG has a distinct mitogenic effect on lymphocytes (Werner *et al.*, 1974). Since cells not only from rabbits and normal mice but also from nude mice were stimulated (Damais *et al.*, 1975), PG was considered a B-cell orientated mitogen. As can be seen from the data collected in Table 4, this proved to hold true for human B-cells as well as mouse or rabbit lymphocytes and for staphylococcal PG as well as for PGs of other bacterial species. However, although polyclonal B-cell activation might be an important property of PG and possibly the basis of its immunological adjuvant activity, it can by no means be considered a very selective or specific effect of PG since a vast number of other biological compounds also display this activity (Cottier, 1980).

Table 4   Polyclonal B-cell Activation by Peptidoglycan

Source of cells	Source of PG	Parameter determined	Reference
Man	*Mycobacterium tuberculosis*	Mitogenic effect	Werner *et al.*, 1974
Rabbit/ mouse	Various bacterial species	Mitogenic effect	Damais *et al.*, 1975
Man/rabbit	*Nocardia rubra*	Mitogenic effect	Ciorbaru *et al.*, 1976
Mouse	Various bacterial species	Mitogenic effect	Takada *et al.*, 1980
Mouse	*Staphylococcus aureus*	Mitogenic effect Ig secretion	Dziarski, 1980a Dziarski, 1980b
Man/mouse/ rat	*Staph. aureus*	Mitogenic effect	Dziarski *et al.*, 1980
Mouse	*Staph. aureus*	Mitogenic effect Autoantibody production	Dziarski, 1982a,b,c
Man	*Bacillus subtilis* *Staph. aureus*	Mitogenic effect Lymphocyte inhibition factor production	Räsänen *et al.*, 1982
Man	*Staph. aureus*	Mitogenic effect Cell differentiation	Levinson *et al.*, 1983

D. Effects of Peptidoglycan on Macrophages

The effect of PG on various types of macrophage populations has been studied for a long time (Heymer *et al.*, 1971, 1973b). Experiments were primarily performed employing *in vitro* assay systems. Some of the data obtained are shown in Table 5. As is evident, except for the inhibition of migration, PG

Table 5   Effects of Peptidoglycan on Macrophages

Source of cells	Source of PG	Phenomenon observed	Reference
Rat	*Streptococcus pyogenes* *S. agalactiae*	Inhibition of migration	Heymer *et al.*, 1971, 1973b
Rat/guinea pig	Various bacterial species	Inhibition of migration	Bültmann *et al.*, 1975
Man	*Staphylococcus aureus*	Secretion of endogenous pyrogen	Oken *et al.*, 1979
Mouse	*Staph. aureus*	Secretion of colony stimulating factor Secretion of interleukin 1 Secretion of prostaglandin	Gold and Mishell, 1981
Mouse	*S. pyogenes*	Inhibition of migration	Caravano and Oberti, 1981
Mouse/ guinea pig	*Listeria monocytogenes*	Increase of tumouricidal activity	Saiki *et al.*, 1982
Man	Various bacterial species	Stimulation of migration	Ogawa *et al.*, 1982
Mouse	*L. monocytogenes*	Increase of tumouricidal activity	Hether *et al.*, 1983

Table 6   Stimulators of Prostaglandin Release by Macrophages

Stimulator	Reference
Corynebacterium parvum	Grimm *et al.*, 1978
Zymosan (yeast cell walls)	Gemsa *et al.*, 1979
Endotoxin (lipopolysaccharide)	Kurland and Bockman, 1978
Water-soluble adjuvant (WSA)	Wahl *et al.*, 1979
Antigen–antibody complexes	Bonney *et al.*, 1979
Aggregated IgG	Passwell *et al.*, 1979
Calcium ionophore A 23187	Weidemann *et al.*, 1978
Colchicine	Gemsa *et al.*, 1980

stimulated macrophage activity inducing the release of numerous macrophage products including endogenous pyrogen (Oken *et al.*, 1979), interleukin 1 and prostaglandins (Gold and Mishell, 1981). Since the latter compounds are nowadays believed to represent important mediators of inflammation (Lewis, 1975; Morley, 1981; Samuelsson, 1982), PG-induced secretion of prostaglandins might well have important implications with respect to the pathogenesis of the inflammatory processes that occur after parenteral application of PG

(Ginsburg *et al.*, 1977). In addition, activation of macrophages may play a role in the immunoadjuvanticity of PG. However, one should keep in mind two facts: (1) PG shares the ability to stimulate prostaglandin production and release by macrophages with a diversity of other agents (Table 6) indicating that this property is not particularly specific for PG. (2) The complex role played by prostaglandins in the pathogenesis of inflammation is far from clear (Brune, 1981). Thus, at present, one primarily has to record that PG activates macrophages similarly to many other cells including human synovial lining cells (Hamilton *et al.*, 1982).

E. Effects of Peptidoglycan on Granulocytes

The effects of PG on polymorphonuclear leucocytes have been studied far less than those on lymphocytes or macrophages. One reason for this divergent interest may be due to the fact that the former primarily represent effector cells while the latter also function as mediator or potentiator cells. In addition, since the analysis of the biological activity of PG originated from the intention to define the target cell of the PG immunoadjuvanticity (Lederer, 1977; Chedid, 1981; Kotani *et al.*, 1981), lymphocytes and macrophages appeared to be more appropriate cell types and more likely candidates for study. Nevertheless — as can be seen in Table 7 — some authors did investigate the effects of PG on granulocytes. Interestingly, PG — in contrast to macrophages — inhibited most granulocyte functions. Taking into account the known differences in structure, life span and function of these two cell types (van Furth *et al.*, 1977; van Furth and Willemze, 1979; Smolen and Weissmann, 1978; Havemann and Janoff, 1978; Baggiolini and Schnyder, 1979; Cottier, 1980) this, on the one hand, may

Table 7   Effects of Peptidoglycan on Polymorphonuclear Leucocytes

Source of cells	Source of PG	Phenomenon observed	Reference
Man/mouse/ guinea pig	*Staphylococcus aureus*	Inhibition of migration	Weksler and Hill, 1969
Guinea pig	*Staph. aureus*	Inhibition of migration	Grov, 1976
Man	*Staph. aureus*	Inhibition of phagocytosis Inhibition of chemotaxis Stimulation of chemiluminescence	Musher *et al.*, 1981
Man	*Streptococcus pyogenes**	Capping of C' receptors	Pryzwansky *et al.*, 1983

*Peptidoglycan–polysaccharide opsonized with C'.

not be surprising. On the other hand, it must be stressed once more that the interaction of PG with polymorphonuclear leucocytes has not yet been studied intensively enough. Therefore, data summarized in Table 7 are far from being complete.

F. Release of Mediators by Peptidoglycan

The number of potential mediators of inflammation known today (Vane and Ferreira, 1978; Haferkamp, 1980b; Cottier, 1980) is so vast and frustrating that the statement: 'to fish for mediators of inflammation could appear to be an international sport' (Ryan and Majno, 1977) is basically justified. Nevertheless, it is possible to name a group of substances which are almost certainly involved in the pathogenesis of inflammatory reactions (Youlten, 1978; Samuelsson, 1982; Vogt, 1982). Most of these factors (listed in Table 8) have been known for quite a long time. Knowledge of their biochemical characteristics and biological activity is so common that there is no need to go into any detail. However, when discussing the potential release of mediators by PG, three points can be

Table 8   Mediators of Inflammation

Vasoactive amines (e.g. histamine)
Complement (e.g. C_{3a}, C_{5a}
Kinins (e.g. bradykinin)
Products of coagulation or fibrinolysis
Lysosomal enzymes (e.g. proteases)
Immunoglobulins (e.g. IgE)
Lymphokines (e.g. MIF, MAF)
Monokines (e.g. LAF)
Prostaglandins (e.g. PGE_2, $PGF_{2\alpha}$)
Leucotrienes (e.g. SRS-A)
Oxygen-derived free radicals (e.g. $O_2^{-\cdot}$)

Note: MIF, Macrophage inhibition factor; MAF, macrophage activation factor; LAF, lymphocyte activation factor

made: (1) As is evident from the foregoing discussion of the biological properties of PG, this bacterial component has been shown to induce several of the mediators mentioned in Table 8. (2) In addition to what has been discussed so far, PG is able to induce the release of histamine from mast cells (Kimura *et al.*, 1981). (3) It should be noted that certain mediators listed in Table 8, such as the vasoactive amines, primarily affect blood vessels, while others, such as the lymphokines and monokines, primarily affect cells. This notion is important since the activity of the former correlates with acute inflammation whereas the activity of the latter more closely correlates with chronic inflammation. Basically, PG appears to be able to induce the release of both types of mediators.

G. Complex Biological Effects of Peptidoglycan

Since PG, as is evident from data presented, can activate potent mediator systems such as the immune, complement and clotting systems and in addition interacts in various ways with macrophages and granulocytes, it is not surprising that rather complex biological effects have also been observed. Some of these phenomena are summarized in Table 9. While properties such as the ability to increase capillary permeability (Ohta, 1981) may be based on PG-induced release of mediators (e.g. histamine), others such as the potentiation of tumouricidal activity are more difficult to explain. Possibly, this activity is related to the immunoadjuvant effect of PG. However, the ambiguity of such a phenomenon is illustrated by the fact that at least in one instance (Goguel *et al.*, 1982) the reverse effect, namely tumour enhancement by PG, was observed. Thus, at present a plausible interpretation of some of the activities listed in Table 9 is not feasible.

Table 9   Complex Biological Effects of Peptidoglycan

Test animal	Source of PG	Phenomenon observed	Reference
Rabbit/ mouse	*Mycobacterium tuberculosis*	Increase of · tumouricidal activity	Werner *et al.*, 1974
Mouse	*Nocardia asteroides*	Induction of circulating interferon	Barot-Ciorbaru *et al.*, 1978, 1981
Guinea pig Rat	*Streptococcus pyogenes*	Increase of capillary permeability	Ohta, 1981
Rat	*Escherichia coli* *Proteus mirabilis*	Activation of bone marrow myelopoietic cells	Monner *et al.*, 1981
Mouse	Various bacterial species	Increase of tumouricidal activity Tumour enhancement	Goguel *et al.*, 1982
Mouse Guinea pig	*Listeria mono- cytogenes*	Increase of tumouricidal activity	Saiki *et al.*, 1982

H. Induction of Inflammation by Peptidoglycan

On the one hand, inflammation represents a most important mechanism of defence without which the mammalian organism cannot survive. On the other hand, inflammatory reactions, in particular if they do not promptly subside when the inducing agent is destroyed, always carry the risk of transient or permanent tissue damage. As already extensively described, PG is able to activate or release many potent mediators of inflammation (e.g. complement, histamine, prostaglandin). Thus, it is by no means surprising that intense inflammatory reactions occur after parenteral injection of PG. A random selection of findings is given in Table 10. It should be noted that reactions can be induced in

Table 10   Induction of Inflammation by Peptidoglycan

Test species	Source of PG	Type of inflammation observed	Reference
Rabbit/rat	Various bacterial species	Necrosis of skin	Abdulla and Schwab, 1965
Guinea pig	*Staphylococcus aureus* *Streptococcus pyogenes*	Acute inflammation of skin	Kowalski and Berman, 1971
Rat	*S. agalactiae*	Acute inflammation of skin	Heymer *et al.*, 1971, 1973b
Guinea pig	*Staph. aureus*	Acute inflammation of skin	Pryjma *et al.*, 1976
Guinea pig Rat	*S. pyogenes*	Acute inflammation of skin	Ohta, 1981
Rat	*S. pyogenes*	Acute inflammation of joints	Fox *et al.*, 1982
Man	Various bacterial species	Acute inflammation of skin	von Mayenburg *et al.*, 1980, 1982

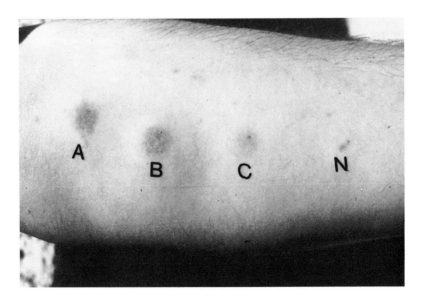

Figure 2. Skin reactions 3 h after intradermal injection of 10 μg of *Streptococcus pyogenes* peptidoglycan (A), *Staphylococcus aureus* peptidoglycan (B), *Staphylococcus epidermidis* peptidoglycan (C), and saline control (N) in a healthy human subject

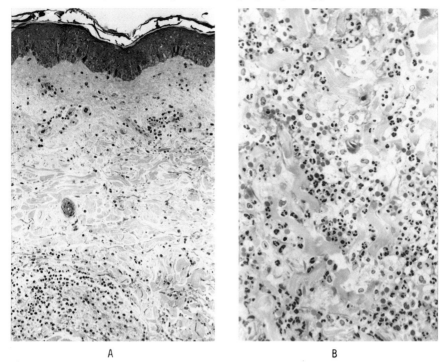

A   B

Figure 3. Skin reaction 3 h after intradermal injection of 10 µg of *Streptococcus pyogenes* peptidoglycan in a healthy human subject. Semithin section, stained with haematoxylin and eosin. Magnification: A, × 120; B, × 285

experimental animals as well as in man and that acute inflammatory reactions occurred in each instance. Taking into account the immunogenicity and the complex biological activity of PG, it is understandable that interpretation of the underlying pathomechanisms has been difficult and controversial from the very outset (Kowalski and Berman, 1971; Heymer *et al.*, 1971, 1973b).

Basically, this also holds true for the inflammatory skin reactions induced by PG in man (Heymer and Rietschel, 1977; von Mayenburg *et al.*, 1980, 1982). Nevertheless, from these studies it is now quite clear that the intradermal injection of sonically solubilized PG in a concentration of > 20 µg in man always induces an acute inflammatory reaction. Macroscopically, such reactions are primarily characterized by erythema and swelling of skin (Figure 2). Histologically, there is oedema and hyperaemia of the dermis and prominent infiltration of the corium by polymorphonuclear leucocytes (Figure 3). Lesions start a few minutes after the injection, reach a maximum at different intervals and then gradually subside within 48 to 72 h. There is complete resolution of reactions without permanent tissue damage. When the PG dose employed is reduced to 1–2 µg, a whole spectrum of skin reactions occurs differing in intensity (from negative to strongly positive), time course (immediate, late or dual type) and histology (granulocytic or lymphocytic infiltrations; von Mayenburg *et al.*, 1980). By electron microscopy, degranulation of mast cells can be observed in many instances. Immunohistologically, deposition of complement (C_3) at the site of reaction is frequently seen in skin specimens excised within the first 6 h after the PG injection (von Mayenburg *et al.*, 1980). Lesions induced under these test conditions (PG dose 1–2 μg) manifest themselves as acute transient inflammatory reactions, disappearing completely within a few days. In particular, when staphylococcal PG is used for injection there is a positive correlation between serum PG antibody titres of probands and the result of PG skin tests (von Mayenburg *et al.*, 1982). This provides indirect evidence that immune factors may be involved in the pathogenesis of the latter reactions. Thus, the findings on inflammation induced by PG in man can be summarized in three statements: (1) Skin reactions induced by intradermal injection of PG in man basically correspond to those produced in experimental animals. However, in a manner similar to the response to endotoxin, man seems to react most intensively. (2) Lesions induced by pure PG represent acute transient inflammatory reactions. There is no chronic inflammation and no permanent tissue damage. (3) Preliminary data indicate that non-immunological as well as immunological mechanisms participate in the PG-induced skin reactions.

VI. BIOLOGICALLY ACTIVE PART OF PEPTIDOGLYCAN

Many attempts have been made to determine whether PG possesses a core structure responsible for its biological activity. The primary stimulus for such efforts came from experiments to isolate the active principle of Freund's complete adjuvant (Adam *et al.*, 1972, 1973; Werner *et al.*, 1974; Lederer, 1977). Thus, most investigations along these lines concentrated on the study of the immunoadjuvant activity (Stewart-Tull, 1983a,b). It was found that muramyl-dipeptide (MDP) represented the smallest subunit of PG still active in this respect (Ellouz *et al.*, 1974; Chedid *et al.*, 1976; Chedid and Audibert, 1977; Kotani *et al.*, 1981; Chedid, 1981). Thereafter, MDP was also studied with regard to other biological activities known from PG. Out of the vast literature that has accumulated on this topic only some of the most recent findings and references are listed in Table 11. Without going into detail (see chapter by Takada and Kotani), the following facts are evident from the data presented: (1) There is a fairly close correlation between the spectrum of biological activities of MDP (Table 11) and PG (Table 1). (2) In spite of the chemical homogeneity of synthetic MDP, its biological properties appear to be as diverse as those of PG. (3) Similarly to PG, there are biological activities attributed to MDP that apparently contradict each other; e.g. stimulation of non-specific resistance to bacterial infection and generation of antigen-specific suppressor T-cells. Furthermore, it was reported (Tanaka *et al.*, 1977; Ogawa *et al.*, 1983) that the biological

Table 11   Biological Activity of Muramyl-dipeptide*

Test species	Phenomenon observed	Reference
Rat	Induction of adjuvant arthritis	Kohashi *et al.*, 1980 Nagao and Tanaka, 1980
Rabbit	Induction of fever	Rotta *et al.*, 1979, 1981
Guinea pig/rat	Formation of epithelioid cell granuloma	Tanaka and Emori, 1980 Tanaka *et al.*, 1982
Rabbit/cat	Promotion of sleep	Krueger *et al.*, 1982
Man	Activation of synovial cells	Hamilton *et al.*, 1982
Rabbit	Secretion of endogenous pyrogen and interleukin 1 by macrophages	Windle *et al.*, 1983
Man	Increase of superoxide production by macrophages[†]	Lopez-Berestein *et al.*, 1983
Man	Stimulation of macrophage chemotaxis	Ogawa *et al.*, 1983
Mouse	Stimulation of non-specific resistance to bacterial infection	Matsumoto *et al.*, 1983
Mouse	Generation of antigen-specific suppressor T-cells	Ferguson *et al.*, 1983
Mouse	Stimulation of chemiluminescence	Masihi *et al.*, 1983

*MDP = N-acetylmuramyl–L-alanyl–D-isoglutamine.
[†]6-O-Stearyl–MDP.

activity of MDP was strictly stereospecific, implying a high degree of dependence on the chemical primary structure. However, in one of these papers (Ogawa *et al.*, 1983) it was also reported that the biological phenomena described as a selective stereospecific property of MDP could also be induced by many other microbial components or even completely different chemical compounds (Windle *et al.*, 1983). While this still may be explained by the possibility that all these factors activate the same mediator system and while differences in activity between PG and MDP could be explained by the assumption that MDP unlike PG might not be effective through activation of preformed endogenous mediators but might mimic such endogenous mediators (e.g. monokines; Fevrier *et al.*, 1978), controversy still exists. Thus, in contrast to the immunoadjuvant effect (Heymer *et al.*, 1978), it was not possible to reproduce (Finger and Wirsing von König, 1980; Heymer, B. and Mohr, W., unpublished observations) other biological activities attributed to MDP such as the stimulation of antibacterial resistance (Matsumoto *et al.*, 1983), the formation of epithelioid cell granulomas (Emori and Tanaka, 1978; Nagao *et al.*, 1981; Tanaka *et al.*, 1982), or induction of adjuvant arthritis (Kohashi *et al.*, 1980, 1982; Chang *et al.*, 1981; Zidek *et al.*, 1982).

VII. METABOLIC FATE OF PEPTIDOGLYCAN

It does not make sense to discuss the biological activity and metabolic fate of isolated PG without asking whether the mammalian organism is ever exposed at all to this structure. Is it not much more likely that tissues, in the course of natural bacterial infections, experience contact with whole microorganisms, their extracellular products, their cellular components, and among these, PG-containing cell wall fragments? Or are there mechanisms that lead to the appearance of isolated PG *in vivo*? Further, is the degradation of PG-containing bacterial components influenced by the inflammatory reaction or by the antibiotic treatment of infections? It is evident that these and similar questions are of fundamental significance.

The issue of the *in vivo* degradation of PG or PG-containing cell wall polymers has been very intensively investigated by Ginsburg and his group (Lahav *et al.*, 1974; Ginsburg and Sela, 1976; Ginsburg *et al.*, 1976, 1977; Ginsburg, 1979). Their findings, which fully agree with our observations (Heymer, 1972; Heymer *et al.*, 1975b; Heymer and Haferkamp, 1980), can be summarized as follows: (1) Isolated PGs of many bacterial species are rapidly degraded after phagocytosis both *in vivo* and *in vitro*. (2) This degradation is primarily due to the action of lysosomal enzymes of phagocytes (granulocytes, macrophages). (3) In contrast to isolated PG, cell walls consisting of PG and polysaccharides resist attack by lysosomal enzymes of the mammalian organism and therefore persist undegraded for prolonged periods. Thus, whereas the half-life of radiolabelled PG after intradermal injection into rats is only about 10 h, the half-life of cell wall fragments containing both PG and polysaccharides is approximately 7 days (Heymer *et al.*, 1975b; Heymer and Rietschel, 1977). Or, as clearly shown by W. C. Schmidt (personal communication), 50% of a given amount of group A streptococcal PG intrinsically labelled with ^{14}C and injected intravenously into mice is degraded within 4–5 days. In contrast, the degradation of ^{14}C-labelled deproteinized cell walls lasts about 100 days. Furthermore, such material is detectable within the liver of experimental animals for at least 400 days. The issue of the metabolic fate of PG *in vivo* becomes even more striking if one remembers that MDP, the presumed biologically active part of PG, after parenteral application into mice, is excreted unchanged in urine within minutes (Tomasic *et al.*, 1980). This is the reason why in most *in vivo* studies MDP has been found to be active only when incorporated into mineral oil (Kohashi *et al.*, 1977a,b,c, 1980, 1982; Lopez-Berestein *et al.*, 1983) or liposomes (Fraser-Smith *et al.*, 1983).

However, it is doubtful whether the data reported on the metabolic fate of isolated PG and MDP are relevant for the conditions of a spontaneous bacterial infection. It is obvious that in natural infections the mammalian organism will hardly be exposed to isolated PG or MDP, but much rather to PG-containing cell wall fragments formed in the course of the degradation of bacteria *in vivo*

Table 12   Biological Properties of Peptidoglycan–cell wall Fragments

1. Induction of humoral and cellular immune responses
2. Activation of lymphocytes (e.g. release of lymphokines)
3. Activation of macrophages (e.g. release of monokines, lysosomal enzymes, prostaglandins)
4. Phagocytosis, transport and storage by macrophages
5. Resistance to degradation (persistence in tissue)
6. Induction of chronic inflammation

(Ginsburg, 1979). Thus, in fact, it might be more important to know the biological activity and metabolic fate of such naturally occurring PG-containing cell wall components than that of artificially produced isolated PGs or MDP. With respect to this important issue, one should first of all state that, as evident from Table 12, such polymers basically display biological activities similar to those of isolated PG (Heymer *et al.*, 1975b). However, if one compares items listed in Table 1 and 12, it is obvious that there are also distinct differences due to the considerably different *in vivo* degradation or elimination rates of isolated PGs and PG-containing cell wall fragments.

The practical significance of this different metabolism is illustrated schematically in Figure 4. Whereas isolated PGs, for example after intradermal injection, produce an acute transient inflammatory reaction which subsides within a short period of time (Heymer *et al.*, 1971, 1973b; von Mayenburg *et al.*, 1980, 1982), PG-containing cell wall fragments parenterally applied induce long-lasting chronic inflammation (Ohanian and Schwab, 1967; Cromartie *et al.*, 1977, 1979; Ginsburg, 1979; Heymer and Haferkamp, 1980). If one assumes

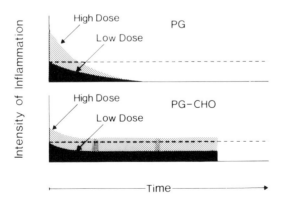

Figure 4. Schematic diagram illustrating the differences in intensity and time course of inflammatory reactions induced by isolated peptidoglycan (PG) or by peptidoglycan–polysaccharide (PG–CHO) polymers. The dotted line indicates the limit of clinical detectability (below the line = subclinical inflammation). Modified from Heymer *et al.* (1982)

that in natural bacterial infections the latter are more likely to occur than isolated PGs, this would imply a potential pathogenic role for such polymers in chronic inflammation. On the other hand, under certain *in vitro* conditions high-molecular-weight soluble PG can be secreted into the surrounding medium (Mirelman *et al.*, 1974; Zeiger *et al.*, 1982; Seidl and Schleifer, 1984). Such material may also be responsible for some of the biological properties of PG *in vivo*.

After this discussion of the metabolic fate and biological activity of isolated PGs and PG-containing cell wall fragments, it seems appropriate to ask what happens with these bacterial components, as far as is known today, in the course of natural bacterial infections. When pathogenic germs invade tissues, phagocytes (granulocytes, macrophages) appear at the site of the inflammatory reaction, and phagocytose and kill the invaders (Wilkinson, 1974; van Furth *et al.*, 1977; Quie *et al.*, 1978; van Furth and Willemze, 1979; Muller, 1981). For this purpose, they possess a rich armoury of highly effective mechanisms (Ginsburg and Sela, 1976; Havemann and Janoff, 1978; Baggiolini and Schnyder, 1979; Haferkamp, 1980a). Earlier studies (Hirsch, 1960; Cohn, 1963; Spector *et al.*, 1970) indicated that phagocytes additionally are able to degrade microorganisms by lysosomal enzymes. However, although mammalian lysosomal enzymes such as N-acetylmuraminidase (lysozyme), N-acetylglucosaminidase and others rapidly split isolated PG, they possess very poor bacteriolytic activity (Chipman and Sharon, 1969; Lahav *et al.*, 1974; Ginsburg, 1979). Interestingly, there is some evidence now that lysozyme may not be effective as a muralytic enzyme but rather as an activator of pre-existing bacterial autolytic wall enzymes (Wecke *et al.*, 1982). Therefore, the *in vivo* degradation of PG — or bacteriolysis in general — might not primarily depend on an 'attack from the outside' (lysosomal enzymes of phagocytes) but rather on an 'attack from the inside' (autolytic enzymes of bacteria). In this case, the fate of microorganisms and of PG would be directed, on the one hand, by the availability of agents capable of activating autolytic wall enzymes in bacteria and, on the other hand, by the presence of inhibitory substances (e.g. polyelectrolytes) which can block bacteriolysis in tissues. Although this new concept (Ginsburg and Lahav, 1983) of the biodegradation of bacteria *in vivo* may considerably modify the view hitherto held of the natural dismantling process, there is little doubt that in the course of spontaneous bacterial infections PG-containing cell wall components in fact do persist in tissues for weeks or even months (Ginsburg and Sela, 1976; Ginsburg, 1979; Heymer and Haferkamp, 1980).

The last aspect of the metabolic fate of PG can be summarized as follows: There is evidence that both the inflammatory reaction and antibiotic treatment profoundly influence the degradation of bacteria, of bacterial cell walls and hence of PG *in vivo* (Ginsburg *et al.*, 1976, 1982; Zeiger *et al.*, 1981, 1982; Ginsburg and Lahav, 1983).

VIII. CONCLUSIONS

When trying to draw some reasonable conclusions from the present discussion of the biological activity of PG one may stress the following facts: (1) PG, with few exceptions, is present in all eubacteria. Therefore, it occurs ubiquitously in the environment of man. Consequently, its pathogenetic potency—even if low grade—must be taken into account. (2) PG is an immunogen. Therefore, some of its biological effects may partially or totally depend on and vary from the immunological state of the host. (3) Although there are slight differences in activity among PGs from different bacterial species, most properties are shared by all PGs, indicating a common biologically active core structure. (4) There are quite a few contradictory findings published in the literature on the biological activity of PG. If one takes into account the complex macromolecular structure of PG (Schleifer and Kandler, 1972) and the difficulties intrinsic in the physicochemical isolation of 'pure' and 'homogeneous' PG preparations (Schleifer, 1975), then such discrepancies are relatively easy to explain (Heymer, 1975b; Heymer and Rietschel, 1977). They by no means prevent a meaningful interpretation of results. (5) When comparing the present state of knowledge with the state 10 years ago (Schleifer and Heymer, 1975), the topic of the biological activity of PG has changed from the description of a vast 'hotch-potch' of diverse properties without a common denominator to a relatively plausible and more unifying concept. In other words, PG has been found to activate important mediator systems of the mammalian organism such as the immune, complement and clotting systems and to release endogenous mediators such as the prostaglandins and interferon. These observations widely explain the, at a first glance, perplexing and frustrating diversity of the biological properties of PG. (6) There is only a preliminary answer to the important question, whether the experimental findings on the biological activity of PG are relevant for man. The pathogenicity of PGs in man—as determined by skin tests—is at least as pronounced as in experimental animals (von Mayenburg *et al.*, 1980). There are several human diseases, in particular chronic inflammatory (Bennett, 1978) or allergic (von Mayenburg *et al.*, 1982) processes, in which PG or PG-containing cell wall components might play a pathogenetic role (Ely, 1980; Heymer and Haferkamp, 1980).

REFERENCES

Abdulla, E. M., and Schwab, J. H. (1965). Immunological properties of bacterial cell wall mucopeptide. *Proc. Soc. Exp. Biol. Med.*, **118**, 359–362.

Adam, A., Ciorbaru, R., Petit, J.-F., and Lederer, E. (1972). Isolation and properties of a macromolecular, water-soluble, immunoadjuvant fraction from the cell wall of *Mycobacterium smegmatis. Proc. Natl. Acad. Sci. USA*, **69**, 851–854.

Adam, A., Ciorbaru, R., Petit, J.-F., Lederer, E., Chedid, L., Lamensans, A., Parant, F., Parant, M., Rosselet, J. P., and Berger, F. M. (1973). Preparation and biological properties of water-soluble adjuvant fractions from delipidated cells of *Mycobacterium smegmatis* and *Nocardia opaca*. *Infect. Immun.*, **7**, 855–861.

Audibert, F., Chedid, L., Lefrancier, P., and Choay, J. (1976). Distinctive adjuvanticity of synthetic analogs of mycobacterial water-soluble components. *Cell. Immunol.*, **21**, 243–249.

Audibert, F., Heymer, B., Gross, C., Schleifer, K. H., Seidl, P. H., and Chedid, L. (1978). 'Absence of binding of MDP, a synthetic immunoadjuvant, to anti-peptidoglycan antibodies. *J. Immunol.*, **121**, 1219–1222.

Baggiolini, M., and Schnyder, J. (1979). Macrophage activation and the mechanisms of tissue destruction. In *Connective Tissue Changes in Rheumatoid Arthritis and the Use of Penicillamine* (Ed. I. L. Bonta), pp.25–38. Birkhäuser-Verlag, Basel, Boston, Stuttgart.

Barot-Ciorbaru, R., Wietzerbin, J., Petit, J.-F., Chedid, L., Falcoff, E., and Lederer, E. (1978). Induction of interferon synthesis in mice by fractions from *Nocardia*. *Infect. Immun.*, **19**, 353–356.

Barot-Ciorbaru, R., Catinot, L., Wietzerbin, J., Petit, J.-F., Chedid, L., and Falcoff, E. (1981). Involvement of a radioresistant cell in the production of circulating interferon induced by *Nocardia* fractions in mice. *J. Reticuloendothelial Soc.*, **30**, 247–257.

Bennett, J. C. (1978). The infectious etiology of rheumatoid arthritis. *Arthritis Rheum.*, **21**, 531–538.

Beveridge, T. J. (1981). Ultrastructure, chemistry, and function of the bacterial wall. *Int. Rev. Cytol.*, **12**, 229–317.

Bokisch, V. A. (1975). Interaction of peptidoglycans with anti-IgGs and with complement. *Z. Immun.-Forsch.*, **149**, 320–330.

Bonney, R. J., Naruns, P., Davies, P., and Humes, J. L. (1979). Antigen-antibody complexes stimulate the synthesis and release of prostaglandins by mouse peritoneal macrophages. *Prostaglandins*, **18**, 605–611.

Boyle, M. D. P., and Borsos, T. (1983). Tissue damage caused by the direct and indirect action of complement.' In *The Reticuloendothelial System*, Vol. 4 (Eds. N. R. Rose and B. V. Siegel), pp.43–76. Plenum Press, New York, London.

Brune, K. (1981). Schmerz, Prostaglandine und Entzündung. *Verh. Dtsch. Ges. Rheumatol.*, **7**, 62–72.

Bültmann, B., Heymer, B., Schleifer, K. H., Seidl, H. P., and Haferkamp, O. (1975). Migration inhibition of peritoneal macrophages by peptidoglycan. *Z. Immun.-Forsch.*, **149**, 289–294.

Caravano, R., and Oberti, J. (1981). Cellular responses of the mouse to the peptidoglycan of a gram-positive bacterium *Streptococcus pyogenes*. *Ann. Immunol. (Paris)*, **132**, 257–274.

Chang, Y.-H., Pearson, C. M., and Chedid, L. (1981). Adjuvant polyarthritis. V. Induction by *N*-acetylmuramyl–L-alanyl–D-isoglutamine, the smallest peptide subunit of bacterial peptidoglycan. *J. Exp. Med.*, **153**, 1021–1026.

Chedid, L. (1981). Immunomodulation by BCG and synthetic bacterial-like adjuvants. In *Immunomodulation by Bacteria and Their Products* (Eds. H. Friedman, T. W. Klein and A. Szentivanyi), pp.151–163. Plenum Press, New York, London.

Chedid, L., and Audibert, F. (1977). Activity in saline of chemically well defined non-toxic bacterial adjuvants. In *Immunopathology, VIIth International Symposium* (Ed. P. A. Miescher), pp.382–396. Schwabe, Basel, Stuttgart.

Chedid, L., Audibert, F., Lefrancier, P., Choay, J., and Lederer, E. (1976). Modulation of the immune response by a synthetic adjuvant and analogs. *Proc. Natl. Acad. Sci. USA*, **73**, 2472–2475.

Chedid, L., Parant, M., Parant, F., Audibert, F., Lefrancier, F., Choay, J., and Sela, M. (1979). Enhancement of certain biological activities of muramyl dipeptide derivatives after conjugation to a multi-poly (L-alanine)–poly(L-lysine) carrier. *Proc. Natl. Acad. Sci.*, **76**, 6557–6561.

Chipman, D. M., and Sharon, N. (1969). Mechanism of lysozyme action. *Science*, **165**, 454–465.

Ciorbaru, R., Petit, J.-F., Lederer, E., Zissman, E., Bona, C., and Chedid, L. (1976). Presence and subcellular localization of two distinct mitogenic fractions in the cells of *Nocardia rubra* and *Nocardia opaca*: preparation of soluble mitogenic peptidoglycan fractions. *Infect. Immun.*, **13**, 1084–1090.

Cohn, Z. A. (1963). The fate of bacteria within phagocytic cells. I. The degradation of isotopically labeled bacteria by polymorphonuclear leucocytes and macrophages. *J. Exp. Med.*, **117**, 27–42.

Cottier, H. (1980). *Pathogenese*, Bd. 1 und 2. Springer-Verlag, Berlin, Heidelberg, New York.

Cromartie, W. J., Craddock, J. G., Schwab, J. H., Anderle, S. K., and Yang, Ch.-H. (1977). Arthritis in rats after systemic injection of streptococcal cells or cell walls. *J. Exp. Med.*, **146**, 1585–1602.

Cromartie, W. J., Anderle, S. K., Schwab, J. H., and Dalldorf, F. G. (1979). Experimental arthritis, carditis and pinnitis induced by systemic injection of group A streptococcal cell walls into guinea-pigs. In *Pathogenic Streptococci* (Ed. M. T. Parker), pp.50–52, Reedbooks Ltd., Chertsey, Surrey.

Damais, C., Bona, C., Chedid, L., Fleck, J., Nauciel, C., and Martin, J. P. (1975). Mitogenic effect of bacterial peptidoglycans possessing adjuvant activity. *J. Immunol.*, **115**, 268–271.

Dziarski, R. (1980a). Modulation of mitogenic responsiveness by staphylococcal peptidoglycan. *Infect. Immun.*, **30**, 431–438.

Dziarski, R. (1980b). Polyclonal activation of immunoglobulin secretion in B lymphocytes induced by staphylococcal peptidoglycan. *J. Immunol.*, **125**, 2478–2483.

Dziarski, R. (1981). Effects of staphylococcal cell wall products on immunity. In *Immunomodulation by Bacteria and Their Products* (Eds. H. Friedman, T. W. Klein and A. Szentivanyi), pp.95–133. Plenum Press, New York, London.

Dziarski, R. (1982a). Studies on the mechanism of peptidoglycan- and lipopolysaccharide-induced polyclonal activation. *Infect. Immun.*, **35**, 507–514.

Dziarski, R. (1982b). Preferential induction of autoantibody secretion in polyclonal activation by peptidoglycan and lipopolysaccharide I. *In vitro* studies. *J. Immunol.*, **128**, 1018–1025.

Dziarski, R. (1982c). Preferential induction of autoantibody secretion in polyclonal activation by peptidoglycan and lipopolysaccharide II. *In vivo* studies. *J. Immunol.*, **128**, 1026–1030.

Dziarski, R., Dziarski, A., and Levinson, A. I. (1980). Mitogenic responsiveness of mouse, rat and human lymphocytes to *Staphylococcus aureus* cell wall, teichoic acid, and peptidoglycan. *Int. Arch. Allergy Appl. Immunol.*, **63**, 383–395.

Eisenberg, R., Fox, A., Greenblatt, J. J., Anderle, S. K., Cromartie, W. J., and Schwab, J. H. (1982). Measurement of bacterial cell wall in tissues by solid-phase radioimmunoassay: correlation of distribution and persistence with experimental arthritis in rats. *Infect. Immun.*, **38**, 127–135.

Ellouz, F., Adam, A., Ciorbaru, R., and Lederer, E. (1974). Minimal structural requirements for adjuvant activity of bacterial peptidoglycan derivatives. *Biochem. Biophys. Res. Commun.*, **59**, 1317–1325.

Ely, P. H. (1980). The bowel bypass syndrome: A response to bacterial peptidoglycans. *J. Am. Acad. Dermatol.*, **2**, 473–487.

Emori, K., and Tanaka, A. (1978). Granuloma formation by synthetic bacterial cell wall fragment: Muramyl dipeptide. *Infect. Immun.*, **19**, 613–620.

Ferguson, T. A., Krieger, N. J., Pesce, A., and Michael, G. (1983). Enhancement of antigen-specific suppression by muramyl dipeptide. *Infect. Immun.*, **39**, 800–806.

Fevrier, M. L., Birrien, J. L., Leclerc, C., Chedid, L., and Liacopoulos, P. (1978). The macrophage, target cell of the synthetic adjuvant muramyl dipeptide. *Eur. J. Immunol.*, **8**, 558–562.

Finger, H., and Wirsing von König C.-H. (1980). Failure of synthetic muramyl dipeptide to increase antibacterial resistance. *Infect. Immun.*, **27**, 288–291.

Fox, A., Brown, R. R., Anderle, S. K., Chetty, C., Cromartie, W. J., Gooder, H., and Schwab, J. H. (1982). Arthropathic properties related to the molecular weight of peptidoglycan–polysaccharide polymers of streptococcal cell walls. *Infect. Immun.*, **35**, 1003–1010.

Franken, N., Seidl, P. H., Kuchenbauer, T., Kolb, H. J., Schleifer, K. H., Weiss, L., and Tympner, K.-D. (1984). Specific immunoglobulin A antibodies to a peptide subunit sequence of bacterial cell wall peptidogylycan. *Infect. Immun.*, **44**, 182–187.

Fraser-Smith, E. B., Eppstein, D. A., Larsen, M. A., and Matthews, T. R. (1983). Protective effect of a muramyl dipeptide analog encapsulated in or mixed with liposomes against *Candida albicans* infection. *Infect. Immun.*, **39**, 172–178.

Gallis, H. A. (1979). Interactions of streptococci with complement and immunoglobulin. In *Pathogenic Streptococci* (Ed. M. T. Parker), pp.78–80. Reedbooks Ltd., Chertsey, Surrey.

Gemsa, D., Seitz, M., Menzel, J., Grimm, W., Kramer, W., and Till, G. (1979). Modulation of phagocytosis induced prostaglandin release from macrophages. *Adv. Exp. Med. Biol.*, **114**, 421–426.

Gemsa, D., Kramer, W., Brenner, M., Till, G., and Resch, K. (1980). Induction of prostaglandin E release from macrophages by colchicine. *J. Immunol.*, **124**, 376–380.

Ginsburg, I. (1979). The role of lysosomal factors of leucocytes in the biodegradation and storage of microbial constituents in infectious granulomas. In *Lysosomes* (Eds. J. T. Dingle, P. J. Jacques and I. H. Shaw), pp.327–406. North-Holland, Amsterdam, New York, Oxford.

Ginsburg, I., and Lahav, M. (1983). Lysis and biodegradation of microorganisms in infectious sites may involve cooperation between leukocyte, serum factors and bacterial wall autolysins: a working hypothesis. *Eur. J. Clin. Microbiol.*, **2**, 186–191.

Ginsburg, I., and Sela, M. N. (1976). The role of leukocytes and their hydrolases in the persistence, degradation and transport of bacterial constituents in tissue: Relation to chronic inflammatory processes in staphylococcal, streptococcal, and mycobacterial infections, and in chronic peridontal disease. *Crit. Rev. Microbiology*, **4**, 249–332.

Ginsburg, I., Neeman, N., Gallily, R., and Lahav, M. (1976). Degradation and survival of bacteria in sites of allergic inflammation. In *Infection and Immunology in the Rheumatic Diseases* (Ed. D. C. Dumonde), pp.43–59, Blackwell Scientific, Oxford, London, Edinburgh, Melbourne.

Ginsburg, I., Zor, U., and Floman, Y. (1977). Experimental models of streptococcal arthritis: Pathogenetic role of streptococcal products and prostaglandins and their modification by anti-inflammatory agents. In *Experimental Models of Chronic Inflammatory Diseases* (Eds. L. E. Glynn and H. D. Schlumberger), pp.256–299. Springer, Berlin, Heidelberg, New York.

Ginsburg, I., Lahav, M., Bergner-Rabinowitz, S., and Ferne, M. (1982). Effect of antibodies on the lysis of staphylococci and streptococci by leukocyte factors, on the production of cellular and extracellular factors by streptococci, and on the solubilization of cell-sensitizing agents from gram-negative rods. In *The Influence of Antibiotics on the Host–Parasite Relationship* (Eds. Eickenberg, Hahn, and Opferkuch), pp.219–227. Springer-Verlag, Stuttgart, Berlin, Heidelberg, New York.

Goguel, A. F., Lespinats, G., and Nauciel, C. (1982). Peptidoglycans extracted from gram-positive bacteria: Expression of antitumor activity according to peptide structure and route of injection. *J. Natl. Cancer Inst.*, **68**, 657–663.

Gold, M. R., and Mishell, R. I. (1981). Membrane receptors on murine macrophages for bacterial peptidoglycans. *Fed. Proc.*, **40**, 1160.

Goldstein, I., Caravano, R. and Parlebas, J. (1973). Immunochemical study of group A streptococcus peptidoglycan solubilized by 8 M urea. *J. Immunol.*, **110**, 1667–1671.

Greenblatt, J., Boackle, R. J., and Schwab, J. H. (1978). Activation of the alternate complement pathway by peptidoglycan from streptococcal cell wall. *Infect. Immun.*, **19**, 296–303.

Grimm, W., Seitz, M., Kirchner, H., and Gemsa, D. (1978). Prostaglandin synthesis in spleen cell cultures of mice injected with *Corynebacterium parvum*. *Cell Immunol.*, **40**, 419–426.

Grov, A. (1976). The effect of specific antibodies on the inhibition of leucocyte migration caused by staphylococcal peptidoglycan. *Acta Pathol. Microbiol. Scand. Sect. B.*, **84**, 315–317.

Grov, A., and Oeding, P. (1971). Serological cross-reactions of tanned erythrocytes sensitized with staphylococcal antigens. *Acta Pathol. Microbiol. Scand. Sect. B.*, **79**, 539–544.

Haferkamp, O. (1980a). Die akute Entzündung und ihre Zellen. *Dtsch. Ärztebl.*, **14**, 895–897.

Haferkamp, O. (1980b). Die akute Entzündung und ihre Mediatoren. *Dtsch. Ärztebl.*, **15**, 957–960.

Hamilton, J. A., Zabriskie, J. B., Lachman, L. B., and Chen, Y.-S. (1982). Streptococcal cell walls and synovial cell activation. *J. Exp. Med.*, **155**, 1702–1718.

Havemann, K., and Janoff, A. (1978). *Neutral Proteases of Human Polymorphonuclear Leukocytes*. Urban and Schwarzenberg, Baltimore, Munich.

Helgeland, S. M., and Grov, A. (1971). Immunochemical characterization of staphylococcal and micrococcal mucopeptides. *Acta Pathol. Microbiol. Scand. Sect. B*, **79**, 819–826.

Helgeland, S. M., and Grov, A. (1975). Estimation of peptidoglycan antibodies by an immunoperoxidase technique. *Z. Immun.-Forsch.*, **149**, 165–167.

Helgeland, S. M., Grov, A., and Schleifer, K. H. (1973). The immunochemistry of *Staphylococcus aureus* mucopeptide. *Acta Pathol. Microbiol. Scand. Sec. B*, **81**, 413–418.

Hether, N. W., Campbell, P. A., Baker, L. A., and Jackson, L. L. (1983). Chemical composition and biological functions of *Listeria monocytogenes* cell wall preparations. *Infect. Immun.*, **39**, 1114–1121.

Heymer, B. (1972). Untersuchungen über die enzymatische Freisetzung bakterieller Antigene. In *Theor. Klin. Med. Einzeldarst.*, **56**, 36–78.

Heymer, B. (1975a). Biologische Aktivität bakterieller Peptidoglycane (Mureine). *Klin. Wochenschr.*, **53**, 49–57.

Heymer, B. (1975b). Biological properties of the peptidoglycan. *Z. Immun.-Forsch.*, **149**, 49–57.

Heymer, B., and Haferkamp, O. (1980). Struktur und Biochemie microbieller Komponenten bei Granulombildung. *Verh. Dtsch. Ges. Pathol.*, **64**, 48–62.

Heymer, B., and Rietschel, E.Th. (1977). Biological properties of peptidoglycans. In *Microbiology 1977* (Ed. D. Schlesinger), pp.344–349. American Society for Microbiology, Washington.

Heymer, B., Bültmann, B., and Haferkamp, O. (1971). Toxicity of streptococcal mucopeptides *in vivo* and *in vitro*. *J. Immunol.*, **106**, 858–861.

Heymer, B., Schachenmayr, W., Bültmann, B., Spanel, R., Haferkamp, O., and Schmidt, W. C. (1973a). A latex agglutination test for measuring antibodies to streptococcal mucopeptides. *J. Immunol.*, **111**, 478–484.

Heymer, B., Bültmann, B., Schachenmayr, W., Spanel, R., Haferkamp, O., and Schmidt, W. C. (1973b). Migration inhibition of rat peritoneal cells induced by streptococcal mucopeptides. Characteristics of the reaction and properties of the mucopeptide preparations. *J. Immunol.*, **116**, 1743–1754.

Heymer, B., Bernstein, D., Schleifer, K. H., and Krause, R. M. (1975a). A radioactive hapten-binding assay for measuring antibodies to the pentapeptide determinant of peptidoglycan. *J. Immunol.*, **114**, 1191–1196.

Heymer, B., Spanel, R., and Haferkamp, O. (1975b). Biologische Aktivität bakterieller Zellwände. *Immun. Infekt.*, **3**, 232–240.

Heymer, B., Schleifer, K. H., Read, S, Zabriskie, J. D., and Krause, R. M. (1976). Detection of antibodies to bacterial cell wall peptidoglycan in human sera. *J. Immunol.*, **117**, 23–26.

Heymer, B., Finger, H., and Wirsing von König, C.-H. (1978). Immunoadjuvant effects of the synthetic muramyl-dipeptide (MDP) *N*-acetylmuramyl-L-alanyl–D-isoglutamine. *Z. Immun.-Forsch.*, **155**, 87–92.

Heymer, B., Spanel, R., and Haferkamp, O. (1982). Experimental models of arthritis. *Curr. Topics. Pathol.* **71**, 123–152.

Hirsch, J. B. (1960). Antimicrobial factors in tissues and phagocytic cells. *Bacteriol. Rev.*, **24**, 133–148.

Hisatsune, K., De Courcy, S. J., and Mudd, S. (1967). The immunologically active cell wall peptide polymer of *Staphylococcus aureus. Biochemistry*, **6**, 595–603.

Hughes, R. C., Thurman, P. F., and Salaman, M. R. (1971). Antigenic properties of *Bacillus licheniformis* cell wall components. *Eur. J. Biochem.*, **19**, 1–8.

Johnson, P. M., Phua, K. K., Perkins, H. R., and Bucknall, R. C. (1982). Antibody to bacterial cell wall peptidoglycan in rheumatic disease. *Ann. Rheum. Dis.*, **41**, 192–209.

Johnson, P. M., Phua, K. K., Perkins, H. R., Hart, C. A., and Bucknall, R. C. (1984). Antibody to streptococcal cell wall peptidoglycan-polysaccharide polymers in seropositive and seronegative rheumatic disease. *Clin. Exp. Immunol.*, **55**, 115–124.

Kandler, O. (1982). Cell wall structures and their phylogenetic implications. *Zentralbl. Bakteriol. Hyg. Abt. 1. Orign. Reihe C*, **3**, 149–160.

Karakawa, W. W., and Krause, R. M. (1966). Studies on the immunochemistry of streptococcal mucopeptide. *J. Exp. Med.*, **124**, 155–171.

Karakawa, W. W., Lackland, H., and Krause, R. M. (1966). An immunochemical analysis of bacterial mucopeptides. *J. Immunol.*, **97**, 797–804.

Karakawa, W. W., Lackland, H., and Krause, R. M. (1967). Antigenic properties of the hexosamine polymer of streptococcal mucopeptides. *J. Immunol.*, **99**, 1179–1182.

Karakawa, W. W., Braun, D. G., Lackland, H., and Krause, R. M. (1968). Immunochemical studies on the cross-reactivity between streptococcal and staphylococcal mucopeptide. *J. Exp. Med.*, **128**, 325–340.

Karakawa, W. W., Maurer, P. H., Walsh, P., and Krause, R. M. (1970). The role of D-alanine in the antigenic specificity of bacterial mucopeptides. *J. Immunol.*, **104**, 230–237.

Kimura, Y., Norose, Y., Kato, T., Furuya, M., Hida, M., and Okabe, T. (1981). Histamine released from mast cells, platelets or isolated intestines by action of peptidoglycan fraction extracted from group-A streptococcal cell walls. In *Basic Concepts of Streptococci and Streptococcal Diseases* (Eds. S. E. Holm and P. Christensen), pp.99–100. Reedbooks Ltd, Chertsey, Surrey.

Koga, T., and Pearson, C. M. (1973). Immunogenicity and arthritogenicity in the rat of an antigen from *Mycobacterium tuberculosis* wax D. *J. Immunol.*, **111**, 599–608.

Kohashi, O., Pearson, C. M., Beck, F. J. W., and Alexander, M. (1977a). Effect of oil composition on both adjuvant-induced arthritis and delayed hypersensitivity to purified protein derivative and peptidoglycans in various rat strains. *Infect. Immun.*, **17**, 244–249.

Kohashi, O., Pearson, C. M., and Koga, T. (1977b). Arthritogenicity of wax D from various mycobacteria related to oil vehicle composition and to the combination with poly I:C, cord factor and acetylated wax D. *Int. Arch. Allergy Appl. Immunol.*, **53**, 357–365.

Kohashi, O., Pearson, C. M., Watanabe, Y., and Kotani, S. (1977c). Preparation of arthritogenic hydrosoluble peptidoglycans from both arthritogenic and non-arthritogenic bacterial cell walls. *Infect. Immun.*, **16**, 861–866.

Kohashi, O., Tanaka, A., Kotani, S., Shiba, T., Kusumoto, S., Yokogawa, K., Kawata, S., and Ozawa, A. (1980). Arthritis-inducing ability of a synthetic adjuvant, *N*-acetylmuramyl peptides, and bacterial disaccharide peptides related to different oil vehicles and their composition. *Infect. Immun.*, **29**, 70–75.

Kohashi, O., Aihara, K., Ozawa, A., Kotani, S., and Azuma, I. (1982). New model of a synthetic adjuvant, *N*-acetylmuramyl–L-alanyl–D-isoglutamine-induced arthritis. *Lab. Invest.*, **47**, 27–36.

Kotani, S., Takada, H., Tsujimoto, M., Ogawa, T., Kato, K., Okunaga, T., Ishihara, Y., Kawasaki, A., Morisaki, I., Kono, N., Shimono, T., Shiba, T., Kusumoto, S., Inage, M., Harada, K., Kitaura, T., Kano, S., Inai, S., Nagai, K., Matsumoto, M., Kubo, T., Kato, M., Tada, Z., Yokogawa, K., Kawata, S., and Inoue, A. (1981). Immunomodulating and related biological activities of bacterial cell walls and their components, enzymatically prepared or synthesized. In *Immunomodulation by Bacteria and their Products* (Eds. H. Friedman, T. W. Klein and A. Szentivanyi), pp.231–273. Plenum Press, New York, London.

Kowalski, J. J., and Berman, D. T. (1971). Immunobiological activity of cell wall antigens of *Staphylococcus aureus*. *Infect. Immun.*, **4**, 205–221.

Krause, R. M. (1975). Immunological activity of the peptidoglycan. *Z. Immun.-Forsch.*, **149**, 136–150.

Krueger, J. M., Pappenheimer, J. R., and Karnovsky, M. L. (1982). The composition of sleep-promoting factor isolated from human urine. *J. Biol. Chem.*, **257**, 1664–1669.

Kurland, J. I., and Bockman, R. (1978). Prostaglandin E production by human blood monocytes and mouse peritoneal macrophages. *J. Exp. Med.*, **147**, 952–957.

Lahav, M., Ne'Eman, N., Adler, E., and Ginsburg, I. (1974). Effect of leukocyte hydrolases on bacteria. I. Degradation of ^{14}C-labeled *Streptococcus* and *Staphylococcus* by leucocyte lysates *in vitro*. *J. Infect. Dis.*, **129**, 528–531.

Lederer, E. (1977). *Natural and Synthetic Immunostimulants Related to the Mycobacterial Cell Wall*. Elsevier, Amsterdam.

Levinson, A. I., Dziarski, A., Zweiman, B., and Dziarski, R. (1983). Staphylococcal peptidoglycan: T-cell-dependent mitogen and relatively T-cell-independent polyclonal B-cell activator of human lymphocytes. *Infect. Immun.*, **39**, 290–296.

Lewis, G. P. (1975). *The Role of Prostaglandins in Inflammation*. Hans Huber Publishers, Bern, Stuttgart, Vienna.

Lopez-Berestein, G., Mehta, K., Mehta, R., Juliano, R. L., and Hersh, E. M. (1983). The activation of human monocytes by liposome-encapsulated muramyl dipeptide analogues. *J. Immunol.*, **130**, 1500–1502.

Masihi, K. N., Azuma, I., Brehmer, W., and Lange, W. (1983). Stimulation of chemiluminescence by synthetic muramyl dipeptide and analogs. *Infect. Immun.*, **40**, 16–21.

Matsumoto, K., Otani, T., Une, T., Osada, Y., Ogawa, H., and Azuma, I. (1983). Stimulation of non-specific resistance to infection induced by muramyl dipeptide analogs substituted in the γ-carboxyl group and evaluation of N^α-muramyl dipeptide–$N\epsilon$-stearoyllysine. *Infect. Immun.*, **39**, 1029–1040.

Mirelman, D., Bracha, R., and Sharon, N. (1974). Penicillin-induced secretion of a soluble, uncross-linked peptidoglycan by *Micrococcus luteus* cells. *Biochemistry*, **13**, 5045–5053.

Monner, D. A., Gmeiner, J., and Mühlradt, P. F. (1981). Evidence from a carbohydrate incorporation assay for direct activation of bone marrow myelopoietic precursor cells by bacterial cell wall constituents. *Infect. Immun.*, **31**, 957–964.

Morley, J. (1981). Role of prostaglandins secreted by macrophages in the inflammatory process. *Lymphokines*, **4**, 377–394.

Muller, H. K. (1981). Mechanisms of clearing injured tissue. In *Tissue Repair and Regeneration* (Ed. L. E. Glynn), pp.145–175. Elsevier North-Holland Biomedical Press, Amsterdam.

Musher, D. M., Verbrugh, H. A., and Verhoef, J. (1981). Suppression of phagocytosis and chemotaxis by cell wall components of *Staphylococcus aureus*. *J. Immunol.*, **127**, 84–88.

Nagao, S., and Tanaka, A. (1980). Muramyl dipeptide-induced adjuvant arthritis. *Infect. Immun.*, **28**, 624–626.

Nagao, S., Ota, F., Emori, K., Inoue, K., and Tanaka, A. (1981). Epithelioid granuloma induced by muramyl dipeptide in immunologically deficient rats. *Infect. Immun.*, **34**, 993–999.

Nguyen-Huy, H., Nauciel, C., and Wermuth, C.-G. (1976). Immunochemical study of the peptidoglycan of gram-negative bacteria. *Eur. J. Biochem.*, **66**, 79–84.

Ogawa, T., Kotani, S., Tsujimoto, M., Kusomoto, S., Shiba, T., Kawata, S., and Yokogawa, K. (1982). Contractile effects of bacterial cell walls, their enzymatic digests, and muramyl dipeptides on ileal strips from guinea pigs. *Infect. Immun.*, **35**, 612–619.

Ogawa, T., Kotani, S., Kusumoto, S., and Shiba, T. (1983). Possible chemotaxis of human monocytes by *N*-acetylmuramyl-L-alanyl-D-isoglutamine. *Infect. Immun.*, **39**, 449–451.

Ohanian, S. H., and Schwab, J. H. (1967). Persistence of group A streptococcal cell walls related to chronic inflammation of rabbit dermal connective tissue. *J. Exp. Med.*, **125**, 1137–1148.

Ohta, M. (1981). Studies on the increased capillary permeability by the intracutaneous administration of peptidoglycan fraction extracted from group A streptococcal cell walls. *Nippon Ika Daigaku Zasshi*, **48**, 402–409.

Oken, M. M., Peterson, P. K., and Wilkinson, B. J. (1979). Peptidoglycan stimulation of endogenous pyrogen secretion by human monocytes. *Clin. Res.*, **27**, 352–361.

Passwell, J. H., Dayer, J.-M., and Merler, E. (1979). Increased postaglandin production by human monocytes after membrane receptor activation. *J. Immunol.*, **123**, 115–120.

Peterson, B. H., and Rosenthal, R. S. (1982). Complement consumption by gonococcal peptidoglycan. *Infect. Immun.*, **35**, 442–448.

Peterson, P. K., Wilkinson, B. J., Kim, Y., and Schmeling, D. (1978). The key role of peptidoglycan in the opsonization of *Staphylococcus aureus*. *J. Clin. Invest.*, **61**, 597–609.

Pope, R. M., Rutstein, J. E., and Strauss, D. C. (1982). Antibodies to the immunodominant portion of streptococcal mucopeptide (pentapeptide) in patients with rheumatic disorders. *Ann. Rheum. Dis.*, **41**, 193.

Pryjma, J., Pryjma, K., Grov, A., and Heczko, P. B. (1976). Immunological activity of staphylococcal cell wall antigens. In *Zentralbl. Bakteriol. Parasitenkd. Infektionskr. Hyg. Abt. 1. Suppl.*, **5**, 873–881.

Pryzwansky, K. B., MacRae, E. K., and Lambris, J. D. (1983). Capping of complement receptors on human neutrophils induced by group A streptococcal cell walls. *J. Immunol.*, **130**, 1674–1677.

Quie, P. G., Mills, E. L., McPhail, L. C., and Johnston, R. B. (1978). Phagocytic defects. *Springer Semin. Immunopathol.*, **1**, 323–337.

Ranu, R. S. (1975). Studies on the immunochemistry of *Staphylococcus aureus* cell wall: Antigenicity of pentaglycine bridges. *Med. Microbiol. Immunol.*, **161**, 53–61.

Räsänen, L., Mustikkamäki, U. P., and Arvilommi, H. (1982). Polyclonal response of human lymphocytes to bacterial cell walls, peptidoglycans and teichoic acids. *Immunology*, **46**, 481–486.

Reichert, C. M., Carelli, C., Jolivet, M., Audibert, F., Lefrancier, P., and Chedid, L. (1980). Synthesis of conjugates containing *N*-acetylmuramyl–L-alanyl–D-isoglutaminyl (MDP). Their use as hapten-carrier systems. *Mol. Immunol.*, **17**, 357–363.

Rogers, H. J. (1974). Peptidoglycans (mucopeptides): structure, function, and variations. *Ann. N.Y. Acad. Sci.*, **235**, 29–51.

Rolicka, M., and Massell, B. F. (1973). Antipeptidoglycan in rheumatic fever: Agreement with carditis. *Proc. Soc. Exp. Biol. Med.*, **144**, 892–895.

Rolicka, M., and Park, J. D. (1969). Antimucopeptide antibodies and their specificity. *J. Immunol.*, **103**, 196–203.

Rotta, J. (1975). Endotoxin-like properties of the peptidoglycan. *Z. Immun.-Forsch.*, **149**, 230–244.

Rotta, J., and Schleifer, K. H. (1974). Pyrogenic activity of bacterial mucopeptides. *J. Hyg. Epidemiol. (Praha)*, **18**, 50.

Rotta, J., Ryc, M., Masek, K., and Zaòral, M. (1979). Biological activity of synthetic subunits of *Streptococcus* peptidoglycan. *Exp. Cell Biol.*, **47**, 258–268.

Rotta, J., Ryc, M., Straka, R., and Zaoral, M. (1981). *Streptococcus* peptidoglycan and its analogues: structure and function relationship. In *Basic Concepts of Streptococci and Streptococcal Diseases* (Eds. S. E. Holm and P. Christensen), pp.96–98. Reedbooks Ltd., Chertsey, Surrey.

Ryan, G. B., and Majno, G. (1977). Acute inflammation. *Am. J. Pathol.*, **86**, 185–249.

Ryc, M., Wagner, B., Wagner, M., and Straka, R. (1982). The nature of the peptidoglycan immunodeterminants of a group A streptococcus strain demonstrable by the immunoferritin technique. *Curr. Microbiol.*, **7**, 187–190.

Saiki, I., Kamisango, K.-I., Tanio, Y., Okumura, H., Yamamura, Y., and Azuma, I. (1982). Adjuvant activity of purified peptidoglycan of *Listeria monocytogenes* in mice and guinea pigs. *Infect. Immun.*, **38**, 58–66.

Samuelsson, B. (1982). Die Leukotriene, superaktive, an Allergie und Entzündung beteiligte Wirkstoffe. *Angew. Chem.*, **94**, 881–889.

Schachenmayr, W., Heymer, B., and Haferkamp, O. (1975). Antibodies to peptidoglycan in the sera from population surveys. *Z. Immun.-Forsch.*, **149**, 179–186.

Schleifer, K. H. (1975). Chemical structure of the peptidoglycan, its modifiability and relation to the biological activity. *Z. Immun.-Forsch.*, **149**, 104–117.

Schleifer, K. H., and Heymer, B. (1975). International workshop on the immunological and biological properties of peptidoglycan and related bacterial cell-wall polymers. *Z. Immun.-Forsch.*, **149**, 103–356.

Schleifer, K. H., and Kandler, O. (1972). Peptidoglycan types of bacterial cell walls and their taxonomic implications. *Bacteriol. Rev.*, **36**, 407–477.

Schleifer, K. H., and Kandler, O. (1983). Primary structure of murein and pseudomurein. In *The Target of Penicillin* (Eds. R. Hakenbeck, J. V. Höltje and H. Labischinski), pp.11–17. Walter de Gruyter, Berlin, New York.

44   *Immunology of the Bacterial Cell Envelope*

Schleifer, K. H., and Krause, R. M. (1971a). The immunochemistry of peptidoglycan. The immunodominant site of the peptide subunit and the contribution of each of the amino acids to the binding properties of the peptides. *J. Biol. Chem.*, **246**, 986–993.

Schleifer, K. H., and Krause, R. M. (1971b). The immunochemistry of peptidoglycan. Separation and characterization of antibodies to the glycan and to the peptide subunit. *Eur. J. Biochem.*, **19**, 471–478.

Schleifer, K. H., and Seidl, P. H. (1974). The immunochemistry of peptidoglycan. Antibodies against a synthetic immunogen cross-reacting with peptidoglycan. *Eur. J. Biochem.*, **43**, 509–519.

Schleifer, K. H., and Seidl, P. H. (1977). Structure and immunological aspects of peptidoglycans. In *Microbiology 1977* (Ed. D. Schlesinger), pp.339–343. American Society for Microbiology, Washington.

Schleifer, K. H., and Seidl, P. H. (1984). Chemical composition and structure of murein. *Soc. Appl. Bacteriol. Symp. Ser.*, **20**, 201–219.

Schleifer, K. H., and Stackebrandt, E. (1983). Molecular systematics of prokaryotes. *Annu. Rev. Microbiol.*, **37**, 143–187.

Schopfer, K., Douglas, S. D., and Wilkinson, B. (1980). Immunoglobulin E antibodies against *Staphylococcus aureus* cell walls in the sera of patients with hyperimmunoglobulinemia E and recurrent staphylococcal infection. *Infect. Immun.*, **27**, 563–568.

Seidl, P. H., and Schleifer, K. H. (1975). Immunochemical studies with synthetic immunogens chemically related to peptidoglycan. *Z. Immun.-Forsch.*, **149**, 157–164.

Seidl, P. H., and Schleifer, K. H. (1977). The immunochemistry of peptidoglycan. Antibodies against a synthetic immunogen cross-reacting with an interpeptide bridge of peptidoglycan. *Eur. J. Biochem.*, **74**, 353–363.

Seidl, P. H., and Schleifer, K. H. (1978a). Specific antibodies to the N-termini of the interpeptide bridges of peptidoglycan. *Arch. Microbiol.*, **118**, 185–192.

Seidl, P. H., and Schleifer, K. H. (1978b). Rapid test for the serological separation of staphylococci from micrococci. *Appl. Environ. Microbiol.*, **35**, 479–482.

Seidl, P. H., and Schleifer, K. H. (1979). The immunochemistry of peptidoglycan. Serological detection of a difference in a single N-terminal amino acid. *Mol. Immunol.*, **16**, 385–388.

Seidl, P. H., and Schleifer, K. H. (1984). Secretion of fragments from bacterial cell wall peptidoglycan. In *Environmental Regulation of Microbial Metabolism* (Eds. I. S. Kualev, A. T. Severin and E. A. Dawes). Academic Press, London.

Seidl, P. H., Franken, N., and Schleifer, K. H. (1983). The immunochemistry of peptidoglycan. In *The Target of Penicillin* (Eds. R. Hakenbeck, J. V. Höltje and H. Labischinski), pp.299–304. Walter de Gruyter, Berlin, New York.

Seltmann, G. (1982). *Die bakterielle Zellwand*. Gustav Fischer Verlag, Stuttgart.

Semeraro, N., Colucci, M., and Vermylen, J. (1979). Complement-dependent and complement-independent interactions of bacterial lipopolysaccharides and mucopeptides with rabbit and human platelets. *Thromb. Haemostas.*, **41**, 392–406.

Smolen, J. E., and Weissmann, G. (1978). The granulocyte: Metabolic properties and mechanisms of lysosomal enzyme release. In *Neutral Proteases of Human Polymorphonuclear Leukocytes* (Eds. K. Havemann and A. Janoff), pp.56–76. Urban und Schwarzenberg, Baltimore, Munich.

Spector, W. B., Reichhold, N., and Ryan, G. B. (1970). Degradation of granuloma-inducing micro-organisms by macrophages. *J. Pathol.*, **101**, 339–354.

Stewart-Tull, D. E. S. (1980). The immunological activities of bacterial peptidoglycans. *Annu. Rev. Microbiol.*, **34**, 311–340.

Stewart-Tull, D. E. S. (1983a). Immunopotentiating products of bacteria. In *Medical Microbiology*, Vol. 2, *Immunization Against Bacterial Disease* (Eds. C. S. F. Easmon and J. Jeljaszewicz), pp.1–42. Academic Press, London.

Stewart-Tull, D. E. S. (1983b). Immunologically important constituents of *Mycobacteria*: Adjuvants. In *Biology of Mycobacteria*, Vol. 2, (Eds. C. Ratledge and J. Stanford), pp.3–84. Academic Press, London.

Takada, H., Nagao, S., Kotani, S., Kawata, S., Yokogawa, K., Kusumoto, S., Shiba, T., and Yano, I. (1980). Mitogenic effects of bacterial cell walls and their components on mureine splenocytes. *Biken J.*, **23**, 61–68.

Tanaka, A., and Emori, K. (1980). Epithelioid granuloma formation by a synthetic bacterial cell wall component, muramyl dipeptide (MDP). *Am. J. Pathol.*, **98**, 733–748.

Tanaka, A., Nagao, S., Saito, R., Kotani, S., Kusomoto, S., and Shiba, T. (1977). Correlation of stereochemically specific structure in muramyl dipeptide between macrophage activation and adjuvant activity. *Biochem. Biophys. Res. Commun.*, **77**, 621–627.

Tanaka, A., Emori, K., Nagao, S., Kushima, K., Kohashi, O., Saitoh, M., and Kataoka, T. (1982). Epithelioid granuloma formation requiring no T-cell function. *Am. J. Pathol.*, **106**, 165–170.

Tomasic, J., Ladesic, B., Valinger, Z., and Hrsak, J. (1980). The metabolic fate of ^{14}C-labeled peptidoglycan monomer in mice. I. Identification of the monomer and the corresponding pentapeptide in urine. *Biochim. Biophys. Acta*, **629**, 77–82.

Uchida, K., and Aida, K. (1977). Acyl type of bacterial cell wall: Its simple identification by colorimetric method. *Appl. Microbiol.*, **23**, 249–260.

Vane, J. R., and Ferreira, S. H. (1978). *Inflammation*, Springer Verlag, Berlin, Heidelberg, New York.

van Furth, R., and Willemze, R. (1979). Phagocytic cells during an acute inflammatory reaction. In *Curr. Top. Pathol.*, **68**, 180–212.

van Furth, R., van Waarde, D., Thompson, J., and Gassmann, A. E. (1977). The regulation of the participation of mononuclear phagocytes in inflammatory responses. In *Experimental Models of Chronic Inflammatory Diseases* (Eds. L. E. Glynn and H. D. Schlumberger), pp.302–326. Springer, Berlin, Heidelberg, New York.

Verbrugh, H. A., van Dijk, W. C., Peters, R., van Erne, M. E., Daha, M. R., Peterson, P. K., and Verhoef, J. (1980). Opsonic recognition of staphylococci mediated by cell wall peptidoglycan: Antibody independent activation of human complement and opsonic activity of peptidoglycan antibodies. *J. Immunol.*, **124**, 1167–1173.

Verbrugh, H. A., Peters, R., Rozenberg-Arska, M., Peterson, P. K., and Verhoef, J. (1981). Antibodies to cell wall peptidoglycan of *Staphylococcus aureus* in patients with serious staphylococcal infections. *J. Infect. Dis.*, **144**, 1–9.

Vogt, W. (1982). Aktivierung und biologische Wirkungen des Komplementsystems. *Funkt. Biol. Med.*, **1**, 189–198.

von Mayenburg, J., Heymer, B., Düngemann, H., Schleifer, K. H., Seidl, H. P., Galle, J., Neiss, A., and Borelli, S. (1980). Hautreaktionen gegen isolierte bakterielle Zellwandkomponenten, insbesondere bakterielle Peptidoglycane. *Z. Hautkr.*, **55**, 710–733.

von Mayenburg, J., Heymer, B., Düngemann, H., Schleifer, K. H., Seidl, P. H., Neiss, A., and Borelli, S. (1982). Studies on bacterial hypersensitivity in man. *Allergy*, **37**, 249–258.

Wadström, T. (1973). Bacteriolytic enzymes from *Staphylococcus aureus*. *Contrib. Microbiol. Immunol.*, **1**, 397–405.

Wagner, M., and Wagner, B. (1978). Die Verwendung von Lysozym-Peroxydase-Konjugaten zum elektronenmikroskopischen Nachweis von Peptidoglycan in der Zellwand von Streptokokken. *Zentralbl. Bakteriol. Hyg. Abt. 1. Orig. Reihe A*, **240**, 302–312.

Wahl, S. M., Wahl, L. M., McCarthy, J. B., Chedid, L., and Mergenhagen, S. E. (1979). Macrophage activation by mycobacterial water soluble compounds and synthetic muramyl dipeptide. *J. Immunol.*, **122**, 2226–2231.

Wecke, J., Lahav, M., Ginsburg, I., and Giesbrecht, P. (1982). Cell wall degradation of *Staphylococcus aureus* by lysozyme. *Arch. Microbiol.*, **131**, 116–123.

Weidemann, M. J., Peskar, B. A., Wrogemann, K., Rietschel, E. Th., Staudinger, H., and Fischer, H. (1978). Prostaglandin and thromboxane synthesis in a pure macrophage population and the inhibition, by E-type prostaglandins, of chemiluminescence. *FEBS Lett.*, **89**, 136–140.

Weksler, B. B., and Hill, M. J. (1969). Inhibition of leukocyte migration by a *Staphylococcus* factor. *J. Bacteriol.*, **98**, 1030–1035.

Werner, G. H., Maral, R., Floch, H. F., Migliore-Samour, D., and Jolles, P. (1974). Activités biologiques des adjuvants hydrosolubles de faible poids moléculaire extraits de *Myobacterium tuberculosis* var. *hominis*. *C.R. Acad. Sci. Paris Ser. D*, **278**, 789–796.

Wheat, L. J., Wilkinson, B. J., Kohler, R. B., and White, A. C. (1983). Antibody response to peptidoglycan during staphylococcal infections. *J. Infect. Dis.*, **147**, 16–22.

Wikler, M. (1975). Isolation and characterization of homogenous rabbit antibodies to *Micrococcus lysodeikticus* with specificity to the peptidoglycan and to the glucose–N-acetylaminomannuronic polymer. *Z. Immun.-Forsch.*, **148**, 193–200.

Wildfeurer, A., Heymer, B., Schleifer, K. H., Seidl, H. P., and Haferkamp, O. (1974). Zur Schockdiagnostik: Der Nachweis von Endotoxin und Mucopeptid mit dem *Limulus polyphemus*-Lysat-Test. *Klin. Wochenschr.*, **52**, 175–178.

Wilhelm, J. A., Matter, L., and Schopfer, K. (1982). IgG, IgA and IgM antibodies to *S. aureus* purified cell walls (PCW) in normal and infected individuals. *Experientia*, **38**, 1375–1376.

Wilkinson, P. C. (1974). *Chemotaxis and Inflammation*. Churchill Livingstone, Edinburgh, London.

Wilkinson, B. J., Kim, Y., and Peterson, P. K. (1981). Factors affecting complement activation by *Staphylococcus aureus* cell walls, their components, and mutants altered in teichoic acid. *Infect. Immun.*, **32**, 216–224.

Williams, T. J., and Jose, P. J. (1981). Mediation of increased vascular permeability after complement activation. *J. Exp. Med.*, **153**, 136–153.

Windle, B. E., Murphy, P. A., and Cooperman, S. (1983). Rabbit polymorphonuclear leukocytes do not secrete endogenous pyrogens or interleukin 1 when stimulated by endotoxin, polyinosine:polycytosine, or muramyl dipeptide. *Infect. Immun.*, **39**, 1142–1146.

Youlten, J. F. (1978). Inflammatory mediators and vascular events. In *Inflammation* (Eds. J. R. Vane and S. H. Ferreira), pp.571–587. Springer Verlag, Berlin, Heidelberg, New York.

Zeiger, A. R., and Maurer, P. H. (1973). Immunochemistry of a synthetic peptidoglycan-precursor pentapeptide. *Biochemistry*, **12**, 3387–3394.

Zeiger, A. R., Tuazon, C. U., and Sheagren, J. N. (1981). Antibody levels to bacterial peptidoglycan in human sera during the time course of endocarditis and bacteremic infections caused by *Staphylococcus aureus*. *Infect. Immun.*, **33**, 795–800.

Zeiger, A. R., Wong, W., Chatterjee, A. N., Young, F. E., and Tuazon, C. U. (1982). Evidence for the secretion of soluble peptidoglycans by clinical isolates of *Staphylococcus aureus*. *Infect. Immun.*, **37**, 1112–1118.

Zidek, Z., Masek, K., and Jiricka, Z. (1982). Arthritogenic activity of a synthetic immunoadjuvant, muramyl dipeptide. *Infect. Immun.*, **35**, 674–679.

Immunology of the Bacterial Cell Envelope
Edited by D. E. S. Stewart-Tull and M. Davies
© 1985 John Wiley & Sons Ltd.

CHAPTER 3

Immunopotentiating Activity of Peptidoglycan and Surface Polymers

Duncan E. S. Stewart-Tull

Department of Microbiology, Alexander Stone Building, University of Glasgow, Garscube Estate, Bearsden, Glasgow G61 1QH, UK

I. INTRODUCTION

Since the 1930s the immunomodulating activity (adjuvant or immuno-potentiating activity) of the mycobacterial outer surface component has been studied extensively. The early chemical studies of Rudolph Anderson and

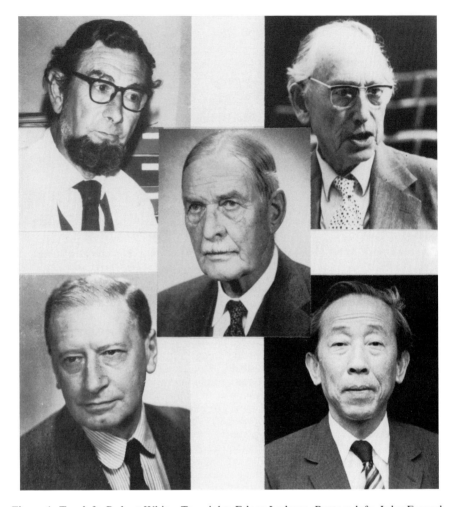

Figure 1. Top left: Robert White. Top right: Edgar Lederer. Bottom left: Jules Freund (reproduced from *J. Immunol.*, **90** (1963)) by permission of Williams & Wilkins Co. Bottom right: Shozo Kotani. Centre: Rudolph Anderson (reproduced from *Journal of Biological Chemistry*, **233** (1958) by permission of the American Society of Biological Chemists)

biological studies of Jules Freund were combined in the search for the component of the cell envelope responsible for a variety of biological effects. The main impetus for such studies came from the groups of Edgar Lederer in Paris, Robert White in London and Shozo Kotani in Osaka, until the early 1970s.

At this time, three major discoveries were announced, namely that (a) *N*-acetylmuramyl–L-Ala–D-isoglutamine (MDP) was the minimal structural component required to effect immunopotentiation (Ellouz *et al.*, 1974), (b) the chemical synthesis of MDP was possible (Merser and Sinay, 1974; Merser *et al.*, 1975), and (c) a cell-mediated immune response was stimulated in guinea-pigs against tumour cells injected with *Mycobacterium bovis* BCG (Zbar *et al.*, 1970, 1971). Since these reports there has been an information explosion on immunopotentiators, albeit that the majority of these papers refer to chemical derivatives of MDP.

It became apparent that, depending on the dose of adjuvant incorporated into an injection mixture, one either potentiated or depressed or caused no effect on the immune response. For this reason, adjuvants are now referred to as immunomodulating agents or immunomodulators.

II. CLASSICAL MYCOBACTERIAL IMMUNOMODULATORS

A. Freund's Complete Adjuvant

The early background to the development of Freund's complete adjuvant (FCA) was detailed by Stewart-Tull (1983a). Most immunologists are familiar with the use of FCA in the stimulation of humoral antibodies against a variety of antigens. Indeed, in many instances the use of Freund's incomplete adjuvant (FIA) will suffice and high levels of antibody are produced.

Freund and his co-workers (Freund and McDermott, 1942; Freund and Bonanto, 1942, 1946) incorporated killed *Mycobacterium tuberculosis* in the mineral oil phase of a water-in-oil emulsion containing a protein antigen; after injection, this mixture stimulated a sustained antibody response in guinea-pigs. In addition, such animals developed a delayed-type hypersensitivity (cell-mediated response) against the protein antigen. This activity was not confined to one species, *M. bovis, M. smegmatis, M. phlei* (Freund, 1947), *M. avium* (White, 1959) and *M. leprae* (Stewart-Tull and Davies, 1972) showing a positive effect. The current commercial FCA contains *M. butyricum* (Sigma, St. Louis, MO, USA).

The biological side-effects associated with the use of the water-in-mineral oil emulsion containing *M. tuberculosis* were often severe in animals and have precluded the extension of the experimental system into vaccines for human use. For example, the subcutaneous injection of *M. tuberculosis* in mineral oil into guinea-pigs stimulates the formation of a local granuloma at the site of injection. The granuloma contains large numbers of epithelioid macrophages, together with giant cells surrounded by an area of infiltrated lymphocytes and macrophages (Rist, 1938; Suter and White, 1954; White *et al.*, 1955) (Figure 2). White (1971) produced some evidence that the granuloma formed in the guinea-pig as the result of a specific immunological stimulus triggered by *M. tuberculosis*, although the mineral oil was a critical factor in the manifestation of this stimulus and an essential prerequisite for maximum immunopotentiation

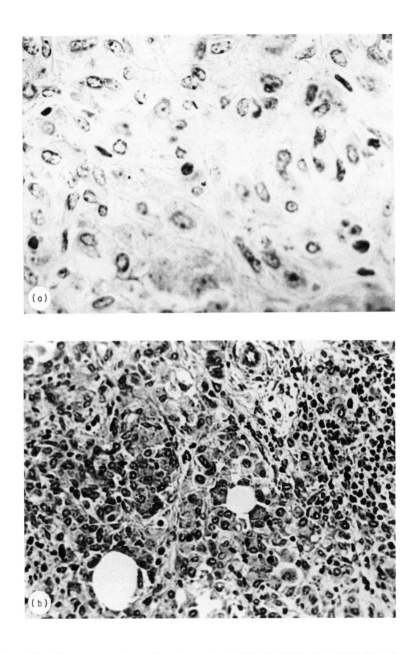

Figure 2. Adjuvant granuloma in guinea-pig. (a) Epithelioid cells. (b) Infiltration of lymphocytes on right

(White, 1976). However, the mineral oil component should not contain short-chain solvent hydrocarbons since these cause intense inflammatory reactions, dissolution of cell membranes, necrosis at the site of injection and an associated immunosuppressive effect (Stewart-Tull *et al.*, 1976). Numerous attempts have been made to find suitable biodegradable hydrocarbons for vaccines (Hilleman, 1966) but without much success. In both *Vibrio cholerae* (Azurin *et al.*, 1967; Ogonuki *et al.*, 1967) and *Clostridium tetani* (MacLennan *et al.*, 1965) severe side-effects were experienced by recipients of an oil-adjuvanted vaccine with the effect that these have fallen into disrepute for human use.

It should be remembered also that the use of FCA in experimental studies can lead to problems for the vaccinator. Stones (1979) described a case where a veterinary surgeon had a finger amputated following accidental self-inoculation with an oil-emulsion adjuvant vaccine that was being used to immunize chickens. Initial symptoms of pain and inflammation at the site of injection were ignored and amputation of a phalanx was required due to the delay in seeking medical attention.

The mycobacterial component of FCA has also been linked to these contraindications and is totally unacceptable for inclusion in human vaccines due to the 'pathogen' label. Unfortunately, the routine administration of mycobacterial organisms in vaccines would be barred also because of sensitization to tuberculin and other protein antigens. However, we should remember that *M. bovis* BCG organisms are inoculated into human beings to stimulate cell-mediated immunity and these contain adjuvant material, so that the use of an adjuvant per se is not necessarily harmful, (see section VIII).

B. Mycobacterial Cell Envelope Adjuvant

In view of the restricted use of FCA, attempts were made to purify the active component in the mycobacterial cell responsible for immunopotentiation. The structure of the mycobacterial outer surface is complex and a number of interpretations have been proposed for the layers revealed by electron microscopy (see Barksdale and Kim, 1977, and Draper, 1982). There is good evidence to show that paired fibres (Takeya *et al.*, 1958, 1961), lying outside the true peptidoglycan layer, extractable with chloroform, contain a peptidoglycolipid (Gordon and White, 1971) (Figure 3). This material was originally referred to as mycobacterial wax D, following the separation of four wax preparations, A–D, from the mycobacterial surface (Aebi *et al.*, 1953; Asselineau and Lederer, 1953). However, the crude wax D could be fractionated into a number of different molecular components by centrifugation in ether at 50 000 *g* (Jollès *et al.*, 1962, 1963), and it was the peptidoglycolipid fraction that proved to be adjuvant-active (White *et al.*, 1964).

The peptidoglycolipid contained a number of amino acids and amino sugars typically associated with the mycobacterial cell-wall peptidoglycan, and it was

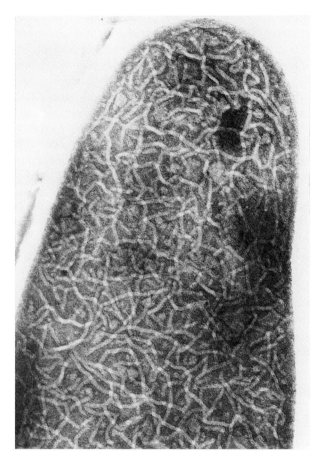

Figure 3. Electron micrograph of *Mycobacterium tuberculosis* showing the characteristic surface peptidoglycolipid filaments. The preparation was negatively stained with ammonium molybdate, × 80 500; the diameter of the filaments is 13 nm. (Kindly provided by Dr. John Gordon, Gartnavel Hospital, Glasgow, UK)

proposed that the structure of these two components might be analogous. The provision of pure muramic acid enabled the complete analogy to be shown (Figure 4) (reviewed by Stewart-Tull, 1983a).

III. PEPTIDOGLYCAN IMMUNOMODULATORS

Meanwhile, studies with other microorganisms indicated that the myco-bacteria were not unique in possessing immunopotentiating activity;

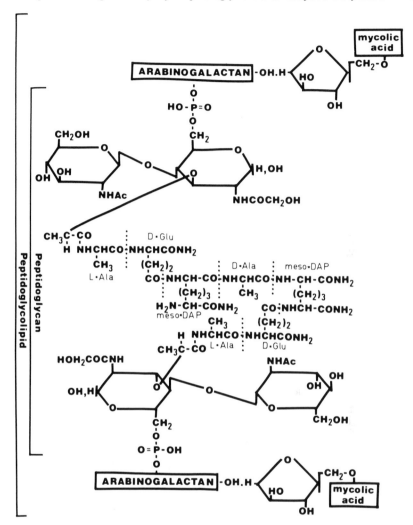

Figure 4. Mycobacterial peptidoglycan and peptidoglycolipid. meso-DAP = meso-diaminopimelic acid. (Reproduced, with permission, from the *Annual Review of Microbiology*, Vol. 34. © 1980 by Annual Reviews Inc.

streptococcal peptidoglycan was active (Holton and Schwab, 1966; see also Chapter 4).

Subsequently, a variety of immunopotentiating activities were shown with cell wall preparations from such widely separated organisms as *Proteus vulgaris, Moraxella glucidolytica, Neisseria perflava* (Nauciel *et al.*, 1973a,b, 1974) *M. bovis* (Nauciel *et al.*, 1974; Stewart-Tull *et al.*, 1975b), *Staphylococcus aureus,*

Micrococcus luteus, Lactobacillus plantarum, Nocardia asteroides, Bacillus megaterium and *Clostridium botulinum* (Kotani *et al.*, 1975a,b,c). Surprisingly, the peptidoglycan preparation of *Micrococcus luteus* (*lysodeikticus*) was inactive. Kotani *et al.* (1977) sought to explain this and suggested that an α-carboxyl group of D-glutamic acid was essential for activity. In the peptidoglycans of the adjuvant-inactive *Corynebacterium poinsettiae, C. betae* and *C. insidiosum*, the amino acid linked to muramic acid, was glycine or L-serine, and not L-alanine. The α-carboxyl group of the second amino acid, either D-glutamic acid or threo-3-hydroxyglutamic acid, was involved in a cross-link to the C-terminal D-alanine of another peptide.

Whereas the cell-wall preparation of *Staphylococcus epidermidis* did not produce an adjuvant effect against the protein antigen, ovalbumin (Kotani *et al.*, 1975a), both the peptidoglycan and the *N*-acetylmuramyl-tetrapeptide (Ellouz *et al.*, 1974) from this organism caused immunopotentiation against the synthetic antigen azobenzenearsonate–*N*-acetyl–L-tyrosine (Fleck *et al.*, 1974). Similarly, a cell-wall endopeptidase digest of the cell-walls of both *Micrococcus luteus* (*lysodeikticus*) and *Staphylococcus epidermidis* contained a component with immunopotentiating activity against ovalbumin (Kotani *et al.*, 1977). From these examples and others reviewed by Stewart-Tull (1980) it is apparent that the assessment of an immunomodulator depends, not only on its chemical structure and conformation, but also on the nature of the antigen, the conditions of administration and the arm of the immune response to be stimulated.

IV. THE PATH TO MURAMYL-DIPEPTIDE

A major disadvantage in the search for good immunomodulators was the insolubility of both the classical peptidoglycolipid and peptidoglycans in water. The former required the presence of a mineral oil for suspension, but as I have mentioned previously, these caused unacceptable adverse reactions; the vaccine was antigen in a water-in-mineral oil emulsion. A significant advance came with the isolation, either from mycobacterial cells of water-soluble adjuvant (Adam *et al.*, 1972; Migliore-Samour and Jollès, 1972), adjuvant anti-tumour factor (Hiu, 1972) and polysaccharide-peptidoglycan, or from spent culture fluid of a Seibert-type glycopeptide (Stewart-Tull *et al.*, 1975b). The water-soluble *N*-acetylglucosamine–*N*-glycolated muramic acid–L-Ala–D-Glu–meso-A$_2$pm–D-Ala was isolated from *M. smegmatis* and shown to have immunopotentiating activity by Adam *et al.* (1974a,b). Ellouz *et al.* (1974) established a new era of research when they removed the terminal D-alanine and *N*-acetylglucosamine from a similar disaccharide–tetrapeptide isolated from *Escherichia coli* and awarded another first to this organism as the resultant muramyl-dipeptide (MDP) was an effective immunomodulator (see Figure 1A, Chapter 5). In France, chemists undertook the task of producing a synthetic MDP and this was achieved by Merser *et al.* (1975). The Japanese groups were also active in this pursuit and reports followed from Kotani *et al.* (1974, 1975b) describing the immunopotentiating activities of these synthetic muramyl-dipeptides. Several major companies realized the potential market for the synthetic immuno-modulator and its derivatives and have produced marketable products. Certainly, one major British company decided not to follow this course of action, so the bulk of research on these compounds has been done in France and Japan. The reader is referred to the Chapter 5 by Takada and Kotani, and also to the following key references to the synthetic product: Adam *et al.*, 1981; Audibert and Chedid, 1980; Azuma *et al.*, 1981; Bahr *et al.*, 1983; Chedid, 1977, 1978, 1983; Chedid and Audibert, 1976, 1977a,b; Chedid and Kotani, 1981; Chedid and Lederer, 1978; Chedid and Parant, 1981; Chedid *et al.* 1977a,b, 1978a,b, 1981, 1982; Lederer, 1980a,b, 1982a,b; Lederer and Chedid, 1982; Lefrancier and Lederer, 1981; Matsumoto *et al.*, 1981; Parant, 1979; Yamamura *et al.*, 1982.

V. POTENTIATION OF HUMORAL ANTIBODY RESPONSE

The characteristic activity of an adjuvant substance is to cause a stimulated immune response, i.e. immunopotentiation. It is curious that so few studies have attempted to define the optimal proportions of antigen and immunopotentiator in a vaccine preparation. In general, White *et al.* (1958, 1964) found that a single injection of a water-in-oil emulsion containing 2.0 mg of ovalbumin in the aqueous phase and 200 μg of whole *M. tuberculosis* cells or the peptidoglycolipid in the oil phase was sufficient to stimulate a prolonged antibody response to the protein antigen. In the guinea-pig, this antibody was usually of the immunoglobulin IgG_1 and IgG_2 classes. Although as little as 40 μg of peptidoglycolipid would stimulate an elevated humoral antibody response, the dose of 200 μg was adopted for comparison, albeit that this amount might be suboptimal or too great, with a resultant immunodepressive effect. The mean levels of anti-ovalbumin precipitating antibodies in the serum expressed as μg N per ml, were greater than 250 for an active preparation; the maximum value was 509. By comparison, Stewart-Tull *et al.* (1975b) obtained a mean value of 865 μg of antibody nitrogen (AbN) per ml following the injection of 200 μg of *M. bovis* BCG cell walls. Following the injection of 100 μg of the cell-wall preparation of *Staphylococcus aureus*, or *Streptococcus pyogenes* in a water-in-oil emulsion containing 1.0 mg of ovalbumin, the levels of anti-ovalbumin were 330 and 480 μg AbN per ml serum, respectively. However, after treatment of the walls with the peptidoglycan-degrading L-11 enzyme from *Flavobacterium* (Kato *et al.*, 1962) the same amount of cell-wall digest stimulated 1103 and 1092 μg AbN per ml serum, respectively (Kotani *et al.*, 1975a). In addition, Kotani *et al.* (1975c) found that 100 μg of the disaccharide–hexapeptide from *Staph. aureus* or the (disaccharide–hexapeptide)-$_n$-ribitol teichoic acid complex stimulated AbN levels of 695 and 770 μg ml, respectively. The

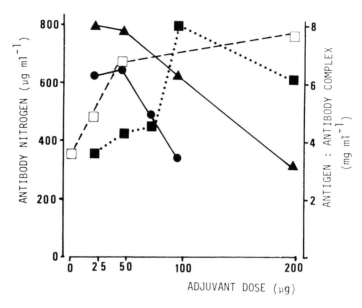

Figure 5. Antibody stimulation in either the guinea-pig with WSA (□ - - - □ , Adam *et al.*, 1972) and a mixture of *N*-acetylmuramyl-tripeptide and -tetrapeptide (▲ —— ▲ , Kotani *et al.*, 1975a), or in the mouse with *M. tuberculosis* (■ . . . . ■) and glycopeptide ST 208 (●——●) (D. E. S. Stewart-Tull, unpublished results)

hexapeptide consisted of *N*-(L-alanyl–D-isoglutaminyl)–*N*-(glycylglycyl)–L-lysyl–D-alanine. In the same study, the immunopotentiating activity of a mixture of *N*-acetylmuramyl-tetrapeptide and *N*-acetylmuramyl-tripeptide was examined. The levels of AbN per ml serum stimulated in the guinea-pig varied according to the dose of adjuvant added to the injection mixture (Figure 5); indeed the potentiation of the immune response decreased with an increase in adjuvant dose. A similar dosage effect was observed by Adam *et al.* (1972) with the water-soluble adjuvant (WSA) from *M. smegmatis*. However, there was a direct relationship between increasing adjuvant dose and potentiation of the antibody response.

In the mouse, I found that a maximum anti-ovalbumin response was obtained with 100 µg of heat-killed, dried *M. tuberculosis* strain DT or with 50 µg of mycobacterial glycopeptide ST208 from the culture filtrate of *M. tuberculosis* strains DT, PN and C (Figure 5). On the other hand, when the stimulation of antibody-forming splenic cells (PFC) was monitored, the optimum amounts of *M. tuberculosis* cells were 50 µg for the IgG response and >200 µg for the IgM response (Figure 6). With 500 µg of *M. tuberculosis* cells or the peptidoglycolipid, Koga *et al.* (1969) detected 16×10^4 IgM-producing spleen cells. Ishibashi *et al.* (1971) also showed that this effect could be obtained if 300 µg of

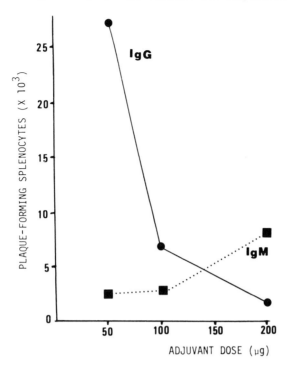

Figure 6. Stimulation of mouse antibody-forming splenic cells with *M. tuberculosis* cells and sheep ertythrocytes. The dosage effect is clearly seen.

peptidoglycolipid were injected 48 h before the injection of the antigen (sheep erythrocytes).

The majority of adjuvant studies in the guinea-pig have been concerned which the stimulation of an IgG response after primary immunization. White *et al.* (1963) noticed that not only was there an elevated immune response, but two classes of IgG antibodies were produced. The IgG_1 class was produced in animals injected with antigen in a water-in-oil emulsion with or without the mycobacterial component. However, the addition of *M. tuberculosis* cells, peptidoglycolipid or glycopeptide stimulates a lymphocyte population which synthesizes the IgG_2 class of antibody. The IgG_1 and IgG_2 antibodies had different biological properties (White *et al.*, 1963; Bloch *et al.*, 1963, Ovary *et al.*, 1963). After electrofocusing sera from guinea-pigs stimulated with FCA and FIA, Stewart-Tull and Arbuthnott (1971) separated pure fractions of IgG_1 and IgG_2. The IgG_1:IgG_2 ratio in stimulated animals was 7.0:1.0 for FCA and 1.0:1.0 for FIA at 21 days (Stewart-Tull, *et al.*, 1975a). Binaghi (1966) also calculated that at this time there was 15.0 mg ml-IgG_1 and 12.3 mg ml-IgG_2 in serum, but like Askonas *et al.* (1965) had used DEAE-cellulose to separate the

IgG components which would provide incomplete recovery of IgG_1 and account for the latter group's conclusion that serum from FCA-stimulated animals contained more IgG_2 than IgG_1.

VI. INDUCTION OF CELL-MEDIATED RESPONSES TO PROTEIN ANTIGENS

Early studies showed that the classical Freund's adjuvant induced a delayed-type hypersensitivity response to the protein antigen, as measured by either skin reaction or corneal reactions (see Stewart-Tull, 1983a,b).

The mycobacterial peptidoglycolipid and glycopeptide were also active in producing a similar effect in the guinea-pig. In addition, Kotani *et al.* (1975a,b) examined the activity of a wide variety of bacterial cell walls in guinea-pigs. As shown in Table 1, many cell-wall preparations were as good as the FCA in producing a cell-mediated immune response; the most effective were those from *Lactobacillus plantarum, Staph. aureus, S. pyogenes, S. salivarius, S. faecalis, S. mutans* and *M. bovis* BCG at the 100 μg dose level. With the N-acetylmuramyl-tri- and -tetra-peptides, significant responses were induced with 25 μg doses. Nauciel *et al.* (1973a,b) had previously shown that 10–50 μg of *Neisseria perflava* and *E. coli* induced cell-mediated immunity to azobenzenearsonate–N-acetyl–L-tyrosine. In view of this, one wonders whether the doses of 400 μg of adjuvant anti-tumour factor (Hiu, 1972), 200 μg of poly-PA (Migliore-Samour and Jollès, 1972), and 500 μg of poly-PA (Werner *et al.*, 1974, 1975) were the optimum amounts to induce cell-mediated immunity. However, it is significant that in all these studies, there was no instance where only one arm of the response was stimulated independently of the other — both humoral and cell-mediated responses were always produced after the injection of the water-in-oil emulsion containing adjuvant and protein antigen. In this respect it is worthwhile to consider the immunological spectrum found in patients suffering from leprosy (see reviews by Turk, 1969; Turk and Bryceson, 1971; Godal, 1978; Navalkar, 1980; and Bloom and Godal, 1983). In the tuberculoid form, patients manifest a cell-mediated response to *M. leprae* while in the lepromatous form they manifest a humoral response to the organism and lack a cell-mediated response. Patients with these extreme forms of the disease may show a shift towards a borderline state in which lowered cell-mediated and humoral responses may be evident. A clear understanding of this immunological balance and the mechanism whereby there is bias towards either a humoral or cell-mediated response in man could prove to be of immense value to those concerned with the design of other specific vaccines and in the possible use of immunopotentiators in cancer immunotherapy (Mathé, 1971; Stanton, 1972. Borsos and Rapp, 1973; Bast *et al.*, 1974a,b; Griffith and Regamey, 1978; Jeljaszewicz *et al.*, 1982; Stewart-Tull, 1983a; Davies, 1984).

Table 1   Immunopotentiating activities associated with bacterial cell walls

Cell walls containing peptidoglycan from:	Stimulation of immunoglobulin production	Induction of cell-mediated immunity
Staphylococcus aureus	+ + +	+ + +
Staphylococcus epidermidis	+	−
Streptococcus mutans	+ + +	+ + +
Streptococcus faecalis	+ + +	+ + +
Streptococcus faecium	+ + +	+ +
Streptococcus lactis	+ + +	+ + +
Streptococcus bovis	+ + +	+ + +
Streptococcus pyogenes	+ +	+ + +
Streptococcus thermophilus	+ + +	+ + +
Mycobacterium bovis BCG	+ + +	+ + +
Mycobacterium smegmatis	+ + +	+ + +
Lactobacillus plantarum	+ + +	+ + +
Nocardia asteroides	+ +	+ + +
Bacillus megaterium	+ + +	+ +
Clostridium botulinum	+ +	+ +
Streptomyces fradiae	+ +	+ +
Streptomyces lavendurae	+ +	+ +
Micrococcus luteus (lysodeikticus)	−	−
Corynebacterium parvum	+ + +	+ +
Corynebacterium poinsettiae	−	−
Corynebacterium betae	−	−
Corynebacterium insidiosum	−	−
Corynebacterium granulosum	+ + +	−
Proteus vulgaris	+ + +	+ + +
Neisseria perflava	+ + +	+ + +
Microbacterium lacticum	−	−
Eubacterium limosum	−	−
Arthrobacter atrocyaneus	−	−

VII. FROM THE LABORATORY ANIMAL MODEL TO MAN

The major contraindications to the incorporation of immunopotentiating substances into human vaccines are: (1) The adverse tissue reactions caused by the suspending medium (e.g. mineral oil). This has already been discussed on p.51 (2) The induction of polyarthritis in rats. (3) The production of experimental autoimmune diseases. The artificiality of these biological phenomena makes it difficult to extrapolate from the laboratory animal to man, but, nevertheless, these experimental manifestations of an adjuvant response are considered to be highly relevant in the debate on the use of immunomodulators. Useful and stimulating reports have appeared (World Health Organization, 1976; Gisler *et al.*, 1979; Edelman, 1980; Edelman *et al.*, 1980; Mizrahi *et al.*, 1980) which have formulated some unofficial guidelines for acceptability (see Table 4).

Studies in the laboratory animal are often of most value in a negative sense. It is essential to know whether a potential immunomodulator is inappropriate because it possesses a harmful activity, such as carcinogenicity or toxicity. However, the lack of such activities in the laboratory animal does not automatically imply acceptability for man, and vice versa.

There is a great need to glean and collate information about the actual effects of microorganisms in man, since these could assist in studies with the chemically synthesized immunomodulators (see Chapter 5). For instance, is there any evidence for an associated polyarthritis or for a higher incidence of autoimmune disease in tuberculous patients? One medical statistician indicated to me that he doubted whether any routine monitoring occurred, but suspected that if there had been a high incidence of one of these diseases in patients suffering from tuberculosis, it would have been noticed. One should be cautious in making the assumption that man will react in a manner similar to that found in the laboratory animal. In this respect it is interesting that antibodies against human brain encephalitogenic factor were detected in the sera of multiple-sclerotic patients. Individuals immunized with *M. bovis* BCG showed the presence of the anti-encephalitogenic antibodies more often than unimmunized subjects (Field *et al.*, 1963).

A. Immunopotentiating Components Contained in Existing Bacterial Vaccines

Information can also be collated from the literature and from manufacturers concerning the adjuvant content of accepted vaccines. The standard *M. bovis* BCG vaccine contains 8×10^6 to 26×10^6 living and 8×10^6 to 26×10^6 dead bacteria per ml, and from the dry weight of these organisms it is possible to obtain an approximation of the weight of peptidoglycan and peptidoglycolipid injected into human individuals (Table 2). The results of small field trials can also be used to calculate acceptable injection doses of immunopotentiator for man. Although acceptable, these may not be the optimal doses. Convit *et al.* (1979) produced an experimental leprosy vaccine which contained 6.4×10^8 *M. leprae* and 5.6×10^7 *M. bovis* BCG per ml. Individuals received 6–8 separate doses of this vaccine in 0.1 ml amounts (6.4×10^7 plus 5.6×10^6 to 8.6×10^6 organisms per 0.1 ml), considerably more organisms and more immunopotentiator than injected with the standard BCG vaccine (16×10^5 to 52×10^5 organisms per 0.1 ml).

With the whooping cough vaccine there are 40×10^9 *Bordetella pertussis* per ml of vaccine and children are given three doses of 0.5 ml. As shown in Table 2, the calculated values of peptidoglycan and lipopolysaccharide and (LPS) are much higher for this vaccine than for the other Gram-negative organisms, *Salmonella typhi, S. paratyphi* A, *S. paratyphi* B, and *V. cholerae*. The dose

Table 2   Calculated quantities of immunopotentiators in existing commercial vaccines

Vaccine	Number of organisms	Number of injections	Total dosage (ml)	Approximate weight (μg of adjuvant administered)		
				Peptidoglycan	Peptidoglycolipid	LPS
Mycobacterium bovis BCG	$\Big\{$ 8×10^6 to 26×10^6 living 8×10^6 to 26×10^6 dead	1	0.1	3.0–5.0	10.0–12.0	–
Mycobacterium leprae	6.4×10^8					
Mycobacterium bovis BCG	5.6×10^7 to 8.6×10^7	6, 8	0.6–0.8	30.0–134.0	25.0–165.0	–
Bordetella pertussis[†]	40×10^9	3	1.5	6.5–50.0	–	6.0–35.0
Salmonella typhi	1.0×10^9	2	0.5–1.0	0.1–1.0	–	0.1–0.6
TAB *Salmonella typhi*	1.0×10^9					
Salmonella paratyphi A	0.5×10^9	2	0.5–1.0	0.2–3.0	–	0.2–1.2
Salmonella paratyphi B	0.5×10^9					
Vibrio cholerae	8.0×10^9	2	0.4–1.5	0.3–12.0	–	0.3–7.0
Vibrio cholerae	2.0×10^{11}	3*	?	1.0–36.0	–	1.0–21.0
Holmgren, J. *et al.*, cited in Levine *et al.*, 1983)	1.0×10^6	1*				

*Oral administration   [†]values calculated from dry weight stated by Novotny and Brookes (1975).

of immunopotentiator is even greater when one calculates the weight in relation to kg per body weight of the child versus the adult. One must ask why it is necessary to inoculate so many organisms and whether the number of *Bordetella pertussis* organisms per ml is, in part, the reason why there are so many reports of adverse effects in young babies (see p.66, and Wardlaw and Parton, 1983). In addition, the *B. pertussis* organism has a heat-labile adjuvant, the histamine-sensitizing leucocytosis-promoting factor (HSF-LPF) and is usually administered with diphtheria and tetanus toxoids adsorbed to mineral adjuvant, e.g. aluminium phosphate or hydroxide (maximum of 1.25 mg of Al (per single human dose). In this instance, the pertussis vaccine contains arbitrary amounts of lipopolysaccharide, peptidoglycan, and HSF-LPF, together with the non-toxic chemical adjuvant. However, we know little about the interaction of these immunopotentiators in a vaccine. Do they cause a synergistic or antagonistic effect? Is it significant that recently Sato *et al.*, (1984) developed a pertussis component vaccine which produced fewer side-effects than the conventional whole-cell vaccine? They stated that they had removed the major portion of LPS from the *B. pertussis* culture supernate vaccine and concluded that LPS should be removed as extensively as possible. Recently, Pollock *et al.* (1984) studied the effects of primary immunization of 10 000 children with the diphtheria–tetanus–pertussis (DTP) or diphtheria–tetanus vaccine. They established that the presence of the adjuvant, alhydrogel, reduced the incidence of post-vaccinal side-effects. In addition, Waight *et al.* (1983) had found pyrexia in children more frequently after plain than adsorbed DTP vaccine.

In an experimental study on cholera immunization, Holmgren and his colleagues (cited in Levine *et al.*, 1983) gave adult volunteers three oral doses of a combination vaccine; each dose contained 5.0 mg of purified *V. cholerae* toxin B subunit and 2×10^{11} killed *V. cholerae* (5×10^{10} classical Inaba, 5x10^{10} classical Ogawa, and 1×10^{11} *el tor* Inaba). The volunteers were challenged one month after the last dose with 1x10^6 living *V. cholerae el tor* Inaba. It is noticeable that the criteria for selecting 2x10^{11} *V. cholerae* organisms were not stated and that at this level of dosage, the volunteers were given both peptidoglycan and LPS immunopotentiators by mouth. In my laboratory we have shown that oral administration of immunopotentiators may stimulate the production of IgG and IgE antibodies to unusual protein antigens added to the diet of experimental animals (Jones, A., and Stewart-Tull, D. E. S., unpublished results). In this respect, some caution should be exercised in such volunteer trials so that individuals predisposed to allergic conditions are not included.

From these few examples, it will be apparent that the amount of immunopotentiator, both in commercial and experimental vaccines, shows marked variation. Difficulties will be encountered in persuading the various ethical committees and licencing authorities to sanction the addition of an immunopotentiator to a commercial vaccine. Nevertheless, the data from small field trials with volunteers may prove to be invaluable in scaling up the vaccination procedures from animals to man. In addition, they will provide the foundation stone for the eventual tests on the incorporation of chemically synthesized muramyl-dipeptide or one of its derivatives into a human vaccine (see also Chapter 5), either as a mixture with the antigen or as an immunopotentiator–antigen conjugate.

B. Adverse Immune Reactions Induced by Immunopotentiators

1. Arthritogenic Activity of Cell Surface Components

The ability of FCA, containing heat-killed mycobacterial organisms, to induce polyarthritis in Lewis rats was observed by Pearson (1956). Subsequently, either mycobacterial peptidoglycolipid (Wood *et al.*, 1969) and cell walls (Azuma *et al.*, 1972; Audibert *et al.*, 1973), or the cell walls or enzymic digests of cell walls from a wide range of bacteria (Koga *et al.*, 1976) produced a similar effect. On the other hand, *M. smegmatis* WSA (Chedid *et al.*, 1972; Audibert *et al.*, 1973) and *M. tuberculosis* glycopeptide ST 208 (Stewart-Tull *et al.*, 1975b) lacked this polyarthritogenic activity.

At that time, Stewart-Tull *et al.* (1975b) proposed that the stimulation of polyarthritis in the Lewis rats was influenced by the length of the glycan chain containing the repeating disaccharide unit of N-acetylmuramic acid–N-acetylglucosamine in the cell-wall component. In addition, these experiments showed that the immunopotentiating and polyarthritogenic activities of the mycobacterial adjuvant were separable. Koga *et al.* (1979) continued to investigate this aspect of glycan chain length in bacterial cell walls and concluded that fractions containing more than (disaccharide)$_5$ were more potent polyarthritogens than those with (disaccharide)$_{2-3}$.

The synthetic N-acetylmuramyl–L-alanyl–D-isoglutamine (MDP), MDP–L-lysyl–D-alanine and MDP–L-lysine all lacked the polyarthritogenic activity at doses up to 500 μg per rat (Kohashi *et al.*, 1976b). However, if 10 μg of MDP were mixed with 100 μg of another potent adjuvant, a copolymer of polyribo-inosinic acid and polycytidylic acid [poly (I:C)] in a water-in-oil emulsion, all rats injected into both inguinal lymph nodes with 0.01 ml of the mixture developed a severe polyarthritis (Kohashi *et al.*, 1979). The rats injected with poly(I:C) alone showed no evidence of polyarthritis. It was suggested that the MDP molecules might be adsorbed on to the poly(I:C) polymer thus artificially creating a molecule with (disaccharide)$_{>3}$ required for a polyarthritogen. This is an example of the possible synergistic interaction between adjuvants referred to previously.

2. Induction of Autoimmune Disease in Animals

A variety of experimental procedures have been used to induce autoimmune disease in animals (Burnet, 1963):

(i)   Administration of serum or cells from animals of another species that have been hyperimmunized with cells or constituents of the recipient species.
(ii)   Immunization with body components from the recipient itself or from syngeneic (isologous) animals usually in FCA.
(iii)   Immunization with cross-reacting antigens which differ by origin or by chemical treatment from those of the organ to be attacked.
(iv)   Administration of allogeneic lymphocytes to an animal that is incapable of rejecting them, either genetically or as a result of irradiation.

The second scheme is relevant to the present discussion and, although the use of FCA is a highly unnatural procedure, the fact that it induces a breakdown in immune homoeostasis is important in the understanding of this normal mechanism. In 1963, Allegranza (personal communication) suggested that the lesions in encephalomyelitis might be due to the passage of adjuvant through the blood–brain barrier. Recently, Daniel *et al.* (1981) monitored the exclusion of mannitol from the brain stem and spinal cord after the intradermal injection of Lewis rats with an homogenate of guinea-pig spinal cord in FCA, as a measure of the effectiveness of the blood–brain barrier. After 14 days, the barrier was breached and there was a two-fold increase in the diffusion of mannitol out of the blood, due to altered permeability of the blood vessels of the central nervous tissue as a result of damage to the vascular endothelium. Changes in the permeability of the barrier were also associated with the degree of mononuclear cell cuffing of the small blood cells.

In experimental autoimmune diseases, it is known that damage to the organ is due to a cell-mediated autoimmune reaction rather than to the cytotoxic effects of autoantibodies. Passive transfer of experimental encephalomyelitis was achieved in rats and guinea-pigs after transplantation of lymphoid cells (Paterson, 1960; Stone, 1961), whereas transfusion of large amounts of anti-encephalitogenic antibodies failed (Batchelor and Lessof, 1964). Ortiz-Ortiz *et al.* (1976) showed conclusively that experimental encephalomyelitis was a T-cell-mediated disease induced after the injection of myelin basic protein. The active encephalitogenic factor of this protein is a hepta- or nonapeptide (Lamoureux *et al.*, 1972; Nagai *et al.*, 1978a,b).

A three-cell model for the activation of autoimmune T effector (T_E) cells was proposed by Killen and Swanborg (1982). The macrophage is a crucial cell in the cellular cascade leading to the stimulation of T_E cells. Removal of macrophages from sensitized donor splenocytes reduced the effectiveness of passive transfer of experimental encephalomyelitis. This activity was restored by the addition of macrophages to the lymph node cell suspension. The antigen-presenting macrophage produces interleukin 1 (IL-1, lymphocyte-activating factor) which activates T helper (T_H) cells. In the Lewis rat, the T_H cells, Lyt-1$^+$2$^-$, W3/25$^+$, produce interleukin 2 (IL-2, T-cell growth factor) which activates the autoreactive T_E cells responsible for the encephalomyelitis (see Figure 7). Although the mycobacterial cells in the FCA stimulate the macrophage to produce IL-1, it has now been established that passive transfer of encephalomyelitis in rats can be achieved with lymphocytes from animals stimulated with myelin protein in FIA (Namikawa *et al.*, 1982; Killen and Swanborg, 1982). The donors did not respond to a subsequent injection of myelin protein in FCA, but their splenic lymphocytes cultured in the presence of myelin protein or concanavalin A transferred encephalomyelitis to recipients. A peculiarity of the induction process is the dose of mycobacterial component required in the mixture. *M. tuberculosis* organisms (100 μg; Nagai *et al.*, 1978a,b), 100 μg of peptidoglycolipid (Freund and Stone, 1959), 12.5 μg of WSA (Lebar and Voisin, 1974) or 1.0 μg of MDP (Nagai *et al.*, 1978a,b) were shown to induce autoimmune encephalomyelitis. Koga *et al.* (1979) found that 20 μg of MDP were inactive and 100 μg of MDP induced encephalomyelitis in 44% of injected Lewis rats. However, 500 μg of MDP were required to induce an orchiepididymitis (Toullet *et al.*, 1977) and was similarly less active for the induction of uveoretinitis in guinea-pigs (Kozak *et al.*, 1979).

For convenience, a number of benchmark references dealing with the induction of a variety of autoimmune diseases are contained in Table 3.

Table 3. The induction of autoimmune diseases with *M. tuberculosis* organisms or components

Experimental autoimmune disease	Animal	Reference
Allergic encephalomyelitis	Monkey, guinea-pig, rat	Morgan 1946, 1947; Kabat *et al.*, 1946, 1947; Wolf *et al.*, 1947; Kopeloff and Kopeloff, 1947; Freund *et al.*, 1947; Allegranza and Rovescalli, 1951a,b; Cazzullo and Allegranza, 1951; Waksman and Adams, 1953; Colover, 1954; Colover and Consden, 1956; Kies *et al.*, 1958; White and Marshall, 1958; Freund and Stone, 1959; Paterson, 1960; Paterson and Bell, 1962
Thyroiditis	Rabbit	Witebsky and Rose, 1956; Rose and Witebsky, 1956; Witebsky *et al.*, 1957; Doniach and Roitt, 1962
Orchitis	Guinea-pig	Freund *et al.*, 1953; Freund and Stone, 1959; Waksman, 1959
Adrenalitis		Colover and Glynn, 1958
Dermatitis	Rabbit, guinea-pig	Wilhemj *et al.*, 1962
Neuritis	Rabbit	Waksman and Adams, 1955

Weigle (1983) described experiments with LPS, a potent B-cell mitogen, in which T-cell-depleted mice were induced to produce antibodies to thymus-dependent antigens. The LPS acted on the B-cells directly, substituting for the T-cell. He postulated that following an infection with a gram-negative organism, an autoimmune response could be induced. In view of these experiments and the comparatively high doses of three bacterial plus one chemical adjuvants administered with the pertussis vaccine, is it possible that the 1 in 110 000 post-vaccinal occurrence of neurological illness could be due to a series of events in which T-cell tolerance is broken?

VIII. AN ACCEPTABLE IMMUNOPOTENTIATOR

With the advent of genetic manipulation technology and procedures for synthesizing peptides, the need for acceptable immunopotentiators will grow. Ultimately, it is envisaged that a derivative(s) of muramyl-dipeptide will be found to meet the rigid criteria proposed for a safe immunopotentiator (Table 4). Although this challenge has been extended to adjuvant researchers and will be answered in time, it is possible that the continued emergence of drug-resistant organisms may stimulate greater urgency.

Arnon (1972, 1979), Sela (1975, 1977), Sela and Arnon (1980) and Lerner *et al.* (1983) have described the recent events in the development of the synthetic vaccine. In many of the published reports, synthetic antigens have been injected in combination with an immunopotentiator because they are low molecular weight peptides and often weakly immunogenic. However, one advantage is that small amounts of the antigen can be used. Maron *et al.* (1978) immunized rabbits with 10 μg of poly(L-Tyr, L-Glu)–poly(DL-Ala)–poly(L-Lys) in FIA

Table 4   Some properties of the ideal immunomodulator

I.   An immunomodulator must not:
 (a) Induce hypersensitivity to host's tissues
 (b) Induce hypersensitivity to the immunomodulator
 (c) Possess (i) cross-reactive antigens
              (ii) carcinogenic activity
              (iii) teratogenic activity
              (iv) abortogenic activity
              (v) toxicity for myelolymphoid cells
              (vi) neoplastic transforming activity for myelolymphoid cells

II. An immunomodulator should:
 (a) Induce either a humoral antibody response or a cell-mediated response
 (b) Biodegrade in the host's tissue
 (c) Improve the immunogenicity of the vaccine antigen
 (d) Retain stability in the vaccine
 (e) Be non-toxic and non-pyrogenic

---

containing WSA. In a critical study, Mozes *et al.* (1980) conjugated this synthetic antigen to MDP and injected the conjugate into mice in saline; a booster injection was given three weeks later. This procedure stimulated high levels of antibody and showed that it was possible to avoid the use of the water in mineral oil emulsion.

An exciting development at the Pasteur Institute, Paris, was the synthesis of a tetradecapeptide sequence of the diphtheria toxin. Anti-toxin antibodies were stimulated in guinea-pigs immunized with this synthetic tetradecapeptide conjugated to bovine serum albumin and administered with MDP (Audibert *et al.*, 1981). These antibodies neutralized the dermonecrotic activity of diphtheria toxin and protected the animals against lethal challenge. Subsequently, an octadecapeptide, composed of the 16 amino acids of the link peptide between diphtheria toxin A and B subunits, plus two alanyl residues at the *N*-terminal end, was synthesized. Both the octadecapeptide and MDP were covalently linked to a synthetic carrier of poly(DL-Ala)–poly(L-Lys) and this conjugate proved to be an efficient vaccine in animals (Audibert *et al.*, 1982). I feel sure that these important and timely studies will provide the foundation stone for the eventual inclusion of immunopotentiators in human vaccines. Many of the natural substances may not reach the required standards mentioned in Table 4. However, the development of the synthetic immunopotentiators should circumvent the problems.

IX. THE EFFECT OF IMMUNOMODULATORS ON CELLS OF THE IMMUNE SYSTEM

It was originally proposed that adjuvant substances exerted their effect by a unitarian mechanism of action, but numerous studies have revealed that several mechanisms operate either independently or simultaneously. Stewart-Tull *et al.* (1977) suggested that the specific (immunological) and non-specific (physiological) stimuli provided by the immunopotentiator required definition, although these may be associated in the adjuvant response.

A. Affinity for Cell Membranes

The majority of immunopotentiators are amphiphiles, such as mycobacterial peptidoglycolipids, lipoteichoic acids (see Chapter 6) and lipopolysaccharides (see Chapter 10). In view of the studies of Middlebrook and Dubos (1948) in which mycobacterial glycopeptides were shown to possess an affinity for erythrocyte membranes, it seemed reasonable to examine the interaction between immunopotentiators and cell membranes. As shown in Figure 7, such interactions may lead to insertion of the hydrophobic moieties of the molecule into the lipid bilayer or attachment of hydrophilic moieties to the membrane through receptors or charge effects. The nature of these interactions has been

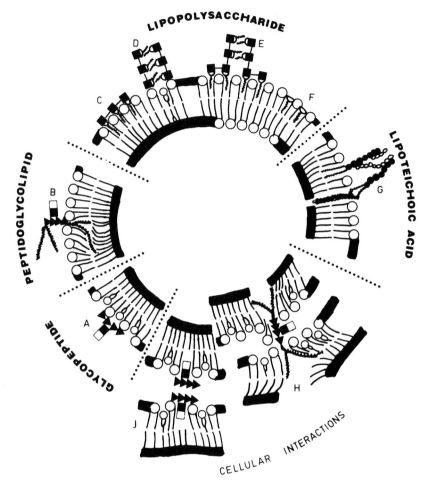

Figure 7. Interactions among amphiphilic immunopotentiators and cell membranes A,C,D, hydrophilic interactions, B,E,F,G, hydrophobic lipid:lipid interactions, H, cell fusion and J, cell bridging initiated by amphipathic molecules.

detailed in Chapter 9. In addition, a molecular interaction was demonstrated between the mycobacterial glycopeptide and guinea-pig IgG (Stewart-Tull *et al.*, 1965; Stewart-Tull and Wilkinson, 1973). Subsequently, we demonstrated that the glycopeptide bound to mammalian cell membranes retained this affinity for the guinea-pig IgG (Davies and Stewart-Tull, 1973). This interaction was suggested as an intermediate step, either in the presentation of antigen molecules to lymphocytes or in B-cell–T_H cell cooperation.

Fleming *et al.* (1984) incorporated immunopotentiators in suboptimally stimulated cultures of normal mouse bone marrow cells. Mycobacterial peptidoglycolipid (100 μg) and glycopeptide (1 μg) increased the responsiveness of colony-forming cells to colony-stimulating factor. They suggested that the response might be related to the amphipathic nature of the molecules acting on the surface of the colony-forming cell, thus making it more responsive to low concentrations of colony-stimulating factor. It is difficult to assess whether this has any direct relevance to the specific adjuvant response, but it could play a part in the responsiveness of antigen-sensitive cells to antigenic stimulation.

B. Activation of Macrophages

As mentioned previously, White (1959) believed that the proliferation of macrophages, many with epithelioid cell morphology, was essential for the initiation of an adjuvant response. In 1976 he stated that the formation of the epithelioid cell granuloma depended upon the use of the mineral oil component in the FCA. Although most workers would agree with the proposition that the macrophage is of great significance in the complex sequence of events that lead to an adjuvant response, recent evidence has dispelled the idea that mineral oil must be present in the injection mixture. For instance, Modolell *et al.* (1974) preincubated macrophages with $0.01 \mu g \ ml^{-1}$ WSA for 24 h. Subsequently, lymphocytes and the antigen (sheep erythrocytes) were added and it was observed that the WSA stimulated an increased immune response *in vitro*. Kelly (1976) found that the presence of the cell walls of *M. bovis* BCG stimulated guinea-pig peritoneal macrophages to incorporate radiolabelled glucosamine, which was a measure of macrophage activation in an aqueous medium. Yarkoni *et al.* (1977) confirmed such macrophage activation in the presence of *M. bovis* BCG cells, both heat-killed and living. Takada *et al.* (1979) examined the effect of a range of bacterial cell-wall preparations on the *in vitro* incorporation of radiolabelled glucosamine by guinea-pig peritoneal macrophages. The cell walls of *M. smegmatis* at a dose of $10 \mu g$ (1.0×10^6 cells) produced maximum activation of the macrophages due to the presence of both peptidoglycan and peptidoglycolipid. The order of activity with other cell walls was $10 \mu g$ *Nocardia corynebacteriodes* $> 10 \mu g$ *Lactobacillus plantarum* $> 1 \mu g$ *Streptomyces gardneri* $> 1 \mu g$ *Corynebacterium diphtheriae*. As might be expected, MDP was shown to activate macrophages (Juy and Chedid, 1975; Fevrier *et al.* 1978). However, Takada *et al.* (1979) made the observation that 6-*O*-(2-tetradecylhexadecanoyl)–MDP and 6-*O*-(3-hydroxy-2-tetradecyloctadecanoyl)–MDP, both insoluble in water and both containing lipophilic acyl groups, were more active than MDP — further evidence of the importance of the amphipathic nature of the immunopotentiator.

Other evidence indicates that immunopotentiators can activate macrophages to inhibit tumour target cells (Juy and Chedid, 1975; Munder *et al.*, 1983). In addition, Fevrier *et al.* (1978) demonstrated the presence of a macrophage lymphokine after MDP stimulation which acted on B-cells through T-cell mediation. Oppenheim *et al.* (1980) induced macrophages to produce IL-1 in the presence of mycobacterial components and proposed that this was part of the adjuvant mechanism. When macrophages were cultured in the presence of MDP > 0.01 μg ml^{-1}, the culture supernate stimulated T-cell activity as measured by the uptake of tritiated thymidine. The T-cell activating factor (TAF) had a molecular weight of 53 000–85 000 whereas that of IL-1 is 12 000–18 000 and its stimulation paralleled the immunopotentiating activity of the adjuvants tested (Iribe *et al.*, 1981). The culture supernate of LPS- or MDP-stimulated macrophages was added to immune T-lymphocytes, from guinea-pigs immunized with *M. tuberculosis*, cultured with 25 μg/ml purified, protein derivative (PPD). If 1×10^3 autologous macrophages per ml were added to the system there was evidence of production of macrophage migration inhibition factor (MIF) by the lymphocytes. This stimulation was not caused either by the culture supernate or the autologous macrophages alone (Yamamoto and Onoue, 1979; Iribe *et al.*, 1981).

Macrophages can also be stimulated to produce interferon and prostaglandin (PGE$_2$) both of which control natural killer (NK) cell activity.

C. Activation of Lymphocytes

The complexity of the adjuvant mechanism is compounded when one considers the additional activity that immunopotentiators exert on B- and T-lymphocytes. Peptidoglycans also exert a pronounced macrophage migration inhibitory effect (Grov *et al.*, 1976; Nagao *et al.*, 1979). The effect was also observed with peptidoglycan fragments containing MDP from the cell walls of *Lactobacillus plantarum* and *Staphylococcus epidermidis* (Nagao *et al.*, 1979). Heymer *et al.* (1973) had previously isolated peptidoglycan fragments from group A and B streptococci ranging from 5000 to 20 000 000 molecular weight. The larger molecular-sized fragments produced migration inhibition reactions with peritoneal macrophages from non-sensitized rats and guinea-pigs; the activity decreased with decreasing molecular weight.

Immunopotentiators may cause some or all of a variety of polyclonal activating effects, e.g. induction of polyclonal lymphokine synthesis and mitogenicity. Nakashima *et al.* (1979, 1980a,b) examined the actions of nine different polyclonal lymphocyte activators, including the capsular polysaccharide of *Klebsiella pneumoniae*, LPS and mycobacterial PPD. They concluded that the polyclonal activation took place at the initiation step of the immune response in which T-cells in the case of T-dependent soluble antigen and B-cells in the case of T-independent antigen play a predominant role. The activation of these lymphocyte populations may be variable. For example, LPS acts on B-cells in the induction of tolerance to T-dependent soluble antigen but on T-cells in the induction of an antibody response to the same antigen. The direct activity on B-cells avoids the requirement for T$_H$ function (Campbell and Kind, 1971; Diamantstein *et al.*, 1971; Jones and Kind, 1972; Diamantstein and Wagner, 1973; Louis *et al.*, 1973; Watson *et al.*, 1973; Ornellas *et al.*, 1974). LPS can also act on T-cells and increase the function of T_H cells which, in turn, stimulate B-cells (Nakashima *et al.*, 1977; Hamaoka and Katz, 1973a,b; Allison and Davies, 1971; Cone and Johnson, 1971).

1. Mitogenic Activity

Numerous studies have demonstrated the mitogenic activity of peptidoglycan immunopotentiators, including the classical mycobacterial peptidoglycolipid (Damais *et al.*, 1975; Ciorbaru *et al.*, 1976; Rook and Stewart-Tull, 1976; Dziarski and Dziarski, 1979; Takada *et al.*, 1979; Banck and Forsgren, 1978; Räsänen *et al.*, 1980).

Damais *et al.* (1975) substituted the mycobacterial component of FCA with the known immunopotentiating peptidoglycans from *E. coli* and *B. megaterium*. Both of these stimulated mouse and rabbit splenic lymphocyte cell suspensions to undergo blast transformation as measured by the incorporation of [^{3}H]-thymidine into the DNA. The inactive adjuvant, *Micrococcus luteus* peptidoglycan did not induce blast transformation and was also non-toxic. The mitogenic peptidoglycans were slightly toxic; at least 100 times less toxic than LPS from *E. coli*. The *E. coli* 707 peptidoglycan was solubilized with lysozyme and the monomer was separated by gel filtration. This fraction, although an active immunopotentiator (Ellouz *et al.*, 1974), was devoid of mitogenic activity. Rook and Stewart-Tull (1976) concluded that mitogenicity was not an essential prerequisite for adjuvant activity because the water-insoluble mycobacterial peptidoglycolipids were mitogenic, but the water-soluble mycobacterial glycopeptides were inactive. Thus, it is apparent that some immunopotentiators are also non-specific mitogens of B-lymphocytes.

Mitogenic peptidoglycans have been obtained from a variety of organisms including *E. coli, Bacillus megaterium, Listeria monocytogenes* (Cohen *et al.*, 1975; Damais *et al.*, 1975; Ciorbaru *et al.*, 1976), *Nocardia corynebacteriodes, Streptomyces gardneri* (Takada *et al.*, 1979) *Staph. aureus* (Dziarski and Dziarski, 1979), and with cells of *Haemophilus influenzae, N. catarrhalis, Bordetella pertussis, M. tuberculosis, Neisseria gonorrhoeae, N. pharyngis* and *Streptococcus pneumoniae* (Banck and Forsgren, 1978). These authors noted that *E. coli, L. monocytogenes, Neisseria meningitidis* and *Staph. aureus* Wood 46 cells were weakly mitogenic. However, Räsänen *et al.* (1980) measured the mitogenic response of mixed human umbilical cord lymphocytes, as measured by the uptake of 5-[^{125}I]iodo-2′-deoxyuridine and recorded activity with *Staph. aureus, N. catarrhalis, M. bovis* BCG and also with *E. coli* and *Staph. aureus* Wood 46, but they noted a dosage effect. With high doses of bacteria, there was less stimulation, possibly due to the bacterial cells hindering cell–cell contact in the mixed cell suspension. In addition, they demonstrated T-lymphocyte proliferation, in the presence of 2.5–10.0% monocytes, with *Staph. aureus, E. coli* and *M. bovis* BCG bacterial cells—a polyclonal lymphocyte response. Clagett and Engel (1978) found polyclonal activation of lymphocytes with *A. viscosus, L. monocytogenes, Serratia piscatorium, Corynebacterium parvum, M. tuberculosis, Staph. aureus, Klebsiella pneumoniae, Brucella abortus* and *E. coli.*

Dziarski *et al.* (1980) compared the mitogenic activity of *Staph. aureus* cell wall, peptidoglycan and teichoic acid at a dose of $400 \mu g$ ml^{-1}. The peptidoglycan was a potent mitogen for mouse, rat and human peripheral blood lymphocytes. However, the cell walls were non-mitogenic for rat lymphocytes and the teichoic acid was non-mitogenic for the lymphocytes from all three species. This study indicates the problems associated with conclusions formulated from the results obtained with a single species. Räsänen *et al.* (1982) examined the mitogenic activity of *Staph. aureus* Wood 46 and *B. subtilis* cell walls, peptidoglycan and teichoic acids against both adult and umbilical cord human blood lymphocytes. Although the mitogenic response was weak, there was once again evidence of the dosage effect with both cell walls and peptidoglycans of both species, such that proliferation was $1 \mu g < 10 \mu g > 100$ or $1000 \mu g$. On the other hand, with teichoic acid, the response was $1 \mu g < 10 \mu g < 100 \mu g > 1000 \mu g$.

In the case of T-dependent antigens, it was shown that the immunopotentiating activity of MDP was mediated by a T_H cell (Specter *et al.*, 1977, 1978; Leclerc *et al.*, 1978). Damais *et al.* (1977) demonstrated the mitogenic activity of MDP against splenic lymphocytes of normal or *nu/nu* mice. Leclerc *et al.* (1979) examined the *in vitro* response to both a T-dependent antigen (sheep erythrocytes) and a T-independent antigen (trinitrophenyl (TNP)–polyacrylamide–(PAA), with spleen cells from *nu/nu* mice cultured in the presence of MDP. With sheep erythrocytes the number of plaque-forming cells increased to a maximum in the presence of $10 \mu g$ of MDP per culture (1293 ± 140) and with TNP–PAA to a maximum with $100 \mu g$ of MDP culture ($11\,273 \pm 144$). The immunopotentiator was able to replace the T_H function but could not replace macrophage function, and it was concluded that MDP acted directly on B-lymphocytes. In the case of LPS, Hoffman *et al.* (1977) noted that it initiated mitosis in cultured mouse B-lymphocytes and facilitated the conversion of antigen-stimulated B-cells to antibody-producing cells, substituting for T_H cells. The helper activity of LPS was dependent upon macrophages, whereas the mitogenic activity was not.

In addition, Davies and Sabbadini (1982) demonstrated that *M. bovis* BCG expanded and activated a population of functionally non-specific T_{H_C} cells in mice.

2. Lymphokine Stimulation

Interleukin 1 (IL-1; Aarden *et al.*, 1979; Oppenheim *et al.*, 1982) is a macrophage-derived protein which modulates many of the responses involved in the process of host defence against bacterial infection. It is involved in numerous non-specific events, including induction of fever and neutrophilia, stimulation of acute-phase protein synthesis and modulation of serum cation concentration. Immunologically IL-1 stimulates antibody production (Wood, 1979a,b), B-lymphocyte differentiation (Hoffmann, 1979) and T-lymphocyte proliferation through the induction of lymphocyte activating factor (Smith, 1980; Shaw *et al.*, 1980; Larsson *et al.*, 1980). Lymphocyte-activating factor is termed interleukin 2 (IL-2; Aarden *et al.*, 1979; Farrar *et al.*, 1982). Räsänen *et al.* (1978) showed that *Staph. aureus* Wood 46, *E. coli*, *N. catarrhalis*, *B. subtilis*, group A *Streptococcus β-haemolyticus*, *Streptococcus α-haemolyticus* and *M. bovis* BCG induced lymphokine synthesis in human B-lymphocytes. Subsequently, Räsänen *et al.* (1982) investigated the activity of *Staph. aureus* Wood 46 and *B. subtilis* cell walls, peptidoglycan and teichoic acids in the stimulation of lymphocytes. There was a progressive increase in the production of leucocyte inhibitory factor (LIF) with an associated increase in the amount of immunopotentiator from 1 to 1000 μg ml^{-1}.

Staruch and Wood (1983) provided the first *in vivo* evidence that IL-1 possessed an immunopotentiating activity. They found that the immuno-potentiating active component was purified in a fraction containing IL-1 (LAF or thymocyte proliferating activity) by gel filtration or gel filtration coupled with isoelectric focusing. Bovine serum albumin (BSA) plus IL-1 (p*I* 7.1; 2000 LAF units), BSA + IL-1 (G75 fraction; 3000 LAF units) and BSA + 100 μg MDP, stimulated 704, 206 and 921 μg of anti-BSA serum antibodies per ml. It was noted that 1000–2000 LAF units stimulated 0.62–0.75 mg anti-BSA serum antibodies per ml but 4000 LAF units only stimulated 0.18 mg ml^{-1}. Once again this reinforced the hypothesis that many immunopotentiators exert their activity by inducing the release of IL-1 from macrophages. Similar findings have been made with LPS (Wood and Cameron, 1978; Mizel, 1980), peptidoglycan (Oppenheim *et al.*, 1980; Vacheron *et al.*, 1983) and MDP (Iribe *et al.*, 1981). Vacheron *et al.* (1983) related the immunopotentiating activity of peptidoglycans from *Bacillus megaterium* and *Staph. aureus*, (both active), and *Micrococcus luteus* and *Corynebacterium poinsettiae* (both inactive) with the induction of IL-1 production by mouse macrophages and human mononuclear cells. Increasing IL-1 activity was found after macrophages were cultured with 10–200 μg ml^{-1} of peptidoglycans from *B. megaterium* or *Staph. aureus*.

Oppenheim *et al.* (1980) incubated C3H/HeJ mouse thymocytes with culture supernates of human mononuclear cells stimulated with either 100 μg ml^{-1} WSA or 10 μg ml^{-1} MDP. They noted an increased uptake of [^{3}H]thymidine by the murine thymocytes due to the production of IL-1 by the mononuclear cells. In addition, with the synthetic derivatives of MDP 1 μg of 6-*O*-stearoyl-MDP was as effective as 1–100 μg of MDP, whereas D-alanine–MDP was less active at the 1–10 μg dose levels.

As Staruch and Wood (1983) pointed out, the IL-1 may activate B-lymphocytes directly and may also enhance the release of IL-2 from T-lymphocytes.

The IL-2 would enhance the proliferation of T_H cells that recognize bacterial antigens and by such means act in the host defence mechanism against infectious agents, as suggested by Räsänen *et al.* (1978).

The non-specific host defence mechanism may also be stimulated by the production of acute phase proteins, notably C-reactive protein (CRP), which are produced following stimulation of hepatocytes with IL-1.

All of these activities of immunomodulators on lymphocytes create a complex situation with respect to a precise mode of action. I am reminded of a senior immunologist, who at retirement said, 'After 40 years, it is still not possible to state *precisely* what happens between the injection of an antigen and the detection of antibodies in the serum'! However, an attempt has been made in Figure 8 to depict the stimulation ('switching on') of immune responses by immunopotentiators based on the various biological studies in animals. It must be stated, however, that these biological activities are often monitored under somewhat artificial conditions in experimental animals. One can only surmise as to whether the same array of activities would occur following the injection of immunomodulators into man.

The mode of action of the immunomodulators becomes even more speculative if some recent studies on suppression and anti-idiotypic immunoregulation are considered. These are included as a possible stimulus to further investigations which might explore depression ('switching off') of the functions of T_S cells or cells producing anti-idiotype or anti-(anti-idiotype) antibodies.

The suppressor system mediated by three types of T-lymphocytes (T_{S1} T_{S2} T_{S3}) fulfils an immune regulatory function (Gershon and Kondo, 1970; Benacerraf, 1983). The immunomodulator may act on macrophages and T- and B-lymphocytes; these cells can function as suppressors of humoral and cell-mediated responses (Horiuchi and Waksman, 1968; Bash and Waksman, 1975; Oehler *et al.*, 1977). In 1965, Stewart-Tull *et al.* proposed that the increased production of antibody in response to an antigen injected in a water-in-oil emulsion containing the mycobacterial peptidoglycolipid was due to a negative feedback inhibition, under the control of antibody molecules. However, it is possible that the immunomodulator may act by diverting T_S cells from their regulatory function and thus a full-blown B-lymphocyte response to the antigen could occur (T. Henry, personal communication, 1981).

In addition, immunoregulatory T_S cells control the expression of a harmful autoimmune response (Swierkosz and Swanborg, 1975, 1977; Welch and Swanborg, 1976; Adda *et al.*, 1977; Bernard, 1977). If the immunomodulator depresses the control exerted by the T_S cells, autoimmunity could result.

Janeway (1982) postulated that a 'beneficial autoimmunity' may control humoral antibody responses by the production of anti-(anti-idiotype) antibodies which are capable of modulating the expression of the original idiotype in an antibody response. Such antibody-specific immunoregulation of B-cell antibody responses has been suggested from a number of studies (Jerne, 1974; Rodkey,

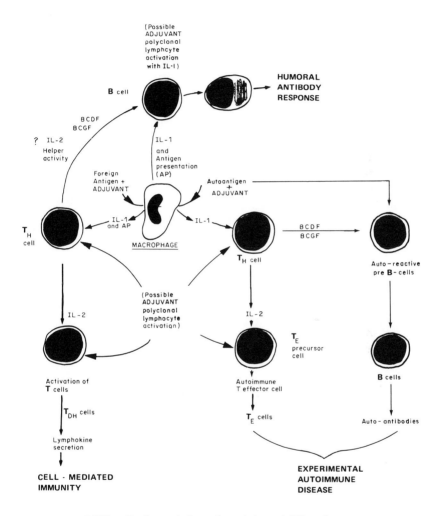

BCGF — B-cell growth factor (now designated PSF · pl)

Figure 8. Experimentally observed immune stimulatory activities of immunopotentiators in humoral, cell-mediated and autoimmune responses. IL-1, Interleukin 1; IL-2, Interleukin 2; BCDF, B-cell differentiation factor; BCGF, B-cell growth factor.

1974; Köhler, 1975; Pierce and Klinman, 1977). Jerne (1974) suggested that the immune system was self-regulated by a network of interacting B- and T-lymphocytes and their idiotypes and anti-idiotypes. Idiotype-recognizing B- and T-lymphocytes have been demonstrated in experimental animals (see Bona and Köhler, 1983, for complete list of references). However, Pierce and Speck (1983) cautioned that the observation of idiotype-specific lymphocytes may be more an artefact of laboratory experiments than a manifestation of an important immune regulatory function. Nevertheless, as McNamara *et al.* (1983) stated 'The elucidation of specific network interactions between the B- and T-cell idiotype repertoires is an essential step towards a more complete understanding of the immune system.' It is interesting to speculate that if the immunomodulator prevented the formation or function of the anti-(anti-idiotype) there would be a continued production of antibody carrying the original idiotype.

Finally, L. Chedid, G. Bahr, G. J. Riveau and J. Krueger (1984, personal communication) have made the fascinating observation that an immunosorbent column containing monoclonal anti-MDP antibody will adsorb IL-1. It appears that the MDP part of IL-1 may be responsible for triggering the latter's activity. Whatever the role of the MDP-like moiety of IL-1, there are many questions to be answered by immunologists before the benefits of immunomodulators can be put to practical use in human vaccines.

ACKNOWLEDGEMENT

I should like to thank Professor D. C. Dumonde for his advice on the presentation of Figure 8.

REFERENCES

Aarden, L. A., Brunner, T. K., Cerottini, J.-C., Dayer, J. M., Weck, A. L., Dinarello, C. A., Sabato, G. D., Farrar, J. J., Gery, I., Gillis, S., Handschumacher, R. E., Henney, C. S., Hoffmann, M. K., Koopman, W. J., Krane, S. M., Lachman, L. B., Lefkowits, I., Mishell, R. I., Mizel, S. B., Oppenheim, J. J., Paetkau, V., Plate, J., Röllinghoff, M., Rosenstreich, D., Rosenthal, A. S., Rosenwasser, L. J., Schimpl, A., Shin, H. S., Simon, P. L., Smith, K. A., Wagner, H., Watson, J. D., Wecker, W., and Wood, D. D. (1979). Revised nomenclature for antigen-nonspecific T-cell proliferation and helper factors. *J. Immunol.*, **123**, 2928–2929.

Adam, A., Ciorbaru, R., Petit, J.-F., and Lederer, E. (1972). Isolation and properties of a macro-molecular, water-soluble, immunoadjuvant fraction from the cell wall of *Mycobacterium smegmatis. Proc. Natl. Acad. Sci. USA*, **69**, 851–854.

Adam, A., Amar, C., Ciorbaru, R., Lederer, E., Petit, J.-F., and Vilkas, E. (1974a). Activité adjuvante des peptidoglycans de mycobactéries. *C. R. Acad. Sci.*, **278**, 799–801.

Adam, A., Ciorbaru, R., Ellouz, F., Petit, J.-F., and Lederer, E. (1974b). Adjuvant activity of monomeric bacterial cell-wall peptidoglycans. *Biochem. Biophys. Res. Commun.*, **56**, 561–567.

Adam, A., Petit, J.-F., Lefrancier, P., and Lederer, E. (1981). Muramyl peptides. Chemical structure, biological activity and mechanism of actions. *Mol. Cell. Biochem.* **41**, 27–47.

Adda, D. H., Berand, E., and Depieds, R. (1977). Evidence for suppressor cells in Lewis rats experimental allergic encephalomyelitis. *Eur. J. Immunol.*, **7**, 620–623.

Aebi, A., Asselineau, J., and Lederer, E. (1953). Sur les lipides de la souche humaine 'Brévannes' de *Mycobacterium tuberculosis. Bull. Soc. Chim. Biol.*, **35**, 661–684.

Allegranza, A., and Rovescalli, A. (1951a). Studi sulla patogenesi dell'encefalomielite sperimentale 'allergica'. *Biol. Lat.*, **4**, 119–128.

Allegranza, A., and Rovescalli, A. (1951b). Studi sulla patogenesi dell'encefalomielite 'allergica' sperimentale. *Biol. Lat.*, **4**, 137–143.

Allison, A. C., and Davies, A. J. S. (1971). Requirement of thymus-dependent lymphocytes for potentiation by adjuvants of antibody formation. *Nature*, **233**, 330–332.

Arnon, R. (1972). Synthetic vaccines—dream or reality. In *Immunity of Viral and Rickettsial diseases* (Eds. A. Kohn and A. M. Klinberg), p.209. Plenum Press, New York.

Arnon, R. (1979). Anti-viral activity induced by synthetic peptides corresponding to regions involved in viral neutralization, *Pharmacol. Ther.*, **6**, 279–289.

Askonas, B. A., White, R. G., and Wilkinson, P. C. (1965). Production of γ1 and γ2-antiovalbumin by various lymphoid tissues of the guinea-pig. *Immunochemistry*, **2**, 329–336.

Asselineau, J., and Lederer, E. (1953). Chimie des lipides bactériens. *Fortschr. Chem. Org. Naturst.*, **10**, 170–273.

Audibert, F., and Chedid, L. (1980). Recent advances concerning the use of muramyl dipeptide derivatives as vaccine potentiators. In *New Developments with Human and Veterinary Vaccines*, (Eds. A. Mizrahi, I. Hertman, M. A. Klingberg and A. Kohn) pp.325–338. Alan R. Liss, New York.

Audibert, F., Parant, M., Petit, J.-F., and Adam, A. (1973). Activité arthrógène de différentes préparations mycobactériennes. *C. R. Acad. Sci.*, **277**, 2097–2100.

Audibert, F., Jolivet, M., Chedid, L., Alouf, J. E., Boquet, P., Rivaille, P., and Siffers, O. (1981). Active antitoxic immunisation by a diphtheria toxin synthetic oligopeptide. *Nature*, **289**, 593–594.

Audibert, F., Jolivet, M., Chedid, L., Arnon, R., and Sela, M. (1982). 'Successful immunization with a totally synthetic diphtheria vaccine' *Proc. Natl. Acad. Sci. USA*, **79**, 5042–5046.

Azuma, I., Kanetsuna, F., Kada, Y., Taskashima, T., and Yamamura, Y. (1972). Adjuvant-polyarthritogenicity of cell walls of *Mycobacteria, Nocardia* and *Corynebacteria. J. J. Microbiol.*, **16**, 333–336.

Azuma, I., Okumura, H., Saiki, I., Kiso, M., Hasegawa, A., Tanio, Y., and Yamamura, Y. (1981). Adjuvant activity of carbohydrate analogs of *N*-acetylmuramyl-L-alanyl-D-isoglutamine on the induction of delayed-type hypersensitivity to azo-benzenearsonate–*N*-acetyl-L-tyrosine in guinea pigs. *Infect. Immun.*, **33**, 834–839.

Azurin, J. C., Cruz, A., Pesigan, T. P., Alvero, M., Camena, T., Suplido, R., Ledesma, L., and Gomez, C. Z. (1967). A controlled field trial of the effectiveness of cholera and cholera El Tor vaccines in the Philippines. *Bull. WHO*, **37**, 703–727.

Bahr, G. M., Eshhar, Z., Ben-Yitzhak, R., Modabber, F. Z., Arnon, R., Sela, M., and Chedid, L. (1983). Monoclonal antibodies to the synthetic adjuvant muramyl dipeptide: characterization of the specificity. *Mol. Immunol.*, **20**, 745–752.

Banck, G., and Forsgren, A. (1978). Many bacterial species are mitogenic for human blood B lymphocytes. *Scand. J. Immunol.*, **8**, 347–354.

Barksdale, L., and Kim, K.-S. (1977). Mycobacterium. *Bacteriol. Rev.*, **41**, 217–372.

Bash, J. A., and Waksman, B. H. (1975). The suppressive effect of immunization on the proliferative responses of rat T cell *in vitro. J. Immunol.*, **114**, 782–787.

Bast, R. C., Zbar, B., Borsos, T., and Rapp, H. J. (1974a). BCG and Cancer. 1. *N. Engl. J. Med.*, **290**, 1413–1420.

Bast, R. C. Zbar, B., Borsos, T., and Rapp, H. J. (1974b). BCG and Cancer. 2. *N. Engl. J. Med.*, **290**, 1458–1469.

Batchelor, J. R., and Lessof, M. H. (1964), Immunological function and auto-immune disease. *Rec. Adv. Med.*, 32–53.

Benacerraf, B. (1983). Suppressor T cells and suppressor factor. In *The Biology of Immunologic Disease* Eds. F. J. Dixon, and D. W. Fisher), pp.49–61. Sinauer Associates Inc., Massachusetts.

Bernard, C. C. A. (1977). Suppressor T-cells prevent experimental allergic encephalomyelitis in mice. *Clin. Exp. Immunol.*, **29**, 100–109.

Binaghi, R. A. (1966). Production of 7S immunoglobulins in immunized guinea-pigs. *J. Immunol.*, **97**, 159–164.

Bloch, K. J., Kourilsky, F. M., Ovary, Z., and Benacerraf, B. (1963). Properties of guinea-pig 7S antibodies III. Identification of anti-bodies involved in complement fixation and hemolysis. *J. Exp. Med.*, **117**, 965–981.

Bloom, B. R., and Godal, T. (1983). Selective primary health care: strategies for control of disease in the developing world. V. Leprosy. *Rev. Infect. Dis.*, **5**, 765–780.

Bona, C., and Köhler, H. (Eds.) (1983). Immune networks. *Ann. N.Y. Acad. Sci.*, **418**, 1–395.

Borsos, T., and Rapp, H. J. (Eds.) (1973). Conference on the use of BCG in therapy of cancer. *Natl. Cancer Inst. Monogr.*, **39**.

Burnet, M. (1963). Experimental production of auto-antibodies or of auto-immune disease. *Br. Med. Bull.*, **19**, 245–250.

Campbell, P. A., and Kind, P. (1971). Bone marrow-derived cells as target cells for polynucleotide adjuvants. *J. Immunol.*, **107**, 1419–1423.

Cazzulo, C. L., and Allegranza, A. (1951). Forme croniche dell'encefalomielite sperimentale 'allergica' nella cavia. *Biol. Lat.*, **4**, 76–108.

Chedid, L. (1977). Therapeutic potential of immunoregulating synthetic compounds. *INSERM*, **72**, 249–262.

Chedid, L. (1978). Immunopharmacological activities of muramyl dipeptide, a synthetic mycobacterial analog. *Adv. Pharmacol. Ther.*, **4**, 187–196.

Chedid, L. (1983). Adjuvants for vaccines. *Adv. Immunopharmacol.*, **2**, 401–406.

Chedid, L., and Audibert, F. (1976). Activity in saline of chemically well-defined non-toxic bacterial adjuvants. In *Immunopathology* (Ed. P. A. Miescher), pp.382–396. Schwabe & Co., Basel.

Chedid, L., and Audibert, F. (1977a). Chemically defined bacterial products with immunopotentiating activity. *J. Infect. Dis.* **136S**, 246–251.

Chedid, L., and Audibert, F. (1977b). Recent advances in the use of the synthetic immunoadjuvants muramyl dipeptide and analogues. *Microbiology*, 388–394.

Chedid, L., and Kotani, S. (1981). Muramyl dipeptide immunoadjuvants. *Adv. Immunopharmacol.*, **1**, 499–506.

Chedid, L., and Lederer, E. (1978). Past, present and future of the synthetic immunoadjuvant MDP and its analogs. *Biochem. Pharmacol.*, **27**, 2183–2186.

Chedid, L., and Parant, M. (1981). Immunostimulatory activity of synthetic polypeptides. Dissociation of anti-infectious activity from adjuvant activity of MDP by various procedures. In *Clinical Immunology and Allergology* (Eds. C. Steffen, and H. Ludwig), pp.199–206. Elsevier North-Holland Biomedical Press, Amsterdam.

Chedid, L., Parant, M., Parant, F., Gustafson, R. H., and Berger, F. M. (1972). Biological study of a non-toxic, water soluble immunoadjuvant from mycobacterial cell walls. *Proc. Natl. Acad. Sci. USA*, **69**, 855–858.

Chedid, L., Parant, M., and Parant, F. (1977a). Augmentation de la résistance non specifique à l'infection de la souris après administration orale de deux glycopeptides synthètiques doués d'activité adjuvant. *C. R. Acad. Sci.*, **284**, 405–408.

Chedid, L., Parant, M., Parant, F., Lefrancier, P., Choay, J., and Lederer, E. (1977b). Enhancement of non-specific immunity to *Klebsiella pneumoniae* infection by a synthetic immunoadjuvant (*N*-acetyl-muramyl-L-analyl-D-isoglutamine) and several analogs. *Proc. Natl. Acad. Sci. USA*, **74**, 2089–2093.

Chedid, L., Audibert, F., and Johnson, A. G. (1978a). Biological activities of muramyl dipeptide, a synthetic glycopeptide analogous to bacterial immunoregulating agents. *Prog. Allergy*, **25**, 63–105.

Chedid, L., Audibert, F., and Parant, M. (1978b). Une nouvelle famille d'immunorégulateurs synthétiques: le muramyl dipeptide et ses analogues. *Pathol. Biol.*, **26**, 527–530.

Chedid, L., Parant, M., and Parant, F. (1981). Immunopharmacologic approaches to bacterial infection. *Adv. Immunopharmacol.*, **1**, 101–107.

Chedid, L. A., Parant, M. A., Audibert, F. M., Riveau, G. J., Parant, F. J., Lederer, E., Choay, J. P., and Lefrancier, P. L. (1982). Biological activity of a new synthetic muramyl peptide adjuvant devoid of pyrogenicity. *Infect. Immun.*, **35**, 417–424.

Ciorbaru, R., Petit, J.-F., Lederer, E., Zissman, E., Bona, C., and Chedid, L. (1976). Presence and subcellular localization of two distinct mitogenic fractions in the cells of *Nocardia rubra* and *Nocardia opaca*: preparation of soluble mitogenic peptidoglycan fractions. *Infect. Immun.*, **13**, 1084–1090.

Clagett, J. A., and Engel, D. (1978). Polyclonal activation: a form of primitive immunity and its possible role in the pathogenesis of inflammatory diseases. *Dev. Comp. Immunol.*, **2**, 235–241.

Colover, J. (1954). Tubercle bacillus fractions in experimental allergic encephalomyelitis. *Brain*, **77**, 435–447.

Colover, J., and Consden, R. (1956). Experimental allergic encephalomyelitis produced by tubercle bacillus residues. *Nature*, **177**, 749–750.

Colover, J., and Glynn, L. E. (1958). Experimental iso-immune adrenalitis. *Immunology*, **2**, 172–176.

Cone, R. E., and Johnson, A. G. (1971). Regulation of the immune system by synthetic polynucleotides. III. Action on antigen-reactive cells of thymic origin. *J. Exp. Med.*, **133**, 665–676.

Convit, J., Aranzazu, N., Pinardi, M., and Ulrich, M. (1979). Immunological changes observed in indeterminate and lepromatous leprosy patients and Mitsuda negative contacts after the inoculation of a mixture of *M. leprae* and BCG. *Clin. Exp. Immunol.*, **36**, 214–220.

Damais, C., Bona, C., Chedid, L., Fleck, J., Nauciel, C., and Martin, J. P. (1975). Mitogenic effect of bacterial peptidoglycans possessing adjuvant activity. *J. Immunol.*, **115**, 268–271.

Damais, C., Parant, M., and Chedid, L. (1977). Non-specific activation of murine spleen cells *in vitro* by a synthetic immunoadjuvant (*N*-acetylmuramyl-L-analyl-D-isoglutamine). *Cell. Immunol.*, **34**, 49–56.

Daniel, P. M., Lam, D. K. C., and Pratt, O. E. (1981). Changes in the effectiveness of the blood–brain and blood–spinal cord barriers in experimental allergic encephalomyelitis. *J. Neurol. Sci.*, **52**, 211–219.

Davies, M. (1984). Bacterial cells as anti-tumour agents in man. *Rev. Environ. Health*, **4**, 31–56.

Davies, M., and Sabbadini, E. (1982). Mechanisms of BCG action. I. The induction of non-specific helper cells during the potentiation of alloimmune cell mediated cytotoxic responses. *Cancer Immunol. Immunother.*, **14**, 46–53.

Davies, M., and Stewart-Tull, D. E. S. (1973). The dual affinity of a mycobacterial glycopeptide for sheep erythrocyte membranes and guinea-pig gamma-globulin. *Immunology*, **25**, 1-9.

Diamantstein, T., and Wagner, B. (1973). The use of polyanions to break immunological tolerance. *Nature*, **241**, 117.

Diamantstein, T., Wagner, B., L'Age-Stehr, J., Beyse, I., Odenwald, M. V., and Schultz, G. (1971). Stimulation of humoral antibody formation by polyanions. III. Restoration of the immune response to sheep red blood cells by polyanions in thymectomized and lethally irradiated mice protected with bone marrow cells. *Eur. J. Immunol.*, **1**, 302-309.

Doniach, D., and Roitt, I. M. (1962). Auto-antibodies in disease. *Annu. Rev. Med.*, **13**, 213-240.

Draper, P. (1982). The anatomy of mycobacteria. In *The Biology of the Mycobacteria*, Vol. I. (Eds. C. Ratledge and J. Stanford), pp.9-52. Academic Press, London.

Dziarski, R., and Dziarski, A. (1979). Mitogenic activity of Staphylococcal peptidoglycan. *Infect. Immun.*, **23**, 706-710.

Dziarski, R., Dziarski, A., and Levinson, A. I. (1980). Mitogenic responsiveness of mouse, rat and human lymphocytes to *Staphylococcus aureus* cell wall, teichoic acid and peptidoglycan. *Int. Arch. Allergy Appl. Immunol.*, **63**, 383-395.

Edelman, R. (1980). Vaccine adjuvants. *Rev. Infect. Dis.*, **2**, 370-383.

Edelman, R., Hardegree, M. C., and Chedid, L. (1980). Summary of an international symposium on potentiation of the immune response to vaccines. *J. Infect. Dis.*, **141**, 103-112.

Ellouz, F., Adam, A., Ciorbaru, R., and Lederer, E. (1974). Minimal structural requirements for adjuvant activity of bacterial peptidoglycan derivatives. *Biochem. Biophys. Res. Commun.*, **59**, 1317-1325.

Farrar, J. J., Benjamin, W. R., Hilfiker, M. L., Howard, M., Farrar, W. L., and Fuller-Farrar, J. (1982). The biochemistry, biology and role of interleukin 2 in the induction of cytotoxic T cell and antibody-forming B cell responses. *Immunol. Rev.*, **63**, 129-166.

Fevrier, M., Birrien, J. L., Leclerc, C., Chedid, L., and Liacopoulos, P. (1978). The macrophage, target cell of the synthetic adjuvant muramyl dipeptide. *Eur. J. Immunol.*, **8**, 558-562.

Field, E. J., Caspary, E. A., and Ball, E. J. (1963). Some biological properties of a highly active encephalitogenic factor isolated from human brain. *Lancet*, **ii**, 11-13.

Fleck, J., Mock, M., Tytgat, F., Nauciel, C., and Minck, R. (1974). Adjuvant activity in delayed hypersensitivity of the peptidic part of bacterial peptidoglycans. *Nature*, **250**, 517-518.

Fleming, W. A., Stewart-Tull, D. E. S., McClure, S. F., and McKee, A. M. (1984). Cellular responsiveness *in vitro*: the effect of mycobacterial glycopeptides, glycolipids and peptidoglycolipids on the *in vitro* growth of haemopoietic colony forming cells. *Immunology*, **51**, 555-561.

Freund, J. (1947). Some aspects of active immunization. *Annu. Rev. Microbiol.*, **1**, 291-308.

Freund, J., and Bonanto, M. V. (1942). Effect of amount of antigen on antitoxin formation during primary and secondary immunizations. *J. Immunol.*, **45**, 71-78.

Freund, J., and Bonanto, M. V. (1946). The duration of antibody-formation after injection of killed typhoid bacilli in water-in-oil emulsion. *J. Immunol.*, **52**, 231-234.

Freund, J., and McDermott, K. (1942). Sensitization to horse serum by means of adjuvants. *Proc. Soc. Exp. Biol.*, **49**, 548-553.

Freund, J., and Stone, S. H. (1959). The effectiveness of tuberculoglycolipid as an adjuvant in eliciting allergic encephalomyelitis and aspermatogenesis. *J. Exp. Med.*, **82**, 560-567.

Freund, J., Stern, E. R., and Pisani, T. M. (1947). Isoallergic encephalomyelitis and radiculitis in guinea-pigs after one injection of brain and mycobacteria in water-in-oil emulsion. *J. Immunol.*, **57**, 179–194.

Freund, J., Lipton, M. M., and Thompson, G. E. (1953). Aspermatogenesis in the guinea-pig induced by testicular tissue and adjuvants. *J. Exp. Med.*, **97**, 711–726.

Gershon, R. K., and Kondo, K. (1970). Cell interactions in the induction of tolerance: the role of thymic lymphocytes. *Immunology*, **18**, 723–737.

Gisler, R. H., Dietrich, F. M., Baschang, G., Brownbill, A., Schumann, G., Staber, F. G., Tarcsay, L., Wachsmuth, E. D., and Dukor, P. (1979). New developments in drugs enhancing the immune response: activation of lymphocytes and accessory cells by muramyl-dipeptides. In *Drugs and Immune Responsiveness* (Eds. J. L. Turk, and D. Parker), pp.133–160. Macmillan, London.

Godal, T. (1978). Immunological aspects of leprosy—present status. *Prog. Allergy*, **25**, 211–242.

Gordon, J., and White, R. G. (1971). Surface peptido-glycolipid filaments on *Mycobacterium leprae. Clin. Exp. Immunol.*, **9**, 539–547.

Griffith, A. H., and Regamey, R. H. (Eds.) (1978). *International Symposium on Biological Preparations in the Treatment of Cancer (Dev. Biol. Stand.*, Vol. 38). S. Karger, Basel.

Grov, A., Helgeland, S., and Endresen, C. (1976). Inhibition of leucocyte migration by peptidoglycan fragments. *Zentralbl. Bakteriol. Parasitenkd. Infektionskr. Hyg. Abt. 1 Suppl.*, **5**, 389.

Hamaoka, T., and Katz, D. H. (1973a). Mechanism of adjuvant activity of poly A:U on antibody responses to hapten-carrier conjugates. *Cell. Immunol.*, **7**, 246–260.

Hamaoka, T., and Katz, D. H. (1973b). Cellular site of action of various adjuvants in antibody responses to hapten-carrier conjugates. *J. Immunol.*, **111**, 1554–1563.

Heymer, B., Bultmann, B., Schachenmayr, W., Spanel, R., Haferkamp, O., and Schmidt, W. C. (1973). Migration inhibition of rat peritoneal cells induced by streptococcal mucopeptide preparations. *J. Immunol.*, **111**, 1743–1754.

Hilleman, M. R. (1966). Critical appraisal of emulsified oil adjuvants applied to viral vaccines. *Prog. Med. Virol.*, **8**, 131–182.

Hiu, I. J. (1972). Water-soluble and lipid-free fraction from BCG with adjuvant and anti-tumour activity. *Nature*, **238**, 241–242.

Hoffmann, M. K. (1979). Control of B cell differentiation by macrophages. *Ann. N.Y. Acad. Sci.*, **332**, 557–563.

Hoffmann, M. K., Galanos, C., Koenig, S., and Oettgen, H. F. (1977). B cell activation by lipopolysaccharide. Distinct pathways for induction of mitosis and antibody production. *J. Exp. Med.*, **146**, 1640–1647.

Holton, J. B., and Schwab, J. H. (1966). Adjuvant properties of bacterial cell wall mucopeptides. *J. Immunol.*, **96**, 134–138.

Horiuchi, A., and Waksman, B. H. (1968). Role of the thymus in tolerance. VIII. Relative effectiveness of non-aggregated and heat-aggregated bovine gamma globulin injected directly into lymphoid organs of normal rats in suppressing immune responsiveness. *J. Immunol.*, **101**, 1322–1332.

Iribe, H., Koga, T., Onoue, K., Kotani, S., Kusumoto, S., and Shiba, T. (1981). Macrophage-stimulating effect of a synthetic muramyl dipeptide and its adjuvant-active and -inactive analogs for the production of T-cell activating monokines. *Cell. Immunol.*, **64**, 73–83.

Ishibashi, T., Kohashi, O., Koga, T., Tanaka, A., Kuwano, T., and Sugiyama, K. (1971). The mode of action of immunological adjuvants. I. A new method to assess the adjuvant effect of substances as represented by mycobacterial adjuvants. *Ann. Rep. Jpn.–US Coop Med. Sci. Prog.*, 119–138.

Janeway, C. (1982). Beneficial autoimmunity? *Nature*, **299**, 396–397.

Jeljaszewicz, J., Pulverer, G., and Roszkowski, W. (Eds.) (1982). *Bacteria and Cancer*. Academic Press, London.

Jerne, N. K. (1974). Towards a network theory of the immune system. *Ann. Immunol. Paris*, **125C**, 373–389.

Jollès, P., Samour, D., and Lederer, E. (1962). Analytical studies on Wax D, a macromolecular peptidoglycolipid fraction from human strains of *Mycobacterium tuberculosis. Arch. Biochem. Biophys. Suppl.*, **1**, 283–289.

Jollès, P., Samour, D., and Lederer, E. (1963). Isolement de fractions peptido-glycolipidiques à partir des cires D de mycobacteries bovines, atypiques, aviaires et saprophytes. *Biochim. Biophys. Acta*, **78**, 342–350.

Jones, J. M., and Kind, P. D. (1972). Enhancing effect of bacterial endotoxins on bone marrow cells in the immune response to SRBC. *J. Immunol.*, **108**, 1453–1455.

Juy, D., and Chedid, L. (1975). Comparison between macrophage activation and enhancement of non-specific resistance to tumors by mycobacterial immuno-adjuvants. *Proc. Natl. Acad. Sci. USA*, **72**, 4105–4109.

Kabat, E. A., Wolf, A., and Bezer, A. E. (1946). Rapid production of acute disseminated encephalomyelitis in rhesus monkeys by injection of brain tissue with adjuvants. *Science*, **104**, 362–363.

Kabat, E. A., Wolf, A., and Bezer, A. E. (1947). The rapid production of acute disseminated experimental allergic encephalomyelitis in rhesus monkeys by injection of heterologous and homologous brain tissue with adjuvant. *J. Exp. Med.*, **85**, 117–130.

Kato, K., Kotani, S., Matsubara, T., Kogami, J., Hashimoto, S., Chimori, M., and Kazekawa, I. (1962). Lysis of *Staphylococcus aureus* cell walls by a lytic enzyme purified from culture supernatants of *Flavobacterium* species. *Biken, J.*, **5**, 127–131.

Kelly, M. T. (1976). Activation of guinea-pig macrophages by cell walls of *Mycobacterium bovis* strain BCG. *Cell. Immunol.*, **26**, 254–263.

Kies, M. W., Alvord, E. C., and Roboz, E. (1958). Production of experimental allergic encephalomyelitis in guinea-pigs with fractions isolated from bovine spinal cord and killed tubercle bacilli. *Nature*, **182**, 104–105.

Killen, J. A., and Swanborg, R. H. (1982). Autoimmune effector cells. III. Role of adjuvant and accessory cells in the *in vitro* induction of autoimmune encephalomyelitis. *J. Immunol.*, **129**, 759–763.

Koga, T., Ishibashi, T., Sugiyama, K., and Tanaka, A. (1969). Immunological adjuvants. III. A preliminary report about the mode of action of mycobacterial adjuvants and further confirmation of adjuvant activity of acetylated wax D. *Int. Arch. Allergy*, **36**, 233–244.

Koga, T., Kotani, S., Narita, T., and Pearson, C. M. (1976). Induction of adjuvant arthritis in the rat by various bacterial cell walls and their water-soluble components. *Int. Arch. Allergy*, **51**, 206–213.

Koga, T., Maeda, K., Onoue, K., Kato, K., and Kotani, S. (1979). Chemical structure required for immuno-adjuvant and arthritogenic activities of cell wall peptidoglycans. *Mol. Immunol.*, **16**, 153–162.

Kohashi, O., Pearson, C. M., Beck, F. W. J., Narita, T., and Kotani, S. (1976a). Arthritogenicity in rats of cell walls from several *Streptococci, Staphylococci* and two other bacteria. *Proc. Soc. Exp. Biol. Med.*, **152**, 156–160.

Kohashi, O., Pearson, C. M., Watanabe, Y., Kotani, S., and Koga, T. (1976b). Structural requirements for arthritogenicity of peptidoglycans from *Staphylococcus aureus* and *Lactobacillus plantarum* and analogous synthetic compounds. *J. Immunol.*, **116**, 1635–1639.

Kohashi, O., Pearson, C. M., Watanabe, Y., and Kotani, S. (1977). Preparation of arthritogenic hydrosoluble peptidoglycans from both arthritogenic and non-arthritogenic bacterial cell walls. *Infect. Immun.*, **16**, 861–866.

Kohashi, O., Kotani, S., Shiba, T., and Ozawa, A. (1979). Synergistic effect of polyriboinosinic acid:polyribocytidylic acid and either bacterial peptidoglycans or synthetic *N*-acetyl-muramyl peptides on production of adjuvant-induced arthritis in rats. *Infect. Immun.*, **26**, 690–697.

Köhler, H. (1975). The response to phosphorylcholine: dissecting an immune response. *Transplant. Rev.*, **27**, 24–56.

Kopeloff, L. M., and Kopeloff, N. (1947). Neurologic manifestations in laboratory animals produced by organ (Adjuvant) emulsions. *J. Immunol.*, **57**, 229–237.

Kotani, S., Narita, T., Stewart-Tull, D. E. S., Shimono, T., Watanabe, Y., Kato, K., and Iwata, S. (1975a). Immunoadjuvant activities of cell-walls and their water-soluble fractions prepared from various Gram-positive bacteria. *Biken J.*, **18**, 77–92.

Kotani, S., Watanabe, Y., Shimono, T., Narita, T., Kato, K., Stewart-Tull, D. E. S., Kinoshita, F., Yokogawa, K., Kawata, S., Shiba, T., Kusumoto, S., and Tarumi, Y. (1975b). Immunoadjuvant activities of cell-walls, their water-soluble fractions and peptidoglycan subunits, prepared from various gram-positive bacteria and of synthetic *N*-acetyl-muramyl peptides. *Z. Immun. Forsch.*, **149**, 302–319.

Kotani, S., Watanabe, Y., Shimono, T., Kinoshita, F., Narita, T., Kato, K., Stewart-Tull, D. E. S., and Morisaki, I. (1975c). Immunoadjuvant activities of peptidoglycan subunits from the cell-walls of *Staphylococcus aureus* and *Lactobacillus plantarum*. *Biken J.*, **18**, 93–103.

Kotani, S., Watanabe, Y., Shimono, T., Kato, K., Kinoshita, F., and Stewart-Tull, D. E. S. (1974). Immunostimulation by muramyl peptides isolated from the enzymatic digests of gram-positive bacterial cell walls or chemically synthesized. Sym. *Les Immunostimulants Bacteriens.* Soc..Chim. Biol., Institut Pasteur, Paris.

Kotani, S., Watanabe, Y., Kinoshita, F., Kato, K., and Perkins, H. R. (1977). Immunoadjuvant activities of the enzymatic digests of bacterial cell walls lacking immunoadjuvancy by themselves. *Biken J.*, **20**, 87–90.

Kozak, Y. de, Audibert, F., Thillaye, B., Chedid, L., and Faure, J. P. (1979). Effets d'adjuvants hydrosolubles d'origine mycobactérienne sur l'induction et al prévention de l'uvéo-rétinite autoimmune expérimentale chez le cobaye. *Ann. Immunol., Paris*, **130**, 29–32.

Lamoureux, G., Thibeault, G., Richer, G., and Bernard, C. (1972). Induction de l'encéphalite allérgique expérimentale avec des encéphalitogènes humains de synthèse. *Union Med. Cana.*, **101**, 674–680.

Larsson, E. L., Iscove, N. N., and Continho, A. (1980). Two distinct factors are required for induction of T-cell growth. *Nature*, **283**, 664–666.

Lebar, R., and Voisin, G. A. (1974). Production d'une encéphalomyélite allergique expérimentale autoimmune (EAE) chez le cobaye a l'aide d'un adjuvant hydrosoluble extrait de *Mycobacterium smegmatis*. *Ann. Immunol.*, Paris **125C**, 911–916.

Leclerc, C., Lowy, I., and Chedid, L. (1978). Influence of MDP and of some analogous synthetic glycopeptides on the *in vitro* mouse spleen cell viability and immune response to sheep erythrocytes. *Cell. Immunol.*, **38**, 286–293.

Leclerc, C., Bourgeois, E., and Chedid, L. (1979). Enhancement by muramyl dipeptide of *in vitro* nude mice responses to a T-dependent antigen. *Immunol. Commun.*, **8**, 55–64.

Lederer, E. (1980a). Combined immunostimulation with synthetic muramyl dipeptide (MDP) and natural and synthetic trehalose diesters. *INSERM*, **97**, 137–145.

Lederer, E. (1980b). Synthetic immunostimulants derived from the bacterial cell wall. *J. Med. Chem.*, **23**, 819–825.

Lederer, E. (1982a). Immunomodulation by muramyl peptides: recent developments. *Clin. Immunol. Newsl.*, **3**, 83–86.

Lederer, E. (1982b). Recent progress in the study of natural and synthetic immunomodulators derived from bacterial cell walls. In *Immunomodulation by*

Microbial Products and Related Synthetic Compounds, (Eds. Y. Yamamura, S. Kotani, I. Azuma, A. Koda and T. Shiba), pp.3–16. Excerpta Medica, Amsterdam.

Lederer, E., and Chedid, L. (1982). Immunomodulation by synthetic muramyl peptides and trehalose diesters. In *Immunological Approaches to Cancer Therapeutics* (Ed. E. Mihich), pp.107–135. Wiley, New York.

Lefrancier, P., and Lederer, E. (1981). Chemistry of synthetic immunomodulant muramyl peptides. *Prog. Chem. Org. Nat. Prod.*, **40**, 1–47.

Lerner, R. A., Green, N., Olson, A., Shinnick, T., and Sutcliffe, J. G. (1983). The development of synthetic vaccines. In *The Biology of Immunologic Disease* (Eds. F. J. Dixon, and D. W. Fisher), pp.331–338. Sinauer Associates Inc., Massachusetts.

Levine, M. M., Kaper, J. B., Black, R. E., and Clements, M. L. (1983). New knowledge on pathogenesis of bacterial enteric infections as applied to vaccine development. *Microbiol. Rev.*, **47**, 510–550.

Louis, J. A., Chiller, J. M., and Weigle, W. O. (1973). The ability of bacterial lipopolysaccharide to modulate the induction of unresponsiveness to a state of immunity. Cellular parameters. *J. Exp. Med.*, **138**, 1481–1495.

MacLennan, R., Schofield, F. D., Pittman, M., Hardegree, M. C., and Barile, M. F. (1965). Immunization against neonatal tetanus in New Guinea. Antitoxin response of pregnant women to adjuvant and plain toxoids. *Bull. WHO*, **32**, 683–697.

Maron, R., Mozes, E., Fuchs, S., Sela, M., and Chedid, L. (1978). The effect of a water-soluble adjuvant on the immune responses to synthetic polypeptides. *Ann. Immunol.*, **129**, 489–497.

Mathé, G. (1971). Active immunotherapy. *Adv. Cancer Res.*, **14**, 1–36.

Matsumoto, K., Ogawa, H., Nagase, O., Kusama, T., and Azuma, I. (1981). Stimulation of non-specific host resistance to infection induced by muramyl dipeptides. *Microbiol. Immunol.*, **25**, 1047–1058.

McNamara, M., Gleason, K., and Köhler, H. (1983). Idiotype-specific T-helper cells. *Ann. N.Y. Acad. Sci.*, **418**, 65–73.

Merser, C., Sinay, P., and Adam, A. (1975). Total synthesis and adjuvant activity of bacterial peptidoglycan derivatives. *Biochem. Biophys. Res. Commun.*, **66**, 1316–1322.

Middlebrook, G., and Dubos, R. J. (1948). Specific serum agglutination of erythrocytes sensitized with extracts of tubercle bacilli. *J. Exp. Med.*, **88**, 521–528.

Migliore-Samour, D., and Jollès, P. (1972). A hydrosoluble adjuvant-active mycobacterial 'polysaccharide-peptidoglycan' prepared by a simple extraction technique of the bacterial cells (strain Peurois). *FEBS Lett.*, **25**, 301–304.

Mizel, S. B. (1980). Lymphocyte-activating factor (interleukin 1) a possible mediator of endotoxin adjuvancy. In *Microbiology* (Ed. D. Schlessinger), pp.40–43. ASM, Washington.

Mizrahi, A., Hertman, I., Klingberg, M. A., and Kohn, A. (Eds.) (1980). *New Developments with Human and Veterinary Vaccines*. Alan R. Liss, New York.

Modolell, M., Luckenbach, G. A., Parant, M., and Munder, P. G. (1974). The adjuvant activity of a mycobacterial water-soluble adjuvant (WSA) *in vitro*. I. The requirement of macrophages. *J. Immunol.*, **113**, 395–403.

Morgan, I. M. (1946). Allergic encephalomyelitis in monkeys in response to injection of normal monkey cord. *J. Bacteriol.*, **51**, 614.

Morgan, I. M. (1947). Allergic encephalomyelitis in monkeys in response to injection of normal monkey nervous tissue. *J. Exp. Med.*, **85**, 131–140.

Mozes, E., Sela, M., and Chedid, L. (1980). Efficient genetically controlled antibody formation to a synthetic antigen (T,G)-a-L covalently bound to a synthetic adjuvant MDP. *Proc. Natl. Acad. Sci. USA*, **77**, 4933–4937.

Munder, P. G., Modolell, M., Andreesen, R., Berdel, W., Pahlke, W., Oepke, R., and Westphal, O. (1983). Generation of tumoricidal macrophages and direct selective destruction of tumor cells by membrane active adjuvants. *Prog. Clin. Biol. Res.*, **132**, 393–402.

Nagai, Y., Akiyama, K., Suzuki, K. Kotani, S, Watanabe, Y., Shimono, T., Shiba, T., Kusumoto, S., Ikuta, F., and Takeda, S. (1978a). Minimum structural requirements for encephalitogen and for adjuvant in the induction of experimental allergic encephalomyelitis. *Cell. Immunol.*, **35**, 158–167.

Nagai, Y., Akiyama, K., Kotani, S., Watanabe, Y., Shimono, T., Shiba, T., and Kusumoto, S. (1978b). Structural specificity of synthetic peptide adjuvant for induction of experimental allergic encephalomyelitis. *Cell. Immunol.*, **35**, 168–172.

Nagao, S., Tanaka, A., Yamamoto, Y., Koga, T., Onoue, K., Shiba, T., Kusumoto, K., and Kotani, S. (1979). Inhibition of macrophage migration by muramyl peptides. *Infect. Immun.*, **24**, 308–312.

Nakashima, I., Nagase, F., and Kato, N. (1977). Adjuvant action of capsular polysaccharide of *Klebsiella pneumoniae* on antibody response. VI. Site of its action. *Z. Immun.-Forsch.*, **153**, 204–216.

Nakashima, I., Nagase, F., Yokochi, T., Ohta, M., and Kato, N. (1979). Adjuvant action of polyclonal lymphocyte activators. I. Comparison and characterization of their action in antibody response to deaggregated bovine serum albumin. *Cell. Immunol.*, **46**, 69–76.

Nakashima, I., Nagase, F., Matsuura, A., and Kato, N. (1980a). Adjuvant actions of polyclonal lymphocyte activators. II. Comparison and characterization of their actions in initiation and potentiation of immune responses to T-dependent and T-independent soluble antigens. *Cell. Immunol.*, **49**, 360–371.

Nakashima, I., Nagase, F., Matsuura, A., Yokochi, T., and Kato, N. (1980b). Adjuvant actions of polyclonal lymphocyte activators. III. Two distinct types of T-initiating adjuvant action demonstrated under different experimental conditions. *Cell. Immunol.*, **52**, 429–437.

Namikawa, T., Richert, J. R., Driscoll, B. F., Kies, M. W., and Alvord, E. C. (1982). Transfer of allergic encephalomyelitis with spleen cells from donors sensitized with myelin basic protein in incomplete Freund's adjuvant. *J. Immunol.*, **128**, 932–934.

Nauciel, C., Fleck, J., Martin, J.-P., and Mock, M. (1973a). Activité adjuvante de peptidoglycanes de bactéries à Gram négatif dans l'hypersensibilité de type retardé. *C. R. Acad. Sci.*, **276**, 3499–3500.

Nauciel, C., Fleck, J., Mock, M., and Martin, J.-P. (1973b). Activité adjuvante de fractions monomériques de peptidoglycanes bactériens dans l'hypersensibilité de type retardé. *C. R. Acad. Sci.*, **277**, 2841–2844.

Nauciel, C., Fleck, J., Martin, J.-P., Mock, M., and Nguyen-Huy, H. (1974). Adjuvant activity of bacterial peptidoglycans on the production of delayed hypersensitivity and on the antibody response. *Eur. J. Immunol.*, **4**, 352–356.

Navalkar, R. G. (1980). Immunology of leprosy. *CRC Crit. Rev. Microbiol.*, **8**, 25–47.

Novotny, P., and Brookes, J. E. (1975). The use of *Bordetella pertussis* preserved in liquid nitrogen as a challenge suspension in the Kendrick mouse protection test. *J. Biol. Stand.*, **3**, 11–29.

Oehler, J. R., Herberman, R. B., Campbell, D. A., and Djeu, J. Y. (1977). Inhibition of rat mixed lymphocyte cultures by suppressor macrophages. *Cell. Immunol.*, **29**, 238–250.

Ogonuki, H., Hashizume, S. O., and Takashashi, B. (1967). Preparation and laboratory tests of oil adjuvant cholera vaccine. *Bull. WHO*, **37**, 729–736.

Oppenheim, J. J., Togawa, A., Chedid, L., and Mizel, S. (1980). Components of mycobacteria and muramyl dipeptide with adjuvant activity induce lymphocyte activating factor. *Cell. Immunol.*, **50**, 71–81.

Oppenheim, J. J., Stadler, B. M., Siraganian, R. P., Mage, M., and Mathieson, B. (1982). Lymphokines: their role in lymphocyte responses. Properties of interleukin 1. *Fed. Proc.*, **41**, 257–262.

Ornellas, E. P., Sanfilippo, F., and Scott, D. W. (1974). Cellular events in tolerance. IV. The effect of a graft-versus-host reaction and endotoxin on hapten- and carrier-specific tolerance. *Eur. J. Immunol.*, **4**, 587–591.

Ortiz-Ortiz, L., Nakamura, R. M., and Weigle, W. O. (1976). T-cell requirement for experimental allergic encephalomyelitis induction in the rat. *J. Immunol.*, **117**, 576–579.

Ovary, Z., Benacerraf, B., and Bloch, K. J. (1963). Properties of guinea-pig 7S antibodies. II. Identification of antibodies involved in passive cutaneous and systemic anaphylaxis. *J. Exp. Med.*, **117**, 951–964.

Parant, M. (1979). Biologic properties of a new synthetic adjuvant, muramyl dipeptide (MDP). *Springer Semin. Immunopathol.*, **2**, 101–118.

Paterson, P. Y. (1960). Transfer of allergic encephalomyelitis in rats by means of lymph node cells. *J. Exp. Med.*, **111**, 119–135.

Paterson, P. Y., and Bell, J. (1962). Studies on induction of allergic encephalomyelitis in rats and guinea pigs without the use of mycobacteria. *J. Immunol.*, **89**, 72–79.

Pearson, C. M. (1956). Development of arthritis, periarthritis and periostitis in rats given adjuvant. *Proc. Soc. Exp. Biol. Med.*, **91**, 95–101.

Pierce, S. K., and Klinman, N. R. (1977). Antibody-specific immunoregulation. *J. Exp. Med.*, **146**, 509–519.

Pierce, S. K., and Speck, N. A. (1983). Antibody-specific regulation of primary and secondary B-cell responses. *Ann. N.Y. Acad. Sci.*, **418**, 177–187.

Pollock, T. M., Miller, E., Mortimer, J. Y., and Smith, G. (1984). Symptoms after primary immunization with DTP and with DT vaccine. *Lancet*, **ii**, 146– 149.

Räsänen, L., Karhumäki, E., and Arvilommi, H. (1978). Bacteria induce lymphokine synthesis polyclonally in human B lymphocytes. *J. Immunol.*, **121**, 418–420.

Räsänen, L., Karhumäki, E., Majuri, R., and Arvilommi, H. (1980). Polyclonal activation of human lymphocytes by bacteria. *Infect. Immun.*, **28**, 368–372.

Räsänen, L., Mustikkamäki, U. P., and Arvilommi, H. (1982). Polyclonal response of human lymphocytes to bacterial cell walls, peptidoglycans and teichoic acids. *Immunology*, **46**, 481–486.

Rist, N. (1938). Les lésions metastatiques produites par les bacilles tuberculeux morts enrobés dans les paraffines. *Ann. Inst. Pasteur*, **61**, 121–171.

Rodkey, L. S. (1974). Studies of idiotypic antibodies. Production and characterization of auto anti-idiotypic antiserum. *J. Exp. Med.*, **139**, 712–720.

Rook, G. A. W., and Stewart-Tull, D. E. S. (1976). The dissociation of adjuvant properties of mycobacterial components from mitogenicity and from the ability to induce the release of mediators from macrophages. *Immunology*, **31**, 389–396.

Rose, N. R., and Witebsky, E. (1956). Studies in organ specificity: V. Changes in the thyroid glands of rabbits following active immunization with rabbit thyroid extract. *J. Immunol.*, **76**, 417–427.

Sato, Y., Kimura, M., and Fukumi, H. (1984). Development of a pertussis component vaccine in Japan. *Lancet*, **i**, 122–126.

Sela, M. (1975). Synthetic vaccines of the future. *Perspect. Virol.*, **IX**, 91–98.

Sela, M. (1977). Synthetic approaches to applied medical aspects of immunology. *Asian J. Infect. Dis.*, **1**, 97–103.

Sela, M., and Arnon, R. (1980). Antiviral antibodies obtained with aqueous solution of a synthetic antigen. In *New Developments with Human and Veterinary Vaccines* (Eds. A. Mizrahi, I. Hertman, M. A. Klinberg and A. Kohn), pp.315–323. Alan R. Liss, New York.

Shaw, J., Caplan, B., Paetkan, V., Pilarski, L. M., Delovitch, T. L., and McKenzie, I. F. C. (1980). Cellular origins of co-stimulator (IL2) and its activity in cytotoxic T-lymphocyte responses. *J. Immunol.*, **124**, 2231–2239.

Smith, K. A. (1980). T cell growth factor. *Immunol. Rev.*, **51**, 337–357.

Specter, S., Friedman, H., and Chedid, L. (1977). Dissociation between the adjuvant vs mitogenic activity of a synthetic muramyl dipeptide for murine splenocytes. *Proc. Soc. Exp. Biol. Med.*, **155**, 349–352.

Specter, S., Cimprich, R., Friedman, H., and Chedid, L. (1978). Stimulation of an enhanced *in vitro* immune response by a synthetic adjuvant, muramyl dipeptide. *J. Immunol.*, **120**, 487–491.

Stanton, M. F. (Ed.) (1972). Conference on Immunology of Carcinogenesis. *Natl. Cancer. Inst. Monogr.*, **35**.

Staruch, M. J., and Wood, D. D. (1983). The adjuvanticity of interleukin I *in vivo*. *J. Immunol.*, **130**, 2191–2194.

Stewart-Tull, D. E. S. (1980). The immunological activities of bacterial peptidoglycan. *Annu. Rev. Microbiol.*, **34**, 311–340.

Stewart-Tull, D. E. S. (1983a). Immunologically important components of mycobacteria. In *The Biology of the Mycobacteria* (Eds. C. Ratledge and J. Standford), pp.3–84. Academic Press, London.

Stewart-Tull, D. E. S. (1983b). Immunopotentiating products of bacteria. In *Medical Microbiology*, Vol. 2, *Immunization Against Bacterial Disease* (Eds. C. S. F. Easmon, and J. Jeljaszewicz), pp.1–42. Academic Press, London.

Stewart-Tull, D. E. S., and Arbuthnott, J. P. (1971). The separation of guinea-pig serum proteins by a preparative isoelectric focusing method. *Sci. Tools*, **18**, 17–21.

Stewart-Tull, D. E. S., and Davies, M. (1972). Adjuvant activity of *Mycobacterium leprae*. *Infect. Immun.*, **6**, 909–912.

Stewart-Tull, D. E. S., and Wilkinson, P. C. (1973). The affinity of mycobacterial glycopeptides for guinea-pig gamma$_2$ immunoglobulin and its fragments. *Immunology*, **24**, 205–216.

Stewart-Tull, D. E. S., Wilkinson, P. C., and White, R. G. (1965). The affinity of a mycobacterial glycopeptide for guinea-pig gamma-globulin. *Immunology*, **9**, 151–160.

Stewart-Tull, D. E. S., Arbuthnott, J. P., and Freer, J. H. (1975a). Some properties of IgG$_1$ and IgG$_2$ globulins from normal and adjuvant stimulated guinea-pigs. *Immunochemistry*, **12**, 941–947.

Stewart-Tull, D. E. S., Shimono, T., Kotani, S., Kato, M., Ogawa, Y., Yamamura, Y., Koga, T., and Pearson, C. M. (1975b). The adjuvant activity of a non-toxic water-soluble glycopeptide present in large quantities in the culture filtrate of *M. tuberculosis* strain DT. *Immunology*, **29**, 1–15.

Stewart-Tull, D. E. S., Shimono, T., Kotani, S., and Knights, B. A. (1976). Immunosuppressive effect in mycobacterial adjuvant emulsions of mineral oils containing low molecular weight hydrocarbons. *Int. Arch. Allergy Appl. Immunol.*, **52**, 118–128.

Stewart-Tull, D. E. S., Davies, M., and Jackson, D. M. (1977). The binding of adjuvant-active mycobacterial peptidoglycolipids and glycopeptides to mammalian membranes and their effect on artificial lipid bilayers. *Immunology*, **34**, 57–67.

Stone, S. H. (1961). Transfer of allergic encephalomyelitis by lymph node cells in inbred guinea-pigs. *Science*, **134**, 619–620.

Stones, P. B. (1979). Self injection of veterinary oil-emulsion vaccines. *Br. Med. J.*, **i**, 1627.

Suter, E., and White, R. G. (1954). Response of reticulo-endothelial system to injection of 'purified wax' and lipopolysaccharide of tubercle bacilli; histologic and immunologic study. *Am. Rev. Tuberc.*, **70**, 793–805.

Swierkosz, J. E., and Swanborg, R. H. (1975). Suppressor cell control of unresponsiveness to experimental allergic encephalomyelitis. *J. Immunol.*, **115**, 631–633.

Swierkosz, J. E., and Swanborg, R. H. (1977). Immunoregulation of experimental allergic encephalomyelitis: conditions for induction of suppressor cells and analysis of mechanism. *J. Immunol.*, **119**, 1501–1506.

Takada, H., Tsujimoto, M., Kotani, S., Kusumoto, S., Inage, M., Shiba, T., Nagao, S., Yano, I., Kawata, S., and Yokogawa, K. (1979). Mitogenic effect of bacterial cell walls, their fragments and related synthetic compounds on thymocytes and splenocytes of guinea-pigs. *Infect. Immun.*, **25**, 645–652.

Takeya, K., Mori, R., Koike, M., and Toda, T. (1958). Paired fibrous structure in mycobacteria. *Biochim. Biophys. Acta*, **30**, 197–198.

Takeya, K., Hisatsune, K., and Nakashima, K. (1961). A cell wall mucopeptide complex obtained from the culture filtrate of tubercle bacilli. *Biochim. Biophys. Acta*, **54**, 595–597.

Toullet, F., Audibert, F., Voisin, G. A., and Chedid, L. (1977). Production d'orchiépididymite aspermatogénique autoimmune chez le cobaye à l'aide de différents adjuvants hydrosolubles. *Ann. Immunol.*, **128**, 267–269.

Turk, J. L. (1969). Cell-mediated immunological processes in leprosy. *Bull. WHO*, **41**, 779–792.

Turk, J. L., and Bryceson, A. D. M. (1971). Immunological phenomena in leprosy and related diseases. *Adv. Immunol.*, **13**, 209–266.

Vacheron, F., Guenounou, M., and Nauciel, C. (1983). Induction of interleukin 1 secretion by adjuvant-active peptidoglycans. *Infect. Immun.*, **42**, 1049–1054.

Waksman, B. H. (1959). A histologic study of the auto-allergic testis lesion in the guinea-pig. *J. Exp. Med.*, **109**, 311–324.

Waksman, B. H., and Adams, R. D. (1955). Allergic neuritis: an experimental disease of rabbits induced by the injection of peripheral nervous tissue and adjuvants. *J. Exp. Med.*, **102**, 213–235.

Waksman, B. H., and Adams, R. D. (1953). Tubercle bacillus lipopolysaccharide as adjuvant in the production of experimental allergic encephalomyelitis in rabbits. *J. Infect. Dis.*, **93**, 21–27.

Waight, P. A., Pollock, T. M., Miller, E., and Coleman, E. M. (1983). Pyrexia after diphtheria/tetanus/pertussis and diphtheria/tetanus vaccines. *Arch. Dis. Child.*, **58**, 921–933.

Wardlaw, A. C., and Parton, R. P. (1983). *Bordetella pertussis* toxins. *Pharmacol. Ther.*, **19**, 1–53.

Watson, J., Epstein, R., Nakoinz, I., and Ralph, P. (1973). The role of humoral factors in the initiation of *in vitro* primary immune responses. *J. Immunol.*, **110**, 43–52.

Weigle, W. O. (1983). Immunologic tolerance and immunopathology. In *The Biology of Immunologic Disease* (Eds. F. J. Dixon, and D. W. Fisher), pp.107–116. Sinauer Associates Inc., Massachusetts.

Welch, A. M., and Swanborg, R. H. (1976). Characterization of suppressor cells involved in regulation of experimental allergic encephalomyelitis. *Eur. J. Immunol.*, **6**, 910–912.

Werner, G. H., Maral, R., Floc'h, F., Migliore-Samour, D., and Jollès, P. (1974). Activités biologiques des adjuvants hydrosolubles de faible poids moléculaire extraits de *Mycobacterium tuberculosis* var. *hominis*. *C. R. Acad. Sci.*, **278**, 789–792.

Werner, G. H., Maral, R., Floc'h, F., Migliore-Samour, D., and Jollès, P. (1975). Adjuvant and immunostimulating activities of water-soluble substances extracted from *Mycobacterium tuberculosis* (var. *hominis*). *Biomedicine*, **22**, 440–452.

White, R. G. (1959). The adjuvant effects of mycobacterial cells and fractions. In *Mechanisms of Hypersensitivity* (Eds. J. H. Shaffer, G. A. Lo Grippo, and M. W. Chase), pp.637–645. Churchill, London.

White, R. G. (1971). Recent attempts at immunotherapy. *Scott. Med. J.*, **16**, 280–289.
White, R. G. (1976). The adjuvant effect of microbial products on the immune response. *Annu. Rev. Microbiol.*, **30**, 579–600.
White, R. G., and Marshall, A. H. E. (1958). The role of various chemical fractions of *M. tuberculosis* and other mycobacteria in the production of allergic encephalomyelitis. *Immunology*, **1**, 111–122.
White, R. G., Coons, A. H., and Connolly, J. M. (1955). Studies on antibody production. IV. The role of a wax fraction of *Mycobacterium tuberculosis* in adjuvant emulsions on the production of antibody to egg albumin. *J. Exp. Med.*, **102**, 83–104.
White, R. G., Bernstock, L., Johns, R. G. S., and Lederer, E. (1958). The influence of components of *M. tuberculosis* and other mycobacteria upon antibody production to ovalbumin. *Immunology*, **1**, 54–66.
White, R. G., Jenkins, G. C., and Wilkinson, P. C. (1963). The production of skin-sensitising antibody in the guinea-pig. *Int. Arch. Allergy*, **22**, 156–165.
White, R. G., Jollès, P., Samour, D., and Lederer, E. (1964). Correlation of adjuvant activity and chemical structure of wax D fractions of mycobacteria. *Immunology*, **7**, 158–171.
Wilhelmj, C. M., Kierland, R. R., and Owen, C. A. (1962). Production of hypersensitivity to skin in animals. *Arch. Dermatol.*, **86**, 161–176.
Witebsky, E., and Rose, N. R. (1956). Studies on organ specificity. IV. Production of rabbit thyroid antibodies in the rabbit. *J. Immunol.*, **76**, 408–416.
Witebsky, E., Rose, N. R., Terplan, K., Paine, J. R., and Egan, R. W. (1957). Chronic thyroiditis and autoimmunization. *J. Am. Med. Assoc.*, **164**, 1439–1447.
Wolf, A., Kabat, E. A., and Bezer, A. E. (1947). Pathology of acute disseminated encephalomyelitis produced experimentally in Rhesus monkey and its resemblance to human demyelinating disease. *J. Neuropathol. Exp. Neurol.*, **6**, 333–357.
Wood, D. D. (1979a). Purification and properties of human B cell activating factor. *J. Immunol.*, **123**, 2395–2399.
Wood, D. D. (1979b). Mechanism of action of human B-cell activating factor. I. Comparison of plaque-stimulating activity with thymocyte-stimulating activity. *J. Immunol.*, **123**, 2400–2407.
Wood, D. D., and Cameron, P. M. (1978). Relationship between bacterial endotoxin and human B cell-activating factor. *J. Immunol.* **121**, 53–60.
Wood, F. D., Pearson, C. M., and Tanaka, A. (1969). Capacity of mycobacterial wax D and its subfractions to induce adjuvant arthritis in rats. *Int. Arch. Allergy*, **35**, 456–467.
World Health Organization (1976). Immunological adjuvants. *Techn. Rep. Ser.*, **595**, pp.3–40. WHO, Geneva.
Yamamoto, Y., and Onoue, K. (1979). Functional activation of immune lymphocytes by antigenic stimulation in cell-mediated immunity. *J. Immunol.*, **122**, 942–948.
Yamamura, Y., Kotani, S., Azuma, I., Koda, A., and Shiba, T. (Eds.) (1982). *Immunomodulation by Microbial Products and Related Synthetic Compounds.* Excerpta Medica, Amsterdam.
Yarkoni, E., Wang, L., and Bekierkunst, A. (1977). Stimulation of macrophages by cord factor and by heat-killed and living BCG. *Infect. Immun.*, **16**, 1–8.
Zbar, B., Bernstein, I., Tanaka, T., and Rapp, H. J. (1970). Tumor immunity produced by the intradermal inoculation of living tumor cells and living *Mycobacterium bovis* (strain BCG). *Science*, **170**, 1217–1218.
Zbar, B., Bernstein, I. D., and Rapp, H. J. (1971). Suppression of tumor growth at the site of infection with living Bacillus Calmette-Guérin. *J. Natl. Cancer Inst.*, **46**, 831–839.

Immunology of the Bacterial Cell Envelope
Edited by D. E. S. Stewart-Tull and M. Davies
© 1985 John Wiley & Sons Ltd.

CHAPTER 4

Immunology of Peptidoglycan–Polysaccharide Polymers from Cell Walls of Group A Streptococci

Ronald E. Esser, John H. Schwab and Robert A. Eisenberg

*Departments of Microbiology and Immunology, and Medicine,
School of Medicine, University of North Carolina at Chapel Hill,
Chapel Hill, NC 27514, USA*

I. INTRODUCTION

Interest in the immune response to the peptidoglycan–polysaccharide complex of group A streptococci (PG–APS) stems from both the clinical significance of this group of organisms and from the use of streptococcal antigens as model systems in the study of the regulation of antibody responses. Clinical interest initially centred on the development of a classification system for the β-haemolytic streptococci based on the antigenic properties of the group-specific polysaccharide (Lancefield, 1941). Most of the streptococci pathogenic for human beings belong to group A, although human disease is caused by members of other groups. Non-pathogenic strains isolated from human beings and strains isolated from other species have antigenically distinct polysaccharides. Clinical interest in the immune response to PG–APS polymers also comes from the possible relationship between the pathogenesis of non-suppurative post-streptococcal sequelae and either hypersensitivity to streptococcal antigens, or autoimmunity induced by the cross-reaction of such antigens with human tissues. Increased levels of antibody, specific for either peptidoglycan (PG) or the group A specific polysaccharide (APS) are present in rheumatic fever, rheumatic carditis, post-streptococcal glomerulonephritis, and in rheumatic and juvenile rheumatoid arthritis (Dudding and Ayoub, 1968; Rolicka and Massell, 1973; Braun and Holm, 1970; Heymer *et al.* 1976. Pope *et al.* 1982). Antibody specific for the APS has been reported to cross-react with thymic epithelium (Lyampert *et al.*, 1976) and with heart glycoproteins (Goldstein *et al.* 1967).

The antibody response to streptococcal carbohydrates has also been studied extensively by investigators interested in the regulation of the antibody response and in the genetics of responsiveness. Some of the important contributions that have come from these studies include the description of the inheritance of antibody V_H regions (Yarmush and Kindt, 1979), the demonstration of the genetic control of both the magnitude and the heterogeneity of the antibody response (Braun and Jaton, 1974), and the demonstration of IgG subclass restriction in the antibody response to carbohydrate antigens (Perlmutter *et al.*, 1978; Der Balian *et al.*, 1980). Analysis of homogenous antibody isolated from rabbits immunized with streptococcal vaccines has also provided important amino acid sequence data for structural studies of immunoglobulins (Braun *et al.*, 1976). The antibody response to PG is of interest because of the numerous biological properties of PG (Heymer, 1975; Heymer and Rietschel, 1977).

As a result of this multidisciplined interest many aspects of the immune response to PG–APS have been studied. In this chapter we will briefly review the literature on the antibody response to the PG and the APS moieties of the streptococcal cell wall and describe some of our recent work on the antibody response of Sprague-Dawley rats to individual immunodeterminant groups of the PG–APS.

II. IMMUNOGENICITY OF PEPTIDOGLYCAN

Abdulla and Schwab (1965), using the quantitative precipitin reaction, showed that immunization of rabbits with either bacterial vaccines or with isolated PG resulted in increasing quantities of serum antibody specific for PG. Other investigators have also shown that PG isolated from streptococci and from other gram-positive bacteria can induce antibody formation (Karakawa and Krause, 1966; Hughes *et al.*, 1971; Helgeland *et al.*, 1973). However, PG is generally considered a poor immunogen, since only low levels of antibody specific for PG develop in most animals immunized with bacterial vaccines (Karakawa *et al.*, 1966b).

Normal serum from human beings and from several species of experimental animals have been shown to contain antibody specific for PG. About 20–40% of serum samples from normal rabbits, rats, mice, and guinea pigs agglutinate PG-coated latex particles (Heymer *et al.*, 1973), and about 80% of normal rabbit sera analysed by the quantitative precipitin reaction contain antibody specific for PG (Abdulla and Schwab, 1965). Schachenmayr *et al.* (1975) examined 961 serum samples from healthy human donors and reported that 32.8% of the samples contained detectable levels of antibody specific for PG. Other studies have demonstrated anti-PG activity in varying percentages of normal human serum samples (Rolicka and Massell, 1973; Braun and Holm, 1970; Heymer *et al.*, 1973; Verbrugh *et al.*, 1981; Pope *et al.*, 1982; Wheat *et al.* 1983). The variations in the percentage of positive samples is related to the sensitivity of the assay system employed, and it is likely that all normal adult human and animal sera contain some antibody specific for PG.

With a radioactive antigen binding assay in which the synthetic peptide L-Ala–D-Glu–L-Lys–D-Ala–D-Ala was used to measure antibody, Heymer *et al.* (1975, 1976, 1979) demonstrated that the majority of the human serum samples tested contained antibody specific for the pentapeptide of PG. Healthy adults were reported to have higher levels of antibody specific for the pentapeptide than were healthy children, and these investigators suggested that this was due to the continued antigenic stimuli from bacteria normally present in the respiratory and gastrointestinal tract, and to the repeated infections which occur throughout life.

Unpublished results from our laboratory indicate that a large proportion of normal rat sera also contain detectable antibody specific for PG, and occasional samples from apparently healthy animals have quite high levels. The nature of the stimulus that results in the formation of the high levels of antibody seen in some animals is not known. It is also not known if these high levels persist or if they are present only transiently. Bolton *et al.* (1977) have reported cyclic fluctuations in the levels of antibody specific for the polyglycerophosphate antigen of *Bacillus* in normal unimmunized Sprague-Dawley rats. The levels of antibody specific for PG could be subject to similar fluctuations.

The level of serum antibody specific for PG has been shown to increase following infection. Patients with uncomplicated streptococcal infections and with non-suppurative post-streptococcal sequelae have detectable levels of antibody specific for PG more frequently than do healthy control subjects (Braun and Holm, 1970; Rolicka and Massell, 1973). Wheat *et al.* (1983) have reported that sera from some patients with endocarditis or complicated bacteraemia caused by either staphylococci or streptococci, as well as the sera of patients with infections caused by gram-negative bacteria, contain IgM and IgG antibody specific for PG. Verbrugh *et al.* (1981) have also reported that patients with deep-tissue staphylococcal infections have increased levels of IgG antibody specific for PG. However, in contrast to the results of Wheat *et al.* (1983), patients with infections caused by other gram-positive or by gram-negative bacteria did not have increased quantities of antibody specific for PG. In addition, IgM antibody specific for PG was present only rarely.

Other investigators have quantitated antibody specific for the pentapeptide determinant of PG in the sera of patients with gram-positive infections. During the acute and convalescent phases of staphylococcal pyoderma, the mean level of serum antibody specific for the pentapeptide determinant is significantly greater than the level present in normal serum (Heymer *et al.*, 1979). Patients with staphylococcal endocarditis and bacteraemia also have increased levels of antibody specific for the pentapeptide determinant of PG (Zeiger *et al.*, 1981). However, no increase is associated with uncomplicated streptococcal pharyngitis (Heymer *et al.*, 1979).

It is surprising that so few of the details of the antibody response to PG following infection have been defined. The results of some studies (Verbrugh *et al.*, 1981; Heymer *et al.* 1979) suggest that formation of increased levels of antibody specific for PG may depend on the species of the infecting organism. Gram-positive bacteria may stimulate the formation of more antibody specific for PG than gram-negative organisms, and staphylococci may stimulate more anti-PG antibody formation than streptococci. It is also possible that the site of infection may be an important variable in the antibody response to PG. Serious deep-tissue infections with *Staphylococcus aureus* stimulate more antibody than superficial infections with the same organism (Verbrugh *et al.*, 1981), and gram-positive infections of the skin stimulate greater quantities of anti-PG antibody than do infections of the throat (Heymer *et al.*, 1979). Antibiotic treatment protocols may also influence the antibody response to PG during infection (Zeiger *et al.*, 1981).

It is not known if anti-PG antibody influences the course of infection. However, if antibody specific for PG is protective, the structural similarities in the PGs of different species and the resulting cross-reactivity (Hughes *et al.*, 1971; Karakawa *et al.*, 1966b; Nguyen-Huy *et al.*, 1976; Schleifer and Krause, 1971a) suggest that antibody formed in response to exposure either to the normal flora or to pathogenic bacteria could contribute to protection (Krause, 1975).

III. IMMUNOCHEMISTRY OF THE ANTIBODY RESPONSE TO PEPTIDOGLYCAN

Streptococcal PG is a complex heteropolymer consisting of a glycan backbone of alternating $\beta(1\rightarrow4)$-linked residues of *N*-acetylglucosamine (NAG) and *N*-acetylmuramic acid (NAMA) (Schleifer and Seidl, 1977; Rogers *et al.*, 1980). The lactyl group of NAMA is substituted with a short peptide of alternating

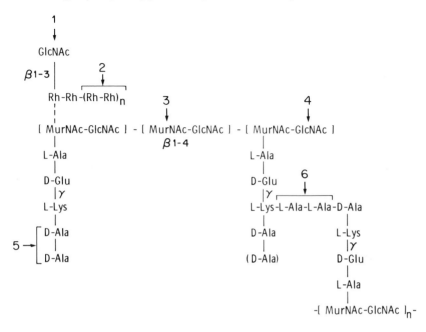

Figure 1. Structure of the peptidoglycan–polysaccharide complex of group A streptococci. The numbers refer to different immunodeterminant groups. See Table 1. (From Eisenberg *et al.*, 1982, reproduced by permission of the American Society for Microbiology)

L- and D-amino acids with the sequence NH_2–L-Ala–D-Glu–L-Lys–D-Ala–D Ala-COOH (Figure 1). Adjacent peptides are often linked by an interpeptide bridge formed between the penultimate D-Ala residue of one peptide and the free amino group of L-Lys of an adjacent peptide. In group A streptococci, the dipeptide L-Ala–L-Ala forms the cross-bridge. Cross-linking of adjacent peptides results in the loss of the terminal D-Ala residue of the pentapeptide. The structure of the glycan backbone and the pentapeptide of staphylococcal PG is identical to that of streptococcal PG. However, cross-linking of staphylococcal PG involves a pentaglycine interpeptide bridge rather than an L-Ala bridge.

Based on the quantitative precipitin reaction between PG and rabbit anti-PG serum, and qualitative tests for antibody and antigen in the supernatant fluids of the precipitin reaction, Abdulla and Schwab (1965) proposed that multiple distinct antigenic groups were present on PG polymers. Subsequently, the results of differential absorption studies of anti-PG serum with PG from several species of bacteria suggested the presence of at least three different antigenic groups on cell wall PG (Schwab and Abdulla, 1968). Other studies by Karakawa *et al.* (Karakawa and Krause, 1966; Karakawa *et al.*, 1967, 1968) indicated that rabbits immunized with group A-variant vaccine formed antibody that reacted with both the glycan backbone and the peptide moieties of PG.

Subsequent work by many researchers has established the existence of at least four different components of the PG that induce antibody formation: (1) the NAG of the glycan backbone (NAG-PG); (2) the NAMA of the glycan backbone (NAMA); (3) the terminal D-Ala–D-Ala residues of the pentapeptide [(D Ala)$_2$]; and (4) the L-Ala–L-Ala cross-bridge [(L-Ala)$_2$]. The remainder of this section will describe the studies that have led to the identification of each of the different immunodeterminant groups. Nearly all of these studies have exploited the large anti-PG response of rabbits immunized with group A-variant vaccine (Karakawa *et al.*, 1966b).

Antibody specific for the glycan backbone of PG was first described by Karakawa *et al.* (Karakawa and Krause, 1966; Karakawa *et al.*, 1967, 1968). Subsequent studies indicated that NAG is the immunodominant sugar of the backbone (Schleifer and Krause, 1971a; Rolicka and Park, 1969; Schleifer and Seidl, 1977). The quantitative precipitin reaction between anti-A-variant antisera and PG from several species of bacteria is inhibited by NAG and chitin, a $\beta(1\rightarrow4)$-linked polymer of NAG, but not by muramic acid, NAMA, *N*-acetylgalactosamine, *N*-acetylmannosamine or several other sugars tested.

These studies clearly indicate that immunization with A-variant vaccine induces antibody specific for the NAG residue of the glycan backbone. Other studies of the antibody response to the PG of *Micrococcus luteus* (formerly *M. lysodeikticus*) have suggested that NAMA is the immunodominant sugar of the glycan backbone (Schleifer and Seidl, 1977; Wikler, 1975). Rabbits immunized with *M. luteus* formed antibody specific for *Micrococcus* PG which was inhibited by NAMA but not by NAG. However, the reaction between PG of non-*Micrococcus* species and either anti-A-variant serum or anti-*Micrococcus* serum was not inhibited by NAMA. Taken together these results suggest that NAMA of *Micrococcus* PG is immunogenic, while NAMA in the PG of other species of bacteria may not be recognized. Presumably this difference is due to the low proportion of NAMA residues that are substituted with peptides in the PG of *M. luteus*. Inhibition of the quantitative precipitin reaction between anti-*Micrococcus* serum and homologous PG by NAMA, but not by the amide of NAMA, where the carboxyl group is blocked, indicates the importance of the unsubstituted carboxyl group of NAMA in antibody binding (Schleifer and Seidl, 1977).

Karakawa *et al.* (Karakawa and Krause, 1966; Karakawa *et al.*, 1968) reported that peptide-rich fractions of enzyme digests of staphylococcal PG inhibit the precipitin reaction between rabbit anti-A-variant serum and staphylococcal PG. Since the pentapeptide side-chain is the only peptide common to the PG of both streptococci and staphylococci, these results suggest that the pentapeptide is immunogenic. In subsequent studies, the effect of a series of synthetic polyamino acids and peptides on the quantitative precipitin reaction between anti-A-variant serum and staphylococcal PG was determined (Karakawa *et al.*, 1970). Synthetic polyamino acids which contained D-Ala and DL-Ala, as well as the dipeptide (DL-Ala)$_2$, inhibited the precipitin reaction. Synthetic polyamino acids which contained L-Ala and the peptide (L-Ala)$_2$ did not affect precipitation.

In a more definitive study, Schleifer and Krause (1971b) analysed a series of synthetic inhibitors which differed in the sequence and configuration of their constituent amino acids for their effect on the quantitative precipitin reaction between anti-A-variant serum and staphylococcal PG. A peptide identical in sequence and configuration to the pentapeptide of streptococcal PG, and to a lesser extent other peptides with carboxy terminal D-Ala–D-Ala residues, were effective inhibitors. Changes in either the sequence or configuration of the carboxy terminal D-Ala–D-Ala residues, were effective inhibitors. Changes in either the sequence or configuration of the carboxy terminal D-Ala–D-Ala residues greatly reduced the ability of peptides to inhibit the precipitin reaction. However, changes at positions removed from the carboxy terminal end had less of an effect on inhibition, and the effect decreased as the distance from the carboxy terminal end increased. These results indicate that the carboxy terminal D-Ala–D-Ala residues represent the immunodominant structure of the pentapeptide, and that L-Ala, D-Glu, and L-Lys contribute little to antibody binding.

Other studies by Schleifer and Seidl (1974, 1977) and Seidl and Schleifer (1975) also indicated that the terminal D-Ala–D-Ala of the pentapeptide induces antibody formation. Serum from rabbits immunized with group A-variant vaccine reacted with proteins to which synthetic peptides terminating in D-Ala–D-Ala had been coupled, Conversely, serum from rabbits immunized with these protein–peptide conjugates was shown to react with isolated PG from staphylococci and streptococci but not with PG from *Bacillus*. In similar studies, Zeiger and Maurer (1973) covalently coupled the synthetic peptide Ala–D-Glu-Lys–D-Ala–D-Ala to the random polypeptide (Glu^{60}Ala^{40})$_n$. Rabbits immunized with this synthetic antigen formed antibody which reacted with PG from group C streptococci. In addition, serum from rabbits immunized with pneumococci reacted with the synthetic polypeptide. Subsequent studies by Zeiger *et al.* (1978) have shown that antibodies from rabbits immunized with this synthetic immunogen also react with soluble PG precursors formed by *M. luteus*.

Helgeland *et al.* (1973) have also shown that the pentapeptide of PG is immunogenic. Rabbit anti-PG serum was fractionated on a Sepharose column to which the synthetic peptide L-Ala–D-Glu–L-Lys–D-Ala–D-Ala had been coupled. Antibody eluted from the column agglutinated staphylococcal PG and erythrocytes coated with staphylococcal extracts.

The L-Ala–L-Ala interpeptide bridge of streptococcal PG as well as the interpeptide bridge of other bacterial PGs also induce antibody formation (Schleifer and Seidl, 1977; Seidl and Schleifer, 1977, 1978). Sera from rabbits injected with A-variant vaccine react with homologous PG and with proteins to which L-Ala terminating peptides have been coupled via either the carboxy or amino terminal ends (Seidl and Schleifer, 1977, 1978). However, the studies of Karakawa *et al.* (1970) indicate that the quantity of antibody present in immune serum specific for the L-Ala–L-Ala cross-bridge may be relatively small compared with the quantity of antibody specific for other immunodeterminants of the PG. In these studies, the quantitative precipitin reaction between anti-A-variant serum and streptococcal PG or staphylococcal PG was compared and shown to be nearly identical, in spite of different cross-linking peptides in the two PGs.

The characterization of the antibody response to individual immuno-determinant groups of the PG as described above has been accomplished largely with the quantitative precipitin reaction and its inhibition by a variety of natural and synthetic compounds. While this approach has provided a great deal of information, it is limited in several ways. First, this assay system measures only antibody with affinity high enough to precipitate antigen. Antibody of high affinity may make up only a small portion of the total antibody response to streptococcal antigens (Stankus and Leslie, 1974; Schalch *et al.*, 1979). Secondly, the reaction can be influenced by rheumatoid factors which are known to be induced by immunization with streptococcal vaccines (Bokisch *et al.*, 1972). Thirdly, it is difficult to relate the inhibition of the precipitin reaction to the quantities of antibody present. Fourthly, the quantitative precipitin reaction lacks the sensitivity of methods currently available.

As mentioned earlier, the identification of different immunodeterminant groups of PG–APS has been accomplished in large part by analysis of the antibody response of rabbits immunized with group A-variant vaccine. It is not known if significant amounts of antibody specific for each of these determinants are also induced by immunization with other forms of PG. It is also not known if other animal species produce antibody specific for each of the immunodeterminant groups identified in the rabbit, although the terminal D-Ala–D-Ala of the pentapeptide has been demonstrated to induce antibody in human beings (Heymer *et al.*, 1975, 1979; Zeiger *et al.*, 1981).

The relative immunogenicity of the individual immunodeterminant groups is also not clear from these studies. Karakawa *et al.* (1967) reported that individual immune sera appeared to vary with respect to the quantity of antibody specific for the glycan backbone and the peptide moieties of PG. With some serum samples from A-variant vaccine-immunized rabbits, the quantitative precipitin reaction with PG was strongly inhibited by peptide-rich fractions of PG digest and only minimally inhibited by hexosamine-rich fractions. The opposite pattern was observed in other serum samples.

Several features of the antibody response to PG should be emphasized. As described earlier, antibody specific for the pentapeptide determinant of PG recognizes primarily the D-Ala–D-Ala residues. The contribution of the internal amino acids of the pentapeptide is negligible, and antibody binding to peptides terminating in a single D-Ala residue is also much less than binding to peptides terminating in D-Ala–D-Ala. However, the D-Ala–D-Ala-terminating pentapeptide is not the predominant form of the peptide in the cell wall. Cross-linking of peptide side-chains results in the loss of the terminal D-Ala residue and in addition the action of carboxypeptidases may remove one or both D-Ala residues (Rogers *et al.*, 1980). Although the frequency of cross-linking varies with different species, and carboxypeptidase activity may also vary, the ratio of D-Ala to D-Glu or glucosamine in bacterial cell walls is usually less than 1.0. Therefore, it is somewhat surprising that the predominant antibody directed toward the pentapeptide is specific for the D-Ala–D-Ala sequence. Antibody specific for the peptide of several species of gram-negative bacteria also react primarily with uncross-linked peptides (Nguyen-Nuy *et al.*, 1976). It has been suggested that preferential stimulation of antibody formation by uncross-linked peptides is due to stereochemical factors and that cross-linked peptides are less accessible (Nguyen-Huy *et al.*, 1976). Unfortunately, the stereochemical orientation of the peptides in relation to the glycan backbone and the orientation of the disaccharide units of the backbone to one another is not known.

Zeiger *et al.* (1981) have recently reported that patients with staphylococcal bacteraemia or endocarditis treated with β-lactam antibiotics have higher levels of antibody specific for the D-Ala–D-Ala immunodeterminant of PG than do patients treated with other antibiotics. These investigators have proposed that soluble PG precursors, which retain the D-Ala–D-Ala sequence, are released from bacterial cells in patients treated with β-lactam antibiotics, and that these precursors stimulate the formation of D-Ala–D-Ala specific antibody. Bacterial cells treated *in vitro* with β-lactam antibiotics have indeed been shown by several groups to release soluble PG (Zeiger *et al.*, 1978; Mirelman *et al.*, 1974; Tynecka and Ward, 1975). In addition, the release of PG fragments also occurs during normal growth of gram-negative bacteria such as *Neisseria gonorrhoeae* (Rosenthal, 1979). Extrapolating from this, it may be that most naturally occurring antibody specific for the D-Ala–D-Ala determinant is induced by PG precursors released during cell wall synthesis.

IV. IMMUNOGENICITY OF THE GROUP A STREPTOCOCCAL POLYSACCHARIDE

The group-specific polysaccharide of group A streptococci, like the cell wall polysaccharides of many bacteria, is immunogenic, and this property is the basis of the Lancefield grouping system for β-haemolytic streptococci (Lancefield, 1941). Analysis of serum from normal human donors shows that the majority of samples have detectable levels of antibody specific for the APS, and that the level of antibody increases following uncomplicated streptococcal pharyngitis

(Schmidt and Moore, 1965; Slade and Hammerling, 1968; Zimmerman *et al.*, 1971; Kaplan *et al.*, 1974; Rabinowitz *et al.*, 1977; Bergner-Rabinowitz *et al.*, 1979; Aasted *et al.*, 1979; Heymer *et al.*, 1979). The level of antibody specific for the APS has also been reported to be elevated in serum samples from patients with non-suppurative post-streptococcal sequelae (Dudding and Ayoub, 1968; Braun and Holm, 1970), and the quantity of serum antibody present in these conditions may exceed that found following uncomplicated streptococcal disease (Schmidt and Moore, 1965; Bergner-Rabinowitz *et al.*, 1979).

V. IMMUNOCHEMISTRY AND IMMUNOBIOLOGY OF THE ANTIBODY RESPONSE TO THE GROUP A STREPTOCOCCAL POLYSACCHARIDE

The discussion in this section will focus primarily on the antibody response to the APS. However, antibody responses specific for the A-variant polysaccharide and for the polysaccharide of group C streptococci will also be discussed where relevant. Each of the three carbohydrates consists of a polyrhamnose backbone of alternating $\alpha(1\rightarrow2)$- and $\alpha(1\rightarrow3)$-linked rhamnose residues (Coligan *et al.*, 1975, 1978). In the APS, NAG is linked $\beta(1\rightarrow3)$ to the rhamnose backbone. In the group C carbohydrate, a disaccharide of N-acetylgalactosamine is linked to the 3-position of the rhamnose backbone. The A-variant polysaccharide also contains both NAG and rhamnose, but the quantity of NAG present is less than the quantity present in the APS. The ratio of rhamnose to NAG in the APS and rhamnose to N-acetylgalactosamine in the group C carbohydrate indicates that the majority of the rhamnose residues with an available 3-position are substituted. In contrast, the majority of rhamnose residues in the A-variant carbohydrate are unsubstituted (Coligan *et al.*, 1978). The group specific carbohydrates are covalently bound to C-6 of NAMA of the glycan backbone of PG by a phosphodiester bond (Rogers *et al.*, 1980).

McCarty and Lancefield (1955) first demonstrated that both the polyrhamnose backbone and the terminal NAG residues of the APS were immunogenic, although antibody specific for the NAG residue is formed in much greater quantities following immunization with group A vaccine. In these studies, the loss of group-specific reactivity by several variant strains of group A streptococci was shown to be associated with a decrease in the quantity of NAG present in the APS. In addition, quantitative precipitin reactions between anti-group A and anti-A-variant sera and the isolated carbohydrates of group A and group A-variant strains of streptococci suggested that two populations of antibody were reacting with two distinct structures. Subsequently, McCarty (1956) reported that enzymatic removal of NAG from the APS resulted in the loss of group-specific reactivity with anti-group A serum, but increased the reactivity of the APS with anti-A-variant serum. This suggests that NAG is responsible for group-specific serological activity and that NAG partially masks the presence of a second specificity. The rhamnose backbone of the APS was identified as the second specificity, since enzymatic hydrolysis of rhamnose bonds eliminated reactivity, and rhamnose oligosaccharides were shown to be potent inhibitors of the quantitative precipitin reaction between anti-A-variant serum and the A-variant carbohydrate.

The identity of the group-A specific marker was confirmed by studies in which NAG was covalently bound to protein carriers (McCarty, 1958). The NAG substituted proteins reacted with anti-group A serum, inhibited the quantitative precipitin reaction between anti-group A serum and the APS, and absorbed 15–30% of the anti-group A activity from immune serum. Differential absorption studies by Karakawa *et al.*, (1965, 1966a) indicated that both human post-streptococcal serum and serum from rabbits injected with group A vaccine contained antibodies specific for the NAG and polyrhamnose immunodeterminants of the APS. Removal of antibody specific for either determinant could be achieved without loss of reactivity for the remaining immunodeterminant.

The immunobiology of the antibody response to the APS has been extensively studied. The impetus for this study has come, in part, from the observation that some rabbits hyperimmunized with streptococcal vaccines produce specific antibody of restricted heterogeneity in quantities sufficient for structural studies. The magnitude of the antibody response to APS has been shown to be under genetic control. Randomly bred rabbits injected with streptococcal vaccine produced highly variable amounts of antibody specific for the APS. However, the progeny of selected high responder or selected low responder parents also tend to be high or low responders, respectively (Braun *et al.*, 1969, 1973; Eichmann *et al.*, 1971). Complete segregation of high and low antibody responses occurred after only two generations of selective breeding, which suggests that the response is regulated by a small number of genes (Eichmann *et al.*, 1971). In mice immunized with group A streptococcal vaccine, Braun and coworkers (Braun *et al.*, 1972; Cramer and Braun, 1974, 1975a) demonstrated that the magnitude of the APS-specific antibody response is controlled by a single autosomal gene which is not linked to either the H-2 or the IgG_H genes. However, studies of additional high and low responder mouse strains have indicated multigene control (Briles *et al.*, 1977). Genes linked to the H-2 and IgG_H gene clusters were shown to exert a moderate effect, while a third locus, which is linked to neither H-2 or IgG_H, exerts a major influence on the magnitude of the response. In rats, Leslie and Carwile (1973) have reported that immunization of the outbred Sprague-Dawley strain with group A vaccine results in hypergammaglobulinaemia in 30–40% of individuals. The quantity of precipitating antibody produced and the kinetics of antibody production were extremely variable. Selective breeding of high and low responders indicated genetic control of responsiveness by a small number of genes (Stankus and Leslie, 1975).

The clonal heterogeneity of the antibody response to group-specific polysaccharides of streptococci is also under genetic control. This topic has recently been reviewed by Braun *et al.* (1980) and will be only briefly discussed here. Genetic control of the heterogeneity of the antibody response to streptococcal carbohydrates was first described in rabbits (Braun and Krause, 1968; Osterland *et al.*, 1966). Immunization of rabbits with group A, group A-variant, and group C streptococcal vaccines has been shown to induce up to 55 mg ml^{-1} of antibody (Braun and Krause, 1968; Braun *et al.*, 1969; Eichmann *et al.*, 1971; Osterland *et al.*, 1966). The bulk of the immunoglobulin produced by some high responders was either homogeneous or of very restricted heterogeneity as indicated by zone electrophoresis and electrophoretic analysis of isolated light chains of affinity-purified antibody (Braun and Krause, 1968; Osterland *et al.*, 1966; Miller *et al.*, 1967; Fleishman *et al.*, 1968). Selective breeding of rabbits with monoclonal or restricted responses greatly increased the proportion of animals with restricted responses. Studies with inbred mice have given similar results (Braun *et al.*, 1972. Cramer and Braun, 1974). The antibody response in some strains was characteristically restricted to a few clones, while other strains gave a heterogeneous response. Cross-breeding of strains that gave heterogeneous responses with strains that gave restricted responses indicated that the restricted response was dominant. In rats, the antibody response to the APS has also been shown to be of restricted heterogeneity (Stankus and Leslie, 1974; Leslie and Carwile, 1973), and selective breeding appears to increase the homogeneity of the responses.

More recently high-resolution analysis by isoelectric focusing techniques has demonstrated that the serum of rabbits previously classified as heterogeneous or homogeneous on the basis of microzone electrophoresis contains a similar number of antibody clonotypes. However, one or a few clonotypes usually dominate the response and account for 60–90% of the total antibody specific for the carbohydrate (Schalch *et al.*, 1979). These results indicate that regulatory mechanisms control clonal expansion during the response, and the existence of a restrictor locus has been proposed (Willcox and Marsh, 1978). Such control is particularly striking in SWR/J mice (Briles and Davie, 1980). Although the SWR/J strain is genetically capable of producing approximately 200 different clonotypes of anti-APS antibody, individual mice normally express only one or a few clones selected at random from the total repertoire.

A potential mechanism for clonal control of the anti-APS response is idiotype–anti-idiotype interaction (Bona and Hiernaux, 1981). Two common idiotypes of anti-APS antibodies have been identified in mice. The A5A idiotype is found in more than 90% of A/J mice making anti-APS (Eichmann, 1973), while in an individual mouse approximately 25% of the anti-APS antibody is A5A idiotype positive (Eichmann and Rajewsky, 1975). The full expression of the A5A idiotype is limited to mouse strains of the Ig-1^e immunoglobulin heavy chain allotype, and breeding experiments have established that the idiotype is indeed linked to this locus. Analysis of recombinant strains further suggests that the idiotype must be coded for by an immunoglobulin heavy chain germ line variable region gene (Eichmann, 1975a). The potential for idiotype-directed control of this system has been clearly demonstrated using heterologous anti-A5A idiotype antisera. Depending on the isotype of the anti-idiotype antibody injected, the A5A idiotype can be completely suppressed by T suppressor cells, or conversely, the anti-APS response can become nearly 100% A5A idiotype positive through induction of an idiotype-positive T helper cell mechanism (Eichmann and Rajewsky, 1975; Eichmann, 1975b; Black *et al.*, 1976). S117 is a similarly shared immunoglobulin heavy chain allotype-linked idiotype in BALB/c mice, although it has been less well studied. In rats, anti-APS antibodies express the Id-1 idiotype. Id-1 does not appear to be allotype restricted (Stankus and Leslie, 1976). Nevertheless, as in the mouse system, idiotypic expression can be profoundly influenced by heterologous anti-idiotypic antibodies (Olson *et al.*, 1982).

The relative quantities of IgG and IgM produced in response to immunization with streptococcal vaccines appear to vary considerably in different strains and species of experimental animals. Immunization of rabbits with streptococcal vaccines has been reported to induce an IgM response initially, but the level of IgM antibody specific for the APS rapidly declines and by six weeks after beginning immunization essentially all of the precipitating antibody is IgG (Bergner-Rabinowitz *et al.*, 1979). Similarly, Cramer and Braun (1975b) have reported that BALB/c mice initially produce IgM antibody in response to intravenous injections of streptococcal vaccine. IgG antibody was detectable by 1–2 weeks and dominated the response by four weeks after the start of immunization. Only trace amounts of IgM were present by six weeks after the start of immunization. However, Briles and Davie (1975) showed that four of the five strains of mice surveyed produced large amounts of both IgM and IgG even after multiple injections of group A vaccine. In one strain, greater than 1% of the total nucleated cells in the spleen secreted IgM antibody specific for the APS following immunization. Such conflicting reports of relative quantities of IgM and IgG may be the result of differences in immunization protocols. Briles and Davie (1975) gave four intraperitoneal injections of increasing doses of group A vaccine. In contrast, Cramer and Braun (1975b) gave three intravenous injections of group A vaccine each week for several weeks. Stankus and Leslie (1974) have reported that the IgG:IgM ratio of antibody specific for the APS in hyperimmunized rats ranges from 0.4 to 6.6. Rats classified as low responders produced smaller quantities of IgG relative to IgM. Larger quantities of IgM were associated with the production of non-precipitating antibody.

Several studies in mice and rats have indicated that production of IgG antibody specific for the APS following immunization with group A vaccine is subclass restricted. Mice produce primarily IgG$_3$ antibody (Perlmutter *et al.*, 1978; Der Balian *et al.*, 1980; Slack *et al.*, 1980) following immunization with group A vaccine, and rats produce primarily IgG$_{2c}$ (Der Balian *et al.*, 1980; Leslie, 1979). Since these subclasses of IgG are typically associated with the response to carbohydrate antigens and do not generally represent a significant component of the antibody response to protein antigens, it has been suggested that the APS is a T-independent (type-2) antigen (Der Balian *et al.*, 1980; Slack *et al.*, 1980). The results of Greenblatt *et al.* (1980) also suggest that both the APS and the PG are thymus-independent antigens in the rat. In these studies, no significant difference was noted in the magnitude of the antibody response of neonatally thymectomized rats and non-thymectomized control rats to the APS or PG antigens following immunization with purified cell wall fragments of group A streptococci. However, studies in mice have indicated that the response to the APS requires T-cells. Nude mice (*nu/nu*) and thymectomized, irradiated bone marrow reconstituted mice immunized with group A vaccine produced very low levels of serum IgM and IgG$_3$ antibody relative to *nu/+* littermates and non-thymectomized controls (Briles *et al.*, 1982). Measurement of isotype-specific plaque forming cells in the spleens of *nu/nu* athymic mice and their littermates also indicated a requirement for T-cells in the response to the APS. The number of plaque forming cells per spleen in *nu/nu* mice was less than 1% of the total present in the spleens of *nu/+* littermates (Slack and Davie, 1982). These more recent observations are consistent with the results of Braun *et al.* (1972), who reported that the response to the APS was T-dependent in mice.

VI. ANTIBODY RESPONSE TO INDIVIDUAL IMMUNODETERMINANT GROUPS OF THE PEPTIDOGLYCAN–POLYSACCHARIDE COMPLEX

As described in the preceding sections, PG–APS is a complex heteropolymer with six defined immunodeterminants. Although the immunogenicity of these determinants in rabbits is established, the relative immunogenicity of the different groups, the isotypes of antibody formed, and the structures which induce antibody formation in other species are not known. Nor is it known if control of the response occurs at the level of the individual determinant or if responses are regulated at the level of the polymer.

In order to address these questions we have developed a solid-phase enzyme-linked immunosorbent assay (ELISA) which allows the measurement of isotype-specific antibody responses to the individual immunodeterminant groups of the PG–APS. In this assay, haptens resembling individual immunodeterminant groups of the PG–APS are covalently coupled to Epoxy-activated Sepharose 6B. The individual immunodeterminant groups and the haptens selected for use in the assay are shown in Table 1. Each of the haptens, with the exception of the group A-variant carbohydrate, is obtained from non-microbial sources to reduce the possibility of cross-contamination. To assay for antibody, immune serum samples are diluted in buffer and incubated with the hapten–Sepharose conjugates in 96-well, U-bottomed microtitre plates. Following incubation at room temperature for 5 h, the beads are washed with buffer to remove unbound serum components and then incubated with affinity-purified alkaline phosphatase conjugated rabbit anti-rat immunoglobulin reagents specific for

Table 1. The Immunodeterminant Groups of PG–APS and the Haptens Used to Assay for Antibody Specific for Each Group

Cell wall structure	Immunodeterminant group	Hapten used to measure antibody	Designation in text	Corresponding number in Fig. 1
Group A polysaccharide	$\beta(1{\to}3)$-linked N-acetyl-D-glucosamine	p-Aminophenyl-N-acetyl-β-D-glucosamine*[†]	NAG-APS	1
Group A polysaccharide	Rhamnose disaccharide	A-Variant polysaccharide[‡]	$(\text{Rham})_n$	2
Glycan backbone of peptidoglycan	N-acetylmuramic acid	N-Acetylmuramic acid[§]	NAMA	3
Glycan backbone of peptidoglycan	$\beta(1{\to}4)$-linked N-acetyl-D-glucosamine	Acid-hydrolysed chitin[¶]	NAG-PG	4
Peptide side-chain of peptidoglycan	D-Ala–D-Ala	$(\text{D-Alanine})_3$[‖]	$(\text{D-Ala})_2$	5
Cross-bridge	L-Ala–L-Ala	$(\text{L-Alanine})_3$[‖]	$(\text{L-Ala})_2$	6

*McCarty, 1958.
[†]Obtained from Vega Biochemicals, Tucson, Arizona.
[‡]Prepared by the method of Krause and McCarty, 1961.
[§]Obtained from Sigma Chemical Co., St. Louis, MO.
[¶]Prepared by the method of Rupley, 1964.
[‖]Schleifer and Seidl, 1977.

the heavy chain of either rat IgG or IgM, or for the Fab fragment of rat immunoglobulins. After overnight incubation with anti-immunoglobulin reagents, the hapten–Sepharose conjugates are again washed with buffer and then incubated with *p*-nitrophenyl phosphate substrate. After 2 h incubation the reaction is stopped by adding sodium hydroxide. The hapten–Sepharose conjugates are centrifuged at 200 *g* for 30 s, and the absorbance of the supernatant fluids is measured at 405 nm. Background is determined by assaying normal rat serum previously absorbed with insoluble PG and PG–APS. A distinctive feature of our method allows the estimation of the weight of antibody bound. Graded standards of purified rat IgG and rat IgM bound to Sepharose beads are incubated with the alkaline phosphatase conjugated anti-immunoglobulin reagents, and the absorbance generated by the standards is used to construct reference curves.

Using this assay system we have examined the IgM and IgG antibody responses to each of the six immunodeterminant groups of the PG–APS in outbred Sprague-Dawley rats immunized with either suspensions of heat-killed, pepsin-treated group A streptococci (group A vaccine) or with fragments of purified PG–APS. Group A vaccine was injected intravenously three times a week for three weeks. Each injection contained approximately 30 μg of rhamnose. Rats immunized with purified PG–APS fragments were given four intraperitoneal injections of 500 μg of rhamnose at approximately 30-day intervals. Blood samples were collected five days after the last injection.

A. Antibody Responses in Rats Immunized with Group A Vaccine

Analysis of a large number of serum samples has indicated that a striking variability occurs in the pattern of antibody responses of individual rats to the six different immunodeterminant groups. To illustrate this variability data from six selected rats immunized with group A vaccine are presented in Table 2. The IgM responses to the individual immunodeterminants of the PG and the APS moieties vary independently. This variation is especially evident in the responses to the NAG-APS and (Rham)$_n$ determinants of the APS. Serum from some rats (R3 and R7) contained relatively high levels of antibody specific for the NAG-APS determinant but no detectable antibody specific for the (Rham)$_n$ determinant. Other samples contained detectable quantities of IgM antibody specific for both the NAG-APS and the (Rham)$_n$ determinants. A comparison by regression analysis of the levels of IgM, IgG, and total serum antibody specific for the NAG-APS and (Rham)$_n$ determinants from groups of rats immunized with group A vaccine indicated that no significant linear relationship existed between the levels of antibody specific for the two determinants. The responses to the different immunodeterminants of the PG also varied independently, and the immunodeterminant which included the greatest quantity of antibody differed from rat to rat. In the sera of some rats (R5 and R7), detectable levels of

Table 2 Variability in the Levels of IgM Antibody Specific for Individual Immunodeterminant Groups in Selected Rats Immunized with Group A Streptococcal Vaccine

Serum number	Immunodeterminant group					
	NAG-APS	(Rham)$_n$	NAG-PG	(D-Ala)$_2$	(L-Ala)$_2$	NAMA
R2	160	23	22	185	ND	ND
R3	560	ND	410	8	4	ND
R5	620	13	50	70	11	8
R7	1010	ND	270	13	4	8
R10	1010	70	202	19	ND	4
R11	2010	13	620	5	ND	ND

Results are expressed as μg IgM antibody per ml of serum.
ND = not detectable.

antibody specific for each of the four PG immunodeterminant groups was present, while other sera contained detectable levels of antibody specific for only some of the determinants. Occasionally, even high levels of antibody specific for one or more determinants of the PG were found in sera that had no detectable antibody specific for other epitopes. These results suggest that the response to the different immunodeterminant groups is controlled at the level of the individual determinant and not at the level of the whole PG or APS polymer. Responsiveness or non-responsiveness to any one determinant is independent of responsiveness to any other determinant. Similar variations in the quantity of total serum antibody (measured using anti-Fab reagents) specific for the different determinants indicates that the differences in IgM responsiveness are not simply due to differences in the ratio of IgM to IgG in individual rats (i.e. differences in IgM to IgG switching).

The mean levels of IgM and IgG antibody specific for each of the six different immunodeterminants in a group of 11 Sprague-Dawley rats immunized with group A vaccine are shown in Figure 2. The most striking feature of the response is the predominance of IgM antibody specific for the NAG-APS and NAG-PG determinants. These antibodies were present in varying quantities in all the serum samples examined. It is possible that a portion of the antibody that reacts with the NAG-APS determinant cross-reacts with the NAG-PG determinant, since regression analysis of antibody levels in the sera of individual rats indicated a significant correlation between the levels of antibody specific for the two epitopes ($r = 0.84$, $P = 0.0006$). However, non-cross-reacting antibody is probably also present, since in several cases the levels of antibody specific for the two determinants did not correspond.

In contrast to the relatively high levels of IgM antibody specific for the NAG-APS and NAG-PG determinants, the other immunodeterminants of the PG–APS induced the formation of only small quantities of IgM antibody. About one-half of the serum samples analysed had detectable amounts of IgM antibody specific

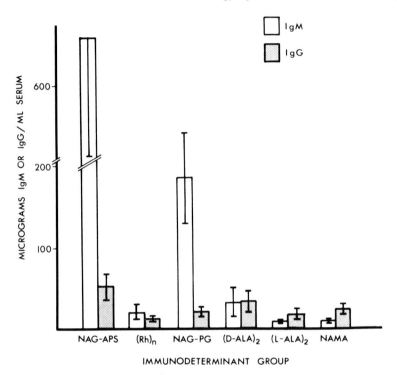

Figure 2. Mean levels of IgM and IgG antibody specific for each of the six different immunodeterminant groups of PG–APS in 11 rats given intravenous injections of group A streptococcal vaccine. Each vertical column shows mean μg of antibody per ml of serum, and bars represent 1 standard error

for the $(Rham)_n$, $(D-Ala)_2$, $(L-Ala)_2$, or the NAMA determinants. Responses to the $(D-Ala)_2$ determinant were especially variable, with a few rats producing relatively large quantities of IgM antibody of this specificity. However, the levels of IgM antibody specific for the $(L-Ala)_2$ and NAMA determinants were uniformly low.

In the majority of serum samples the total amount of IgM antibody specific for the APS moiety was 3–7 times greater than the total amount of IgM antibody specific for the PG moiety. However, one of 11 rats formed larger amounts of antibody specific for the PG moiety than for the APS moiety.

Rats immunized with group A vaccine also formed IgG antibody specific for each of the six different immunodeterminant groups. However, in contrast to the pattern of IgM responses where the NAG-APS and NAG-PG determinants dominated the response, IgG responses to each of the determinants were roughly comparable (see Figure 2). Mean levels of IgG antibody specific for the NAG-APS and NAG-PG determinants were less than 10% of the mean quantities of IgM antibody specific for these determinants. The relative amount of IgG antibody specific for each of the determinants differed from the relative amount of IgM antibody formed. Antibody specific for the (L-Ala)$_2$ and NAMA determinants, which represented only a small part of the total IgM response, comprised a much larger component of the IgG response. The relative response to the (D-Ala)$_2$ and NAG-PG determinants also differed. However, as in the IgM response, IgG antibody specific for the NAG-APS epitope was present in the greatest quantity.

B. Antibody Responses in Rats Immunized with PG–APS Fragments

The mean levels of IgM and IgG antibody in Sprague-Dawley rats immunized with PG–APS fragments are shown in Figure 3. As in the antibody response following immunization with streptococcal vaccines, IgM antibody specific for the NAG-APS determinant was present in greater quantities than antibody of any other specificity, although the extent of its immunodominance was not as striking. Total IgM antibody specific for the four PG determinants was equal to or greater than the quantity of antibody specific for the APS determinants in eight of 10 rats immunized with PG–APS fragment. In contrast, comparable levels of antibody specific for the PG and APS moieties were observed in only two of 11 rats immunized with streptococcal vaccine. In addition, IgG antibody represented a larger proportion of the total antibody produced in the response to PG–APS fragments compared to streptococcal vaccines. In some rats immunized with PG–APS fragments, levels of IgG antibody specific for the NAG-APS and NAG-PG determinants exceeded the levels of IgM specific for these determinants, but this was never observed in rats immunized with streptococcal vaccines.

The results of these studies indicate that rats immunized with either streptococcal vaccines or with PG–APS fragments can form antibody specific for each of the five different immunodeterminant groups of the PG–APS previously identified in the rabbit. In addition, detectable levels of both IgM and IgG antibody specific for NAMA were found in the serum of some rats. As described earlier, antibody specific for NAMA has been reported in the serum of rabbits immunized with *M. luteus* (Schleifer and Seidl, 1977; Wikler, 1975) but not following immunization with streptococcal vaccines. Our ability to detect antibody specific for NAMA is presumably due to the more sensitive methodology used in this study.

In several respects the antibody response of Sprague-Dawley rats to group A vaccine is similar to that of rabbits. In both species, vaccine immunization results in the formation of antibody specific for both the APS and PG moieties, although antibody specific for the APS moiety is usually present in larger amounts. Sera from vaccine-immunized rats contain 3–7 times more antibody specific for the APS moiety than for the PG moiety, and in rabbits greater than

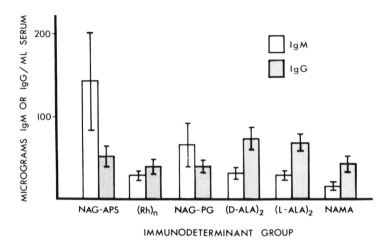

Figure 3. Mean levels of IgM and IgG antibody specific for each of the six different immunodeterminant groups of PG–APS in 10 rats given intraperitoneal injections of PG–APS fragments. Each vertical column shows mean μg antibody per ml of serum, and bars represent 1 standard error

90% of the total antibody formed following immunization with group A vaccine may be specific for the APS (Osterland *et al.*, 1966; Braun *et al.*, 1969). The majority of rats studied here formed detectable quantities of antibody specific for both the NAG-APS and the $(Rham)_n$ determinants of the APS, although antibody specific for the $(Rham)_n$ determinant was present in smaller amounts. Other investigators have reported that human post-streptococcal sera and sera from rabbits immunized with group A vaccine also contain antibody specific for both determinants, and that antibody to the NAG-APS determinant predominates (McCarty and Lancefield, 1955; Karakawa *et al.*, 1965, 1966a).

Immunization with group A vaccine stimulates the formation of only small quantities of antibody specific for the epitopes of PG. In our studies only about one-half of the sera tested contained detectable quantities of antibody specific for the $(D-Ala)_2$, NAMA, and $(L-Ala)_2$ determinants. Other investigators have also reported that antibody specific for PG determinants is present in relatively small amounts following immunization with streptococcal vaccines (Karakawa *et al.*, 1966b; 1970; Rolicka and Park, 1969; Schleifer and Seidl, 1977). The larger amounts of antibody specific for the NAG-PG determinants of PG may be the result of cross-reactivity between antibody specific for the NAG-APS and NAG-PG determinants (Karakawa *et al.*, 1967).

The finding that rats produce primarily IgM antibody specific for the APS following immunization with group A vaccine differs from the results of others. Antibody specific for the APS in rabbits (Bergner-Rabinowitz *et al.*, 1979)

and mice (Cramer and Braun, 1975b) immunized with group A vaccine is primarily IgG antibody. In addition, Leslie and Carwile (1973) have reported that 30–40% of outbred Sprague-Dawley rats also form high levels of IgG antibody specific for the APS moiety following immunization with group A vaccine. Since the IgG antibody response to the APS has been shown to be under genetic control (Braun *et al.* 1969; Cramer and Braun, 1975a; Eichmann *et al.*, 1971; Stankus and Leslie, 1975), the low levels of IgG antibody relative to IgM reported here may be due to the genetic background of the rats used in this study. Two of 11 rats examined here had distinctly higher levels of IgG antibody specific for each of the six different immunodeterminants than did the other members of the group. In these two rats, IgG antibody concentrations were three- to 12-fold greater than the mean IgG antibody levels in the remainder of the group. These high responder animals may represent a genetically distinct subgroup of the outbred Sprague-Dawley population. However, we have never observed the extremely high levels of IgG antibody specific for the APS moiety that have been reported by others in Sprague-Dawley rats (Leslie and Carwile, 1973). In addition, this dichotomy was not seen in the pattern of IgM responses, where individual values were evenly distributed over the entire range of values. It is possible that the technique used to measure antibody levels in this study detects only high affinity antibody and therefore underestimates the total amount of IgG produced. Immunization with streptococcal vaccines is known to induce low affinity anti-APS antibody in rabbits (Schalch *et al.*, 1979), mice (Briles and Davie, 1975), and rats (Stankus and Leslie, 1974).

The antibody response to PG–APS fragments differed from the response to streptococcal vaccines in two ways. First, greater mean quantities of IgG antibody were produced following immunization with PG–APS fragments, and a larger proportion of the total antibody response with IgG. Secondly, following immunization with PG–APS fragments, a much greater proportion of the total antibody produced was specific for PG determinants. The majority of rats immunized with streptococcal vaccines formed more antibody specific for the APS moiety than for the PG moiety. However, five of 10 rats immunized with PG–APS fragments formed greater quantities of antibody specific for the PG moiety than for the APS moiety. The reason for these differences is not known but may be the result of the dissimilar dose of PG–APS and routes of immunization in the two groups. The increased response to PG determinants in PG–APS fragment-immunized rats may be due to the greater availability of PG determinants on the PG–APS fragments. Schalch *et al.* (1979) have recently suggested a similar explanation for the presence of two different populations of antibody specific for the polysaccharide of the A-variant streptococcus. The majority of antibody formed was specific for the more available terminal rhamnose determinant of the carbohydrate. Less accessible determinants of the rhamnose oligosaccharide induced only small amounts of high affinity antibody. Such considerations may be especially important in antibody responses to antigens such as PG–APS, which resist degradation and persist in mammalian tissues (Ohanian and Schwab, 1967; Smialowicz and Schwab, 1977; Ginsburg and Sela, 1976; Eisenberg *et al.*, 1982). The orientation of determinants in the native molecule may not influence the antibody response to immunogens which can be readily degraded, since determinant selection and presentation are not limited to the native conformation. However, when enzymatic degradation is not efficient, the orientation and accessibility of determinants on the antigen may strongly influence which determinants induce antibody formation.

An important aspect of the studies presented here is the extreme variability in the pattern of responses to the different immunodeterminant groups by individual rats. Some rats formed detectable levels of antibody specific for each of the immunodeterminant groups of PG–APS, while others formed detectable levels of antibody specific for only some of the epitopes. Similar variability in the responses to the APS and PG moieties of the PG–APS has also been observed by others. Karakawa *et al.* (1968) have reported that rabbits immunized with group A-variant vaccine exhibited great variability in the relative amounts of antibody specific for the PG and for the group A-variant carbohydrate. Some rabbits formed large amounts of antibody specific for the carbohydrate moiety, while others responded primarily to PG determinants. Other studies (Karakawa and Krause, 1966; Karakawa *et al.*, 1967) have indicated similar variability in response to the different determinants of the PG. These results suggest that the responses to different immunodeterminant groups on the PG–APS are independently regulated.

An unexplored aspect of the variability in responsiveness to PG–APS antigens is the persistence of the pattern of responses seen in individual rats. In our studies, serum samples were collected at a single time point following multiple immunizations. It is not known if the same pattern of responses to individual immunodeterminants is present following the initial injection and is maintained throughout the course of immunizations or if the pattern changes with repeated exposure to antigen. Studies by others on the IgM and IgG responses to the APS moiety have indicated that expression of clonotypes in mice and rabbits immunized with streptococcal vaccines is a stable trait which is first apparent early after the onset of immunization (Eichmann *et al.*, 1970; Cramer and Braun, 1975b; Briles and Davie, 1980).

VII. CONCLUSIONS

PG is one of the few native glycopeptide antigens for which the immunodeterminant groups are known with precision. Since PG is present in the walls of all bacteria and has many biological activities, the immune response against this structure and associated polysaccharides assumes potential clinical importance. The studies reviewed here demonstrate that individual animals vary widely in the relative antibody response to the different immunodeterminants and in the isotypes of antibody specific for each determinant. Further studies are needed to establish the significance of these antibodies in infection and in chronic inflammatory diseases which may be a consequence of bacterial colonization (Schwab, 1979; Cromartie, 1981).

ACKNOWLEDGEMENTS

The studies presented in this chapter were supported by research grants AM25733 and AM28574, from the National Institute of Arthritis, Diabetes, Digestive and Kidney Disease.

REFERENCES

Aasted, B., Bernstein, D., Klapper, D. G., El Kholy, A., and Krause, R. M. (1979). Detection of antibodies in human sera to streptococcal groups A and C carbohydrates by a radioimmunoassay. *Scand. J. Immunol.*, **9**, 61–67.

Abdulla, E. M., and Schwab, J. H. (1965). Immunological properties of bacterial cell wall mucopeptides. *Proc. Soc. Exp. Bio. Med.*, **118**, 359–362.

Bergner-Rabinowitz, S., Ferne, M., and Karshai, H. (1979). Immune response to the group-A polysaccharide. In *Pathogenic Streptococci* (Ed. M. T. Parker), p.89. Reedbooks Ltd., Chertsey, Surrey.

Black, S. J., Hammerling, G. J., Berek, C., Rajewsky, K., and Eichmann, K. (1976). Idiotypic analysis of lymphocytes *in vitro* I. Specificity and heterogeneity of B and T lymphocytes reactive with anti-idiotypic antibody. *J. Exp. Med.*, **143**, 846–860.

Bokisch, V. A., Bernstein, D., and Krause, R. M. (1972). Occurrence of 19S and 7S anti-IgGs during hyperimmunization of rabbits with streptococci. *J. Exp. Med.*, **136**, 799–815.

Bolton, R. W., Rozmiarek, H., and Chorpenning, F. W. (1977). Cyclic antibody formation to polyglycerophosphate in normal and injected rats. *J. Immunol.*, **118**, 1154–1158.

Bona, C., and Hiernaux, J. (1981). Immune response: idiotype antiidiotype network. *CRC Crit. Rev. Immunol.*, **2**, 33–81.

Braun, D. G., and Holm, S. E. (1970). Streptococcal anti-group precipitin in sera from patients with rheumatic arthritis and acute glomerulonephritis. *Int. Arch. Allergy Appl. Immunol.*, **37**, 216–224.

Braun, D. G., and Jaton, J.-C. (1974). Homogeneous antibodies: Induction and value as a probe for the antibody problem. *Curr. Top. Microbiol. Immunol.*, **66**, 29–76.

Braun, D. G., and Krause, R. M. (1968). The individual antigenic specificity of antibodies to streptococcal carbohydrates. *J. Exp. Med.*, **128**, 969–989.

Braun, D. G., Eichmann, K., and Krause, R. M. (1969). Rabbit antibodies to streptococcal carbohydrates. Influence of primary and secondary immunization and of possible genetic factors on the antibody response. *J. Exp. Med.*, **129**, 809–830.

Braun, D. G., Kindred, B., and Jacobson, E. B. (1972). Streptococcal group A carbohydrate antibodies in mice: Evidence for strain differences in magnitude and restriction of the response, and for thymus dependence. *Eur. J. Immunol.*, **2**, 138–143.

Braun, D. G., Kjems, E., and Cramer, M. (1973). A rabbit family of restricted high responders to the streptococcal group A-variant polysaccharide. Selective breeding narrows the isoelectric focusing spectra of dominant clones. *J. Exp. Med.*, **138**, 645–658.

Braun, D. G., Huser, H., and Riesen, W. F. (1976). Variability patterns of anti-polysaccharide antibodies. In *The Generation of Antibody Diversity: A New Look* (Ed. A. J. Cunningham), pp.31–51. Academic Press, New York.

Braun, D. G., Schalch, W., and Schmid, I. (1980). The restricted antibody response to streptococcal group antigens in animals and man: a complex trait. In *Streptococcal Diseases and the Immune Response* (Eds. S. E. Read and J. B. Zabriskie), pp.317–333. Academic Press, New York.

Briles, D. E., and Davie, J. M. (1975). Clonal dominance I. Restricted nature of the IgM antibody response to group A streptococcal carbohydrate in mice. *J. Exp. Med.*, **141**, 1291–1307.

Briles, D. E., and Davie, J. M. (1980). Clonal nature of the immune response II. The effect of immunization on clonal commitment. *J. Exp. Med.*, **152**, 151–160.

Briles, D. E., Krause, R. M., and Davie, J. M. (1977). Immune response deficiency of BSVS mice I. Identification of Ir gene differences between A/J and BSVS mice in antistreptococcal group A carbohydrate response. *Immunogenetics*, **4**, 381–392.

Briles, D. E., Nahm, M., Marion, T. N., Perlmutter, R. M., and Davie, J. M. (1982). Streptococcal group A carbohydrate has properties of both a thymus-independent (TI-2) and thymus-dependent antigen. *J. Immunol.*, **128**, 2032–2035.

Coligan, J. E., Schnute, W. C., and Kindt, T. J. (1975). Immunochemical and chemical studies on streptococcal group-specific carbohydrates. *J. Immunol.*, **114**, 1654–1658.

Coligan, J. E., Kindt, T. J., and Krause, R. M. (1978). Structure of the streptococcal groups A, A-variant, and C carbohydrates. *Immunochemistry*, **15**, 755–760.

Cramer, M., and Braun, D. G. (1974). Genetics of restricted antibodies to streptococcal group polysaccharides in mice I. Strain differences of isoelectric focusing spectra of group A hyperimmune antisera. *J. Exp. Med.*, **139**, 1513–1528.

Cramer, M., and Braun, D. G. (1975a). Genetics of restricted antibodies to streptococcal group polysaccharides in mice II. The Ir-A-CHO gene determines antibody levels, and regulator genes influence the restriction of the response. *Eur. J. Immunol.*, **5**, 823–830.

Cramer, M., and Braun, D. G. (1975b). Immunological memory: Stable IgG patterns determine *in vivo* responsiveness at the clonal level. *Scand. J. Immunol.*, **4**, 63–70.

Cromartie, W. J. (1981). Arthropathic properties of peptidoglycan–polysaccharide complexes of microbial origin. In *Arthritis Models and Mechanisms* (Eds. H. Deicher, and L. Cl. Schultz), pp.24–38. Springer-Verlag, Berlin.

Der Balian, G. P., Slack, J., Clevinger, B. L., Bazin, H., and Davie, J. M. (!980). Subclass restriction of murine antibodies III. Antigens that stimulate IgG_3 in mice stimulate IgG_{2c} in rats. *J. Exp. Med.*, **152**, 209–218.

Dudding, B. A., and Ayoub, E. M. (1968). Persistence of streptococcal group A antibody in patients with rheumatic valvular disease. *J. Exp. Med.*, **128**, 1081–1098.

Eichmann, K. (1973). Idiotype expression and the inheritance of mouse antibody. *J. Exp. Med.*, **137**, 603–621.

Eichmann, K. (1975a). Genetic control of antibody specificity in the mouse. *Immunogenetics*, **2**, 491–506.

Eichmann, K. (1975b). Idiotype suppression II. Amplification of a suppressor T cell with anti-idiotypic activity. *Eur. J. Immunol.*, **5**, 511–517.

Eichmann, K., and Rajewsky, K. (1975). Induction of T and B cell immunity by anti-idiotypic antibody. *Eur. J. Immunol.*, **5**, 661–666.

Eichmann, K., Braun, D. G., Feizi, T., and Krause, R. M. (1970). The emergence of antibodies with either identical or unrelated individual antigenic specificity during repeated immunization with streptococcal vaccines. *J. Exp. Med.*, **131**, 1169–1189.

Eichmann, K., Braun, D. G., and Krause, R. M. (1971). Influence of genetic factors on the magnitude and the heterogeneity of the immune response in the rabbit. *J. Exp. Med.*, **134**, 48–65.

Eisenberg, R., Fox, A., Greenblatt, J. J., Anderle, S. K., Cromartie, W. J., and Schwab, J. H. (1982). Measurement of bacterial cell wall in tissues by solid-phase radioimmunoassay: correlation of distribution and persistence with experimental arthritis in rats. *Infect. Immun.*, **38**, 127–135.

Fleishman, J. B., Braun, D. G., and Krause, R. M. (1968). Streptococcal group-specific antibodies: occurrence of a restricted population following secondary immunization. *Proc. Natl. Acad. Sci. USA*, **60**, 134–139.

Ginsburg, I., and Sela, M. (1976). The role of leukocytes and their hydrolases in the persistence, degradation and transport of bacterial constituents in tissues. *CRC Crit. Rev. Microbiol.*, **4**, 249–332.

Goldstein, I., Halpern, B., and Robert, L. (1967). Immunological relationship between streptococcus A polysaccharide and the structural glycoproteins of heart valve. *Nature*, **213**, 44–47.

Greenblatt, J. J., Hunter, N., and Schwab, J. H. (1980). Antibody response to streptococcal cell wall antigens associated with experimental arthritis in rats. *Clin. Exp. Immunol.*, **42**, 450–457.

Helgeland, S., Grov, A., and Schleifer, K. H. (1973). The immunochemistry of *Staphylococcus aureus* mucopeptide I. Antigenic specificity of the peptide subunits. *Acta Pathol. Microbiol. Scand.*, **81B**, 413–418.

Heymer, B. (1975). Biological properties of peptidoglycan. *Z. Immun.-Forsch.*, **149S**, 245–257.

Heymer, B., and Rietschel, E.Th. (1977). Biological properties of peptidoglycans. In *Microbiology 1977* (Ed. D. Schlessinger), pp.344–349. American Society for Microbiology, Washington, DC.

Heymer, B., Schachenmayr, W., Bultman, B., Spanel, R., Haferkamp, O., and Schmidt, W. C. (1973). A latex agglutination test for measuring antibodies to streptococcal mucopeptides. *J. Immunol.*, **111**, 478–484.

Heymer, B., Bernstein, D., Schleifer, K. H., and Krause, R. M. (1975). A radioactive hapten binding assay for measuring antibodies to the pentapeptide determinant of peptidoglycan. *J. Immunol.*, **114**, 1191–1196.

Heymer, B., Schleifer, K., Read, S., Zabriskie, J., and Krause, R. (1976). Detection of antibodies to bacterial cell wall peptidoglycan in human serum. *J. Immunol.*, **117**, 23–26.

Heymer, B., Hauck, R., Oltersoorf, T., Unz, A., and Haferkamp, O. (1979). Antibodies to streptococcal peptidoglycan and A-carbohydrate in human sera. In *Pathogenic Streptococci* (Ed. M. T. Parker), pp.85–87. Reedbooks Ltd., Chertsey, Surrey.

Hughes, R. C., Thurman, P. F., and Salaman, M. R. (1971). Antigenic properties of *Bacillus licheniformis* cell wall components. *Eur. J. Biochem.*, **19**, 1–8.

Kaplan, E. L., Ferrieri, P., and Wannamaker, L. W. (1974). Comparison of the antibody response to streptococcal cellular and extracellular antigens in acute pharyngitis. *J. Pediat.*, **84**, 21–28.

Karakawa, W. W., and Krause, R. M. (1966). Studies on the immunochemistry of streptococcal mucopeptide. *J. Exp. Med.*, **124**, 155–171.

Karakawa, W. W., Osterland, C. K., and Krause, R. (1965). Detection of streptococcal group-specific antibodies in human sera. *J. Exp. Med.*, **122**, 195–205.

Karakawa, W. W., Lackland, H., and Krause, R. M. (1966a). The production of streptococcal group-specific antibodies in rabbits I. The identification of groups A and A-variant agglutinins in group A antisera. *J. Immunol.*, **96**, 204–209.

Karakawa, W. W., Lackland, H., and Krause, R. M. (1966b). An immunological analysis of bacterial mucopeptides. *J. Immunol.*, **97**, 797–804.

Karakawa, W. W., Lackland, H., and Krause, R. M. (1967). Antigenic properties of the hexosamine polymer of streptococcal mucopeptide. *J. Immunol.*, **99**, 1178–1182.

Karakawa, W. W., Braun, D. G., Lackland, H., and Krause, R. M. (1968). Immunochemical studies on the cross-reactivity between streptococcal and staphylococcal mucopeptide. *J. Exp. Med.*, **128**, 325–340.

Karakawa, W. W., Maurer, P. H., Walsh, P., and Krause, R. M. (1970). The role of D-alanine in the antigenic specificity of bacterial mucopeptides. *J. Immunol.*, **104**, 230–237.

Krause, R. M. (1975). Immunological activity of the peptidoglycan. *Z. Immun.-Forsch.*, **149S**, 136–150.

Krause, R. M., and McCarty, M. (1961). Studies on the chemical structure of streptococcal cell wall I. The identification of mucopeptide in the cell walls of groups A and A-variant streptococci. *J. Exp. Med.*, **114**, 127–140.

Lancefield, R. C. (1941). Specific relationship of cell composition to biological activity of hemolytic streptococci. *Harvey Lectures*, **36**, 251–290.

Leslie, G. A. (1979). Expression of a cross-reactive idiotype on the IgG_{2c} subclass of rat anti-streptococcal carbohydrate antibody. *Mol. Immunol.*, **16**, 281–285.

Leslie, G. A., and Carwile, H. F. (1973). Immune response of rats to group A streptococcal vaccine. *Infect. Immun.*, **7**, 781–785.

Lyampert, I. M., Beletskaya, L. V., Borodiyuk, N. A., Gnezditskaya, E. V., Rassokhina, I. I., and Danilova, T. A. (1976). A cross-reactive antigen of thymus and skin epithelial cells common with the polysaccharide of group A streptococci. *Immunology*, **31**, 47–55.

McCarty, M. (1956). Variation in the group-specific carbohydrate of group A streptococci II. Studies on the chemical basis of serological specificity of the carbohydrates. *J. Exp. Med.*, **104**, 629–643.

McCarty, M. (1958). Further studies on the chemical basis for serological specificity of group A streptococcal carbohydrate. *J. Exp. Med.*, **108**, 311–323.

McCarty, M., and Lancefield, R. C. (1955). Variation in the group-specific carbohydrate of group A streptococci I. Immunochemical studies on the carbohydrate of variant strains. *J. Exp. Med.*, **102**, 11–28.

Miller, E. J., Osterland, C. K., Davie, J. M., and Krause, R. M. (1967). Electrophoretic analysis of polypeptide chains isolated from antibodies in the serum of immunized rabbits. *J. Immunol.*, **98**, 710–715.

Mirelman, D., Bracha, R., and Sharon, N. (1974). Penicillin-induced secretion of a soluble, uncross-linked peptidoglycan by *Micrococcus luteus* cells. *Biochemistry*, **13**, 5045–5053.

Nguyen-Nuy, H., Nauciel, C., and Wermuth, C.-G. (1976). Immunochemical study of the peptidoglycan of Gram-negative bacteria. *Eur. J. Biochem.*, **66**, 79–84.

Ohanian, S. H., and Schwab, J. H. (1967). Persistence of group A streptococcal cell walls related to chronic inflammation of rabbit dermal connective tissue. *J. Exp. Med.*, **125**, 1137–1148.

Olson, J. C., Wagner, C. R., and Leslie, G. A. (1982). The assessment of anti-idiotypic antibodies as effective immunoregulatory probes *in vivo*. *Clin. Exp. Immunol.*, **48**, 458–468.

Osterland, C. K., Miller, E. J., Karakawa, W. W., and Krause, R. M. (1966). Characteristics of streptococcal group-specific antibody isolated from hyperimmune rabbits. *J. Exp. Med.*, **123**, 599–614.

Perlmutter, R. M., Hansburg, D., Briles, D. E., Nicolotti, R. A., and Davie, J. M. (1978). Subclass restriction of murine anti-carbohydrate antibodies. *J. Immunol.*, **121**, 566–571.

Pope, R. M., Rutstein, J. E., and Straus, D. C. (1982). Detection of antibodies to streptococcal mucopeptide in patients with rheumatic disorders and normal controls. *Int. Arch. Allergy Appl. Immunol.*, **67**, 267–274.

Rabinowitz, K., Bergner-Rabinowitz, S., Ferne, M., Fleiderman, S., and Beck, A. (1977). Antibody response to group A streptococci in an epidemic of streptococcal pharyngitis. *J. Lab. Clin. Med.*, **90**, 466–474.

Rogers, H. J., Perkins, H. R., and Ward, J. B. (1980). Structure of peptidoglycan. In *Microbial Cell Walls and Membranes*, pp.190–214. Chapman and Hall, London.

Rolicka, M., and Massell, B. F. (1973). Antipeptidoglycan in rheumatic fever: Agreement with carditis. *Proc. Soc. Exp. Bio. Med.*, **144**, 892–895.

Rolicka, M., and Park, J. T. (1969). Antimucopeptide antibodies and their specificity. *J. Immunol.*, **103**, 196–203.

Rosenthal, R. S. (1979). Release of soluble peptidoglycan from growing gonococci: hexaminidase and amidase activities. *Infect. Immun.*, **24**, 869–878.

Rupley, J. A. (1964). The hydrolysis of chitin by concentrated hydrochloric acid, and the preparation of low-molecular-weight substrates for lysozyme. *Biochim. Biophys. Acta*, **83**, 245–255.

Schachenmayr, W., Heymer, B., and Haferkamp, O. (1975). Antibodies to peptidoglycan in the sera from population surveys. *Z. Immun.-Forsch.*, **149S**, 179–186.

Schalch, W., Wright, J. K., Rodkey, L. S., and Braun, D. G. (1979). Distinct functions of monoclonal IgG antibody depend on antigen-site specificities. *J. Exp. Med.*, **149**, 923–937.

Schleifer, K. H., and Krause, R. M. (1971a). The immunochemistry of peptidoglycan. Separation and characterization of antibodies to the glycan and to the peptide subunit. *Eur. J. Biochem.*, **19**, 471–478.

Schleifer, K. H., and Krause, R. M. (1971b). The immunochemistry of peptidoglycan I. The immunodominant site of the peptide subunit and the contribution of each of the amino acids to the binding properties of the peptides. *J. Biol. Chem.*, **246**, 986–993.

Schleifer, K. H., and Seidl, P. H. (1974). The immunochemistry of peptidoglycan. Antibodies against a synthetic immunogen cross-reacting with peptidoglycan. *Eur. J. Biochem.*, **43**, 509–519.

Schleifer, K. H., and Seidl, P. H. (1977). Structure and immunological aspects of peptidoglycans. In *Microbiology 1977* (Ed. D. Schlessinger), pp.339–343. American Society for Microbiology, Washington, DC.

Schmidt, W. C., and Moore, D. J. (1965). The determination of antibody to group A streptococcal polysaccharide in human sera by hemagglutination. *J. Exp. Med.*, **121**, 793–806.

Schwab, J. H. (1979). Acute and chronic inflammation induced by bacterial cell wall structures. In *Microbiology 1979* (Ed. D. Schlessinger), pp.204–214. American Society for Microbiology, Washington, DC.

Schwab, J. H., and Abdulla, E. M. (1968). Antigenic properties of bacterial cell wall mucopeptides. In *Current Research on Group A Streptococcus* (Ed. R. Caravano), pp.124–129. Excerpta Medica, Amsterdam.

Seidl, P. H., and Schleifer, K. H. (1975). Immunochemical studies with synthetic immunogens chemically related to peptidoglycans. *Z. Immun.-Forsch.*, **149S**, 157–164.

Seidl, P. H., and Schleifer, K. H. (1977). The immunochemistry of peptidoglycan. Antibodies against a synthetic immunogen cross-reacting with an interpeptide bridge of peptidoglycan. *Eur. J. Biochem.*, **74**, 353–363.

Seidl, P. H., and Schleifer, K. H. (1978). Specific antibodies to the termini of the interpeptide bridges of peptidoglycan. *Arch. Microbiol.*, **118**, 185–192.

Shulman, S. T., and Ayoub, E. M. (1979). Antibody response to streptococcal group-A carbohydrate: influence of site of infection in patients with nephritis. In *Pathogenic Streptococci* (Ed. M. T. Parker), pp.87–88. Reedbooks Ltd., Chertsey, Surrey.

Slack, J. H., and Davie, J. M. (1982). Subclass restriction of murine antibodies V. The IgG plaque-forming cell response to thymus-independent and thymus-dependent antigens in athymic and euthymic mice. *Cell. Immunol.*, **68**, 139–145.

Slack, J., Der Balian, G. P., Nahm, M., and Davie, J. M. (1980). Subclass restriction of murine antibodies II. The IgG plaque-forming cell response to thymus-independent type 1 and type 2 antigens in normal mice and mice expressing an X-linked immunodeficiency. *J. Exp. Med.*, **151**, 853–862.

Slade, H. D., and Hammerling, U. (1968). Detection by hemagglutination of antibodies to group A and group E streptococci by the use of *O*-stearoyl derivatives of their cell wall carbohydrate-grouping antigens. *J. Bacteriol.*, **95**, 1572–1579.

Smialowicz, R. J., and Schwab, J. H. (1977). Processing of streptococcal cell walls by rat macrophages and human monocytes *in vitro. Infect. Immun.*, **17**, 591–598.

Stankus, R. P., and Leslie, G. A. (1974). Non-precipitating and electrophoretically restricted antibodies to carbohydrate of group A streptococcus in the rat. *J. Infect. Dis.*, **130**, 169–173.

Stankus, R. P., and Leslie, G. A. (1975). Genetic influences on the immune response of rats to stretococcal A carbohydrate. *Immunogenetics*, **2**, 29–38.

Stankus, R. P., and Leslie, G. A. (1976). Rat interstrain antibody response and crossidiotypic specificity. *Immunogenetics*, **3**, 65–73.

Tynecka, A., and Ward, J. B. (1975). Peptidoglycan synthesis in *Bacillus licheniformis*: the inhibition of cross-linking by benzylpenicillin and cephaloridine *in vivo* accompanied by the formation of soluble peptidoglycan. *Biochem. J.*, **146**, 253–267.

Verbrugh, H. A., Peters, R., Rozenberg-Arska, M., Peterson, P. K., and Verhoef, J. (1981). Antibodies to cell wall peptidoglycan of *Staphylococcus aureus* in patients with serious staphylococcal infections. *J. Infect. Dis.*, **144**, 1–9.

Wheat, L. J., Wilkinson, B. J., Kohler, R. B., and White, A. C. (1983). Antibody response to peptidoglycan during staphylococcal infections. *J. Infect. Dis.*, **147**, 16–22.

Wikler, M. (1975). Isolation and characterization of homogeneous rabbit antibodies to *Micrococcus lysodeikticus* with specificity to the peptidoglycan and to the glucose-*N*-acetylaminomannuronic acid polymer. *Z. Immun.-Forsch.*, **149S**, 193–200.

Willcox, H. N. A., and Marsh, D. G. (1978). Genetic regulation of antibody heterogeneity: Its possible significance in human allergy. *Immunogenetics*, **6**, 209–225.

Yarmush, M. L., and Kindt, T. J. (1979). Idiotypes of rabbit antistreptococcal antibodies. Probes for inheritance and immune regulation. In *Immunology of Bacterial Polysaccharides* (Eds. J. A. Rudbach, and P. J. Baker), pp.41–65. Elsevier/North-Holland, New York.

Zeiger, A. R., and Maurer, P. H. (1973). Immunochemistry of a synthetic peptidoglycan-precursor pentapeptide. *Biochemistry*, **12**, 3387–3394.

Zeiger, A. R., Eaton, S. M., and Mirelman, D. (1978). Antibodies against a synthetic peptidoglycan-precursor pentapeptide cross-react with at least two distinct populations of uncross-linked soluble peptidoglycan secreted by *Micrococcus luteus* cells. *Eur. J. Biochem.*, **86**, 235–240.

Zeiger, A. R., Tuazon, C. U., and Sheagren, J. N. (1981). Antibody levels to bacterial peptidoglycan in human sera during the time course of endocarditis and bacteremic infections caused by *Staphylococcus aureus. Infect. Immun.*, **33**, 795–800.

Zimmerman, R. A., Auernheimer, A. H., and Taranta, A. (1971). Precipitating antibody to group A streptococcal polysaccharide in humans. *J. Immunol.*, **107**, 832–841.

Immunology of the Bacterial Cell Envelope
Edited by D. E. S. Stewart-Tull and M. Davies
© 1985 John Wiley & Sons Ltd.

CHAPTER 5

Immunopharmacological Activities of Synthetic Muramyl-peptides

Haruhiko Takada and Shozo Kotani
*Department of Microbiology and Oral Microbiology,
Osaka University Dental School, 1-8 Yamadaoka, Suita, Osaka 565, Japan*

I. INTRODUCTION

The examination of the biological activities of bacterial cell walls, and especially of the peptidoglycan moiety, has followed two lines. (1) to identify the active principle responsible for the marked immunoadjuvant activities of Freund's complete adjuvant (FCA) (Stewart-Tull, 1980), and (2) to elucidate the role of the cell wall in the pathogenesis of various bacterial infections and their sequelae (Rotta, 1975; Heymer and Rietschel, 1977; Schwab, 1979). These studies resulted in the discovery of an extremely diverse spectrum of biological response modifying (BRM) activities of cell wall peptidoglycans from both indigenous and parasitic bacteria. The prominent BRM activities of cell wall peptidoglycan are similar to those of endotoxic lipopolysaccharide (Morrison and Ryan, 1979; Chapters 8 and 10), and are based on the characteristic chemical composition and structure of the molecule. It may not be unreasonable to suppose that the unique chemical and BRM properties of peptidoglycans have arisen as a result of mutation and selection, on the assumption that BRM activities of peptidoglycans have survival value for both the host and the bacteria.

It is now well established that most, if not all, of the BRM activities of peptidoglycans can be attributed to the N-acetylmuramyl–L-alanyl–D-isoglutamine moiety (MDP) (Fig. 1a) (Chedid *et al.*, 1978; Adam *et al.*, 1981; Kotani *et al.*, 1981, 1982, 1983), which is a key structure common to essentially all bacterial species associated with mammals (Schleifer and Kandler, 1972).

Extensive studies on the BRM activities of cell walls, synthetic MDP and related compounds have been made in an attempt to utilize the beneficial BRM activities, such as the potentiation of antigen-specific and-non-specific host defence mechanisms. This chapter will examine a few selected activities of various natural and synthetic preparations in clinical and preventive medicine.

II. IMMUNOPHARMACOLOGICAL ACTIVITIES OF MURAMYL-PEPTIDES

A. Activities of Muramyl-peptides Detected by *in vivo* Assays

1. Adjuvant Activities

MDP has been identified as the active compound responsible for the immuno-stimulating activities of FCA, which contains mycobacterial cells as an active principle in a water-in-mineral oil (w/o) emulsion. This is particularly true for the induction of delayed-type hypersensitivity (DTH), the characteristic adjuvant activity associated with FCA. However, the use of the w/o emulsion accompanied as it is by severe injurious reactions at both the injection site and in the regional lymph nodes, makes it unsuitable for use as a vehicle for human vaccination.

However, in order to overcome these inherent difficulties, numerous synthetic MDP derivatives were synthesized and their activities in potentiating host

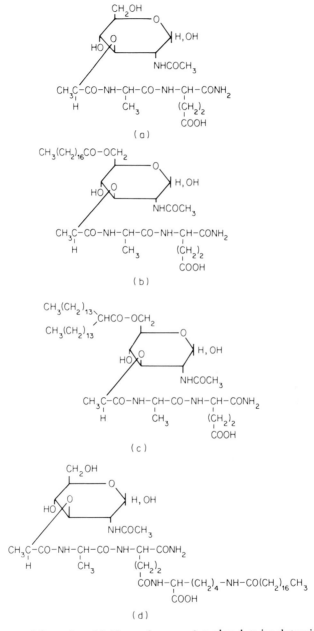

Figure 1. Structural formulae: (a) *N*-acetylmuramyl–L-alanyl–D-isoglutamine (MDP); (b) 6-*O*-stearoyl–MDP (L18–MDP); (c) 6-*O*-(2-tetradecylhexadecanoyl)–MDP (B30–MDP); and (d) N^{α}-(*N*-acetylmuramyl–L-alanyl–D-isoglutaminyl)–N^{ϵ}-stearoyl–L-lysine [MDP–Lys(L18)]

immune responses, especially cell-mediated ones, were examined in combination with various administration vehicles other than w/o emulsion. As a result, some of 6-*O*-acyl derivatives of MDP, especially 6-*0*-stearoyl–MDP (L18–MDP) (Figure 1b), are able to induce DTH against ovalbumin when administered to guinea pigs sequestered in liposomes without causing noticeable local reactions (Kotani *et al.*, 1977a). Further studies showed that 6-*O*-(2-tetradecylhexadecanoyl)–MDP (B30–MDP) (Figure 1c) could also induce DTH against ovalbumin when administered with an immunogen in phosphate-buffered saline (PBS) as well as in liposomes (Kotani *et al.*, 1978). A noticeable side-effect was a mild and transient swelling of the local lymph nodes. The stimulation of serum anti-ovalbumin antibody production in guinea pigs by these compounds in liposomes or PBS is significantly stronger than that stimulated by Freund's incomplete adjuvant (FIA) and comparable to that of FCA. Similar results were obtained with 1-*O*-(MDP–L-Ala)–glycerol-3-mycolate both in liposome and in saline (Parant *et al.*, 1980a; Jolivet *et al.*, 1981).

To increase serum antibody levels against protein antigens, the unsubstituted MDP does not necessarily require the help of the w/o emulsion, since an aqueous solution of MDP is definitely active (Audibert and Chedid, 1976; Chedid *et al.*, 1976). However, the extent of the stimulatory effect is at most comparable to that of FIA but far less than that of the classical FCA or MDP in a w/o emulsion. Further, Chedid *et al.* (1976) showed that MDP enhanced serum antibody production in mice against bovine serum albumin (BSA) when administered by the oral route (BSA by the subcutaneous route). This finding was confirmed in the authors' laboratory by showing that some bacterial cell walls, including mycobacterial cell walls, stimulated antibody production against subcutaneously injected ovalbumin or BSA (I. Morisaki and S. Kotani, unpublished results). The study along this line was recently extended to demonstrate that an oral vaccine consisting of cariogenic *Streptococcus mutans* serotype *g* carbohydrate and the lipophilic MDP derivatives, especially L18–MDP, incorporated into liposomes induced a specific salivary IgA immune response which was protective against challenge with virulent *S. mutans* in rats (Michalek *et al.*, 1983; Kotani *et al.*, 1984) and that N^{α}-(*N*-acetylmuramyl–L-alanyl–D-isoglutaminyl)–N^{ϵ}-stearoyl–L-lysine [MDP–Lys(L18)] (Figure 1d) orally administered together with BSA in liposomes significantly increased serum anti-BSA antibody production in mice (T. Ogawa, H. Shimauchi and S. Kotani, unpublished results). These results clearly suggest that lipophilic MDP derivatives are effective oral adjuvants at least when incorporated into liposomes.

2. Stimulation of Reticuloendothelial System (RES)

Tanaka *et al.* (1977) demonstrated that carbon clearance in mice was significantly enhanced by pretreatment with simultaneous intravenous and intraperitoneal injections of MDP in PBS. Further study with various MDP analogues and derivatives demonstrated that there was a correlation between RES-stimulating and adjuvant activities and structure (Tanaka *et al.*, 1979). This observation suggested that phagocytic cells might be one of the primary targets for immunomodulating activities of muramyl-peptides, and led to a number of studies examining the activation of macrophages by muramyl-peptides (reviewed by Tanaka, 1982). The effective enhancement of carbon clearance by oral administration of MDP was later demonstrated by Waters and Ferraresi (1980). Fraser-Smith *et al.* (1982) found that there was a close correlation with the various MDP analogues between the activity to increase non-specific resistance against *Pseudomonas* and *Candida* infections and the enhancement of carbon clearance.

3. Effects on Blood Leucocytes

Kotani *et al.* (1976) found that an intravenous injection of an aqueous solution of MDP into rabbits first caused leucocytopaenia (for 1–3 h after the injection), which was succeeded by leucocytosis lasting several hours or longer in a manner similar to that observed after the injection of streptococcal cell wall peptidoglycans or their enzymatic digests (Hamada *et al.*, 1971). Later, Kato *et al.* (1982) demonstrated after intravenous injection of MDP, B30–MDP or the cell walls of *Listeria monocytogenes* or their enzymatic lysates induced monocytosis in mice, which appeared after 18 h and persisted for several days. Wuest and Wachsmuth (1982) found in mice that low doses of MDP ($0.1–1$ mg kg^{-1}) provoked lymphocytosis, while larger doses of MDP (10 mg kg^{-1} upwards) resulted in lymphocytopaenia with an increase of young stab neutrophils and monocytes. MDP also induced a dose-dependent increase of bone-marrow macrophage progenitor cells.

The findings described above suggested that MDP stimulated proliferation of macrophage progenitor cells in bone marrow and induced monocytosis, which thus may result in the stimulation of host defence mechanisms.

4. Epithelioid Cell Granuloma Formation

In the course of investigation of macrophage activation by MDP and related compounds, Tanaka and coworkers found that MDP, but not adjuvant-inactive analogues, produced massive epithelioid granulomas, indistinguishable from those induced by tubercle bacilli, in guinea pigs, rats and rabbits (Emori and Tanaka, 1978; Tanaka and Emori, 1980). MDP had to be administered in a w/o emulsion to produce a granuloma, but B30-MDP, in 1% Tween 80–PBS, could evoke granulomas without the help of the w/o emulsion (Tanaka, 1982). Recent studies with nude rats and neonatally thymectomized plus anti-thymocyte serum-injected rats (Nagao *et al.*, 1981b; Tanaka *et al.*, 1982a) revealed that granuloma formation by MDP did not require

T-cell participation, and seemed to be due to the direct macrophage-activating effects of the molecule.

5. Other Activities

Cummings *et al.* (1980) showed that cultured macrophages from MDP-treated mice displayed increased spreading on a solid surface and enhanced lysosomal enzyme activities when compared with those from non-treated control mice. They also demonstrated that macrophages from MDP-treated mice under stimulation with phorbol myristate acetate generated over five times the level of superoxide anion with macrophages from BCG-infected mice. This effect of MDP was observed in athymic nude mice as well as in normal mice, and indicated a non-involvement of mature T lymphocytes. They further revealed that macrophages, stimulated by subcutaneous administration of MDP, killed twice the number of *Candida albicans in vitro* than did cells from untreated animals, although the phagocytosis of *C. albicans* was only slightly enhanced by the MDP injection. Osada *et al.* (1982c) reported that peritoneal polymorphonuclear cells from mice that had received a subcutaneous injection of a lipophilic MDP derivative, MDP–Lys(L18) (Figure 1d), showed an increase in chemotactic mobility, phagocytic activity and superoxide anion production. Pyrogenicity and slow-wave sleep inducing activity of MDP will be described in sections III. C.2 and IV, respectively.

B. *In vitro* Activities and Target Cells of Muramyl-peptides

1. Macrophage Activation and Monokine Release

Current evidence has revealed that MDP or its lipophilic derivatives can stimulate many types of cells. However, many *in vitro* studies strongly suggest that macrophages are the prime, though not exclusive, 'initial target cells' responsible for many of the BRM activities of muramyl-peptides (Tanaka, 1982; Leclerc and Chedid, 1982).

Recent studies (Ogawa *et al.*, 1982a, 1983) have revealed that the chemotactic activity of MDP for human blood monocytes was independent of complement activity and was strictly dependent on the chemical structure of the molecule, since those analogues lacking most of the BRM activities of MDP were also devoid of the chemotactic activity. However, it has also been observed that MDP inhibited the migration of guinea pig peritoneal exudate macrophages induced by irritation with liquid paraffin (Yamamoto *et al.*, 1978; Nagao *et al.*, 1979; Adam *et al.*, 1978). MDP enhanced the attachment and spreading of induced peritoneal guinea pig macrophages on solid surfaces (Tanaka *et al.*, 1980), and this did not need participation of lymphocytes (Nagao *et al.*, 1981a). Tanaka's group concluded that the mode of macrophage migration inhibition by MDP was different from that caused by lymphokines or a purified macrophage migration inhibitory factor (MIF) for the following reasons: (i) the inhibition by MIF but not MDP was reduced when macrophages were pretreated by L-fucose-binding lectin (Homma *et al.*, 1981); (ii) a number of macrophages at the periphery of an aggregated mass of cells stimulated with MIF spread on a solid surface, while only a few macrophages around the cell mass spread in tests with MDP (or lipopolysaccharide, LPS); (iii) macrophages whose migration was inhibited by MIF, exhibit enhanced migration at day 3, unlike those treated with MDP (Nagao *et al.*, 1982b). These findings suggest that MDP acts directly upon macrophages and not through the formation or release of chemical mediators by coexisting lymphocytes. Scanning electron microscopy further revealed that MDP, like MIF, induced characteristic cell surface changes in macrophages, namely the formation of petal-like ruffles (Fukutomi *et al.*, 1981).

MDP and related compounds have been shown to increase or stimulate the following biochemical or metabolic activities of macrophages: glucosamine uptake (Takada *et al.*, 1979a; Imai *et al.*, 1980; Nagao and Tanaka, 1983a), glucose oxidation (Imai *et al.*, 1980), lysosomal enzyme release (Imai and Tanaka, 1981), ornithine decarboxylase level (Nichols and Prosser, 1980), collagenase and prostaglandin E_2 synthesis and intracellular level of cyclic AMP (Wahl *et al.*, 1979). With regard to DNA synthesis, Tanaka *et al.* (1980, 1982b) and Nagao and Tanaka (1983a) found that MDP strongly suppressed DNA synthesis in liquid paraffin-induced peritoneal macrophages but did not cause the suppression in resident macrophages. Schindler *et al.* (1982), however, observed the reverse effect; namely that MDP increased [^{3}H]thymidine incorporation into oil-induced peritoneal macrophages of guinea pigs. Akagawa and Tokunaga (1980) examined the stimulatory effects of MDP on differentiation of murine macrophage cell lines in terms of the induction of Fc receptors and phagocytic activity, and found that MDP could stimulate mature macrophages but not immature ones. This finding suggested the importance of the stage of differentiation of the macrophages used to evaluate the *in vitro* stimulatory activities of MDP. This is particularly important since most of the above effects of MDP on macrophages were hardly detected when resident macrophages were used as the target cells; this situation is contrary to that observed with LPS.

In vitro effects of MDP-activated macrophages on microbes and tumour cells have been the subject of many studies. In 1975, Juy and Chedid showed that MDP activated murine macrophages, from (CBA/2 × C57B1)F1 hybrids, to inhibit P815 (DBA/2) mastocytoma cells *in vitro*. It should also be mentioned that in the above *in vitro* assay system, a conjugate of MurNAc–D-Ala–D-isoGln (an MDP analogue inactive in antigen-specific adjuvant activity) with multi-poly(DL-alanyl)–poly(L-lysine) was reported to induce in macrophages the P815 growth inhibiting activity (Galelli *et al.*, 1980). The augmentation of tumouricidal activity against RBL-5 cells by MDP was reported by Taniyama and Holden

(1979) with murine macrophages isolated from the tumour mass and by murine macrophage cell lines. Sone and Fidler (1980), on the other hand, reported that MDP and macrophage activating factor (MAF) derived from rat lymphocytes acted synergistically to induce rat alveolar macrophages to become cytotoxic against syngeneic as well as allogeneic and xenogeneic tumour cells. The synergistic effects could be increased if the MDP and MAF were encapsulated in liposomes. These *in vitro* studies were followed by *in vivo* assays for anti-tumour activity of MDP encapsulated in liposomes, which will be described in section III. B.2.

With regard to acquisition or increase of antimicrobial activities of macrophages under the action of MDP, Hadden and his colleagues (1978, 1979) reported increased phagocytosis and bactericidal activity of MDP-activated guinea pig peritoneal macrophages on *Listeria monocytogenes*. We also observed that MDP stimulated phagocytosis of *Streptococcus pyogenes* cells by guinea pig peritoneal macrophages, while an adjuvant-inactive analogue, MurNAc–L-Ala–L-isoGln, did not (Takada *et al.*, 1982). On the other hand, Nozawa *et al.* (1980) showed the increase in candidacidal activity of MDP-activated murine macrophages was only observed when the medium conditioned by growth of L-929 fibroblasts was used as a culture fluid.

The increased cytocidal activity against microbes by MDP-activated macrophages seems to be partly explained by the enhanced generation of superoxide anion. Pabst *et al.* (1980b) first demonstrated that resident mouse peritoneal macrophages when exposed to MDP *in vitro* were primed to display the enhanced generation of superoxide anion in response to stimulation by phorbol myristate acetate (PMA) or opsonized zymosan. They further showed that B30–MDP was more active than MDP in priming macrophages (Pabst *et al.*, 1980a), and found that the ability of human blood monocytes to produce superoxide anion, which was gradually lost *in vitro* in the absence of MDP, could be maintained more than four days when MDP was added to monocyte culture (Pabst *et al.*, 1982). Similar enhancement of superoxide anion release by treatment with MDP was reported by Kaku *et al.* (1983) with liquid paraffin-induced peritoneal macrophages of guinea pigs; they showed that MDP enhanced the NADPH oxidase activity of the macrophages. Wilson *et al.* (1982) similarly found enhanced release of superoxide anion of human monocytes treated with MDP, but could not detect any increase of antimicrobial activity of the treated macrophages. Finally, Hotta *et al.* (1982) observed that the culture of murine peritoneal macrophages for three days in the presence of B30-MDP significantly enhanced dengue-2 virus replication in cultured macrophages in a similar manner to those treated with cell walls or peptidoglycans (Hotta *et al.*, 1983).

The last topic discussed in this section concerns the liberation of various mediators influencing other cells, namely monokines, by MDP-activated macrophages. Staber *et al.* (1978) reported that culture supernates of murine adherent peritoneal cells incubated with MDP showed colony stimulating activity on bone-marrow cell cultures. This work was followed by the study of Oppenheim *et al.* (1980), which showed that human adherent mononuclear cells, murine adherent peritoneal cells and macrophage cell lines, which had been stimulated with MDP, produced a factor mitogenic for murine thymocytes, namely lymphocyte-activating factor (LAF; currently termed interleukin 1). They isolated two fractions of low (16 000–20 000) and high (60 000–70 000) molecular weight from the culture supernate from MDP-activated cells. Tenu *et al.* (1980) found that MDP stimulated murine peritoneal macrophages, elicited by intraperitoneal injection of trehalose dimycolate or thioglycolate, but not resident macrophages, to secrete a thymocyte mitogenic protein. The ability of MDP to stimulate rabbit peritoneal exudate cells or human peripheral blood mononuclear cells to produce LAF, was shared by MurNAc–L-Ala–D-Glu–α-*n*-butyl ester (murabutide) (Figure 2), a non-pyrogenic derivative of MDP (Damais *et al.*, 1982). The product stimulated the proliferative response of

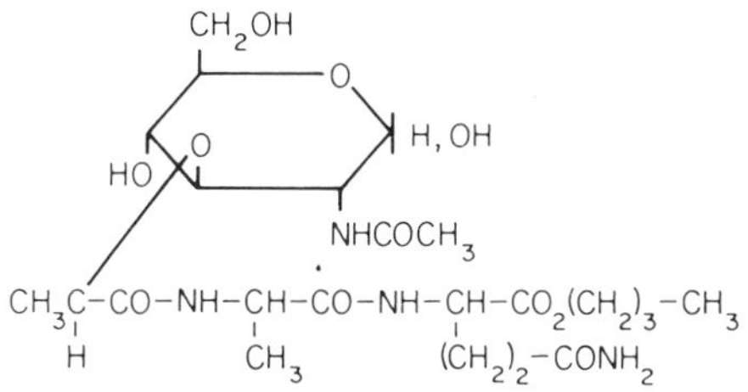

Figure 2. Structural formula of *N*-acetylmuramyl–L-alanyl–D-isoglutanine–α-*n*-butyl ester (murabutide)

murine thymocyte to PHA. Similarly, Iribe *et al.* (1981, 1982) found that MDP stimulated peritoneal macrophages from guinea pigs to release T-cell activating monokines, which (a) increased the proliferative response of a T lymphocyte-enriched fraction of guinea pig lymph nodes to PHA, and (b) caused the antigen-specific activation of immune T lymphocytes, in the absence of macrophages, to produce macrophage migration inhibitory factor. They found that soluble monokines were recovered after gel filtration in both high (50 000–90 000) and low (10 000–30 000) molecular weight fractions. There seem to be some discrepancies among the experimental results reported by the above two groups of investigators, but both sets of findings support the hypothesis that macrophages are one of the initial target cells of MDP. It may be added here that there are reports on the liberation of a mediator that triggers quiescent fibroblasts into active proliferation (Wahl *et al.*, 1979; Rutherford *et al.*, 1982) and the formation of a chemoattractant for fibroblasts, identified as fibronectin (Tsukamoto *et al.*, 1981).

The hypothesis that macrophages are the initial target cells of MDP seems to be valid if one also considers the enhancement of non-specific resistance, namely the augmentation of host defence mechanisms against microbial infection and tumour growth. However, this does not seem to be necessarily true with antigen-specific immunostimulation by MDP, although there are some reports suggesting that macrophages are the primary target cells. For example, Fevrier *et al.* (1978) reported that MDP stimulated macrophages to release factors that acted on B-cells to promote antigen-specific PFC responses through T-cell mediation. Recently, Souvannavong *et al.* (1983) also revealed that MDP alone was unable to induce any *in vitro* primary immune response to sheep red blood cells (SRBC) in macrophage-depleted murine splenocyte cultures, but it was able to enhance the anti-SRBC antibody response of these cultures reconstituted with interleukin 1 obtained from a murine macrophage cell line or a monokine from murine peritoneal resident macrophages. At any rate, these findings have not yet been confirmed in *in vivo* assays. By contrast, there are many reports to show that MDP exerts its antigen-specific adjuvant activity via the stimulation of lymphocytes, especially T-cells (see following section).

2. Lymphocyte Activation

Studies in this field started with the assay for mitogenicity of MDP. In 1977, Takada *et al.* first demonstrated that MDP was mitogenic for murine and guinea pig splenocytes, and this mitogenicity was strictly dependent on the chemical structure of the molecule; i.e. stereoisomers of MDP, inactive with regard to antigen-specific immunoadjuvancy, lacked mitogenic activity. The mitogenic activity of MDP, however, was far less than that of natural peptidoglycans (Takada *et al.*, 1979b, 1980). Damais *et al.* (1977) also showed that MDP induced blast transformation of splenocytes cultured with 2-mercaptoethanol for 4–5 days, and no activity was found on thymocytes from normal mice under the same assay conditions. There are, however, distinct strain differences for the B-cell mitogenicity of MDP; for example, the strain DBA/2 mouse is a high responder, and C57B1/6 is a low responder, while BALB/c is intermediate (Damais *et al.*, 1978). Specter *et al.* (1977, 1978), on the other hand, showed that MDP acted on murine splenocytes as a polyclonal B-cell activator and strongly enhanced the anti-SRBC PFC response to an extent equal to or greater than that by bacterial LPS, although MDP was found to be scarcely mitogenic on splenocytes. Watson and Whitlock (1978) showed that the PFC response of nude mice splenocytes cultured *in vitro* with SRBC and MDP was significantly higher than those sensitized with SRBC alone. They concluded that MDP exhibited T-cell-replacing activity. Leclerc *et al.* (1979) also revealed that MDP could exert its *in vitro* adjuvant activity and polyclonal B-cell activating effect on splenocytes of nude mice toward both T-independent trinitrophenyl–polyacrylamide and T-dependent SRBC antigens. A study of Löwy *et al.* (1980a), on the other hand, demonstrated that MDP increased non-specific PFC responses of murine splenocytes against syngeneic, bromelain-treated red blood cells (br-MRBC) and an autoantigen, mouse albumin. In their study, the non-specific stimulation of anti-br-MRBC PFC by MDP was observed in spleen cell cultures of nude mice and LPS-low-responding C3H/He Orl mice, and also with splenocytes which were depleted of macrophages. Wood and Staruch (1981) showed that macrophage-depleted lymphocytes responded only poorly to the B-cell mitogenicity of MDP, but the responsiveness could be reconstituted by the addition of either fresh macrophages or 2-mercaptoethanol. They also showed that the genes controlling mitogenic responses to LPS and MDP were neither identical nor closely linked. By comparing the *in vitro* mitogenicity and *in vivo* adjuvant activity of MDP in several different genetic strains of mice, they finally concluded that the ability of MDP to act as a mitogen made little or no contribution to its adjuvancy. Thus, although there are many studies showing direct stimulation of B-cells by MDP *in vitro*, there seems to be no conclusive evidence that B-cells are the primary target cells of MDP for the manifestation of its antigen-specific immunostimulating activity *in vivo*.

The consensus among investigators is that MDP is devoid of T-cell mito-genicity. In spite of this, there are a number of studies which infer that MDP exerts its immunopotentiating activity *in vivo* via its effect on T-lymphocytes. Löwy *et al.* (1977) first demonstrated by a cell transfer system in mice that MDP increased the efficacy of antigen-specific education of T-cells against SRBC, while macrophages pretreated with SRBC and MDP did not increase an anti-SRBC immune response in recipient mice. Sugimoto *et al.* (1978) also revealed in their study with a hapten-carrier system that MDP exerted its adjuvant activity by the enhanced stimulation of helper T-cell function. This study was extended by Löwy *et al.* (1980b), showing that MDP was able to prime the carrier-specific T-cells but not the hapten specific B-cells. However, Sugimura *et al.* (1979) analysed the mechanism of potentiation of primary anti-SRBC PFC response by MDP by cell separation procedures, and demonstrated that this was due to direct interaction between antigen-stimulated T- and B-lymphocytes. They further showed that there was no macrophage requirement for MDP to exhibit its adjuvant activity *in vitro*. The ability of MDP to promote the education of helper T-cells by antigen was also demonstrated by Prunet *et al.* (1978). They showed in both *in vivo* and *in vitro* assays that MDP promoted the recovery of a specific anti-pigeon erythrocyte (PRBC) response in murine splenocytes which had been depleted by immunoabsorbent columns of cells specifically responsive to PRBC. The induction of cytotoxic effector T-cells by MDP against mastocytoma P815–X2 cells *in vitro* was also reported (Igarashi *et al.*, 1977). However, Azuma *et al.* (1976) found that whilst the administration of MDP with P815-X2 cells in PBS did not induce antigen-specific cytotoxic effector T-cells, some of the hydrophobic derivatives of MDP, notably 6-*O*-'mycoloyl'–MDPs and quinonyl–MDP-66 (Figure 3), were found to be active under the same experimental conditions (Azuma *et al.*, 1979b; Yamamura and Azuma, 1982).

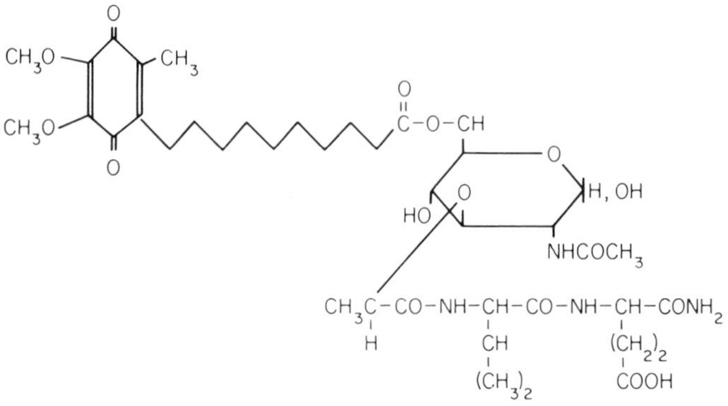

Figure 3. Structural formula of quinoyl–MDP-66

The stimulation of suppressor T-cells following exposure to muramyl-peptides has also been observed. In 1979, Kishimoto *et al.* showed that muramyl-tripeptide (MurNAc–L-Ala–D-isoGln–L-Lys) or 6-*O*-mycoloyl–MDP conjugated with antigen significantly induced antigen-specific suppressor T-cells. Immuno-suppression observed after repeated injections of high doses of MDP was also shown to be mediated by T-lymphocytes (Leclerc *et al.*, 1982).

The findings mentioned in this section indicate quite convincingly that T-cells are target cells in the antigen-specific immunopotentiation by MDP. It should be pointed out, however, that this does not necessarily rule out the possibility of participation of other cells in the manifestation of an antigen-specific adjuvant response by MDP. In fact, Kiyono *et al.* (1982) recently demonstrated that MDP required the presence of macrophages for augmentation of immune responses in murine Peyer's patch cell cultures. No information is available about the target cells of MDP required for the induction of a DTH.

In passing, MDP can induce murine natural killer (NK)-cells *in vivo* and *in vitro* (Sharma *et al.*, 1981).

3. Effects on Cells and Systems other than Macrophages and Lymphocytes

The first demonstration of the stimulatory effect of MDP on polymorphonuclear leucocytes (PMNL) was made by Ishihara *et al.* (1982), who showed that MDP and B30–MDP stimulated phagocytosis of heat-killed *Streptococcus pyogenes* by guinea pig peritoneal PMNL. Subsequently, Osada *et al.* (1982c) showed that treatment of murine peritoneal PMNL with a lipophilic derivative of MDP, MDP-Lys(L18), caused an increase in chemotactic mobility, phagocytic activity, and superoxide anion production in their *in vitro* assay system. However, Ogawa *et al.* (1982a) showed that MDP did not work as a chemoattractant for human blood PMNL but did for blood monocytes. In this connection, Roch-Arveiller *et al.* (1982) found that pretreatment of rat normal PMNL (pleural cells collected after the injection of isologous serum) with MDP resulted in migration inhibition toward chemotactic agents, while the same treatment of inflammatory PMNL (induced by injection of calcium pyrophosphate) restored the impaired chemotactic responsiveness. Kaku *et al.* (1983), on the other hand, did not demonstrate an increase in superoxide anion release from guinea pig peritoneal PMNL by MDP treatment.

With basophilic leucocytes, Ogawa *et al.* (1982c) showed that MDP increased [^{14}C]histidine uptake (a characteristic trait of basophils; Stewart *et al.*, 1979) by guinea pig peripheral blood leucocytes.

It was recently shown by Iribe *et al.* (1983) that MDP stimulated guinea pig skin fibroblasts to produce a thymocyte-activating factor which augmented the proliferative response of thymocytes to phytohaemagglutinin; the active principle was recovered in fractions of molecular weight 30 000–60 000.

Osteoclasts of the rat seem to be another type of target cell for MDP, and these cells are stimulated by MDP to cause bone resorption in organ cultures (Dewhirst, 1982; Dziak *et al.*, 1982; Raisz *et al.*, 1982). Rotta *et al.* (1979) reported that MDP caused lysis of rabbit blood platelets, while Harada *et al.* (1982) showed that a lipophilic MDP derivative, BH48–MDP–L-Lys–D-Ala, stimulated serotonin release by rabbit platelets, but MDP was inactive in this respect. It was also found that B30–MDP and BH48–MDP-L-Lys-D-Ala activated the human complement system by the classical pathway (probably by a direct action on the C1 component, and not by antigen–antibody reaction) and by the alternative route, respectively (Kotani *et al.*, 1981; Kawasaki, 1982). The activities of these synthetic compounds were significantly lower than those of cell walls isolated from various bacterial species, their peptidoglycans and a polymer of peptidoglycan subunits prepared from an enzymatic digest of *Staph. epidermidis* cell walls (Kotani *et al.*, 1981; Kawasaki, 1982). Finally, it was observed that MDP and its 6-*O*-acyl derivatives caused a slow and long-lasting contraction of guinea pig ileal strips suspended in Tyrode's solution in a manner similar to that seen with adjuvant-active cell walls and peptidoglycans, while the BH48–MDP-L-Lys-D-Ala caused relaxation of the strips (Ogawa *et al.*, 1982b).

The findings described above strongly suggest the possibility that under appropriate conditions MDP is able to stimulate a wide variety of mammalian cell types. But it should be borne in mind that it is often difficult to decide whether the observed effects of MDP are due to a direct action on affected cells and systems or an indirect one through mediators formed by appropriate cells.

III. POSSIBLE USE OF MURAMYL-PEPTIDE IN CLINICAL AND PREVENTIVE MEDICINE

A. Vaccines

There have been many attempts to use synthetic muramyl-peptides to potentiate the protective power of various vaccines. This topic has been reviewed by Kotani *et al.* (1982, 1983), Chedid and Audibert (1982) and Chedid (1983a), so we will only mention some recent developments. L18–MDP and B30–MDP incorporated into liposomes increased the potency of *Plasmodium falciparum* merozoite vaccine in owl monkeys (Siddiqui *et al.*, 1978; Siddiqui, 1982), and potentiated the efficacy of a split virus vaccine (Okunaga, 1980) and highly purified HA–NA (haemagglutinin–neuraminidase) (Kotani *et al.*, 1982) preparation from influenza A and B viruses, in terms of the enhanced production of haemagglutinin-inhibiting and virus-neutralizing antibodies.

The second approach which has progressed rapidly during the past few years is the development of totally synthetic vaccines for the induction of immunity against microbial and non-microbial antigens. Audibert and Chedid (1980) and Audibert *et al.* (1981, 1982) synthesized a polypeptide antigen composed of 14 amino acids which held the antigenicity of diphtheria toxin and conjugated it to a synthetic carrier, poly(L-Tyr, L-Glu)–poly(DL-Ala)–poly(L-Lys) (abbreviated to A–L) (Mozes *et al.*, 1980). It was demonstrated that administration of this synthetic antigen with MDP in PBS to guinea pigs stimulated the production of diphtheria antitoxin. They have subsequently succeeded in inducing protective antitoxic immunity by immunizing guinea pigs with a completely synthetic conjugate comprising both MDP and an analogue of the above tetradecapeptide (an octadecapeptide) covalently attached to the synthetic carrier, A–L (Audibert *et al.*, 1983). Arnon *et al.* (1980) also prepared a totally synthetic vaccine against coliphage MS-2 by chemically conjugating MDP to a synthetic fragment (P_2) of the virus coat protein attached to the A–L (MDP–P_2–A–L), and revealed that this completely synthetic material, when administered in aqueous solution to rabbits, yielded highly neutralizing antiserum with a titre similar to that obtained with FCA in the absence of MDP and much higher than that given by a simple mixture of MDP and P_2–A–L. This achievement may lead to the development of totally synthetic vaccines effective against viral infections in human beings and animals.

Carelli *et al.* (1982) prepared a synthetic vaccine for non-microbial antigen. Mice which were immunized with a conjugate (in saline) of a synthetic decapeptide, similar to the hypothalamic, luteinizing hormone releasing hormone (LHRH), together with MDP-L-Lys (without intervention of synthetic carriers), produced higher levels of antibody than the control mice receiving LHRH in FCA. The former mice also showed a strong degeneration of the seminiferous epithelium accompanied by absence of spermatogenesis. In this connection, Nagai *et al.* (1978a,b) found that an injection of a mixture (not a conjugate) of a synthetic encephalitogenic heptapeptide and MDP induced allergic encephalomyelitis in guinea pigs without the use of high-molecular-weight carriers. This finding strongly suggests the possibility that totally synthetic 'vaccines' could induce cell-mediated immune responses, although it should be pointed out that a w/o emulsion whose chemical nature was ill-defined was used as the vehicle in these experiments.

Binz *et al.* (1981), on the other hand, showed that T-lymphocytes, which had been blastoformed by mixed lymphocyte culture, showed a distinct immunogenicity in mice syngeneic to the mice from which T-cells were derived, when the membrane of the T lymphoblasts was covalently coupled with MDP or norMDP (*N*-acetylnormuramyl–L-alanyl–D-isoglutamine) *N*-hydroxysuccinimide ester. This study suggests the possibility that anti-syngeneic tumour cell vaccines could be developed by the use of modified tumour cells conjugated with muramyl-peptide derivatives.

B. Increase of Non-specific Resistance

1. Anti-infectious Activity

The increase of non-specific host resistance to microbial infections by peptidoglycan was first demonstrated by Misaki *et al.* (1966). This was followed by Chedid and his colleagues (1977) who showed that MDP was responsible for the above activity of peptidoglycan. They found that pretreatment of mice with MDP and several analogues non-specifically enhanced the resistance of the treated animals against infection with *Klebsiella pneumoniae* by various administration routes, including oral, and also showed that under suitable conditions the resistance was demonstrable even when the administration was made after the infection. This area has been extensively reviewed, and detailed descriptions are to be found in review articles (Chedid *et al.*, 1978; Kotani *et al.*, 1982, 1983), but a few of the more recent studies will be mentioned here. Parant *et al.* (1980a) showed that some desmuramyl-peptidolipids, 1-*O*-(L-Ala–D-isoGln–L-Ala)–glycerol-3-mycolate and its analogues, which were devoid of antigen-specific immunostimulating activities, significantly increased the resistance of mice against *Klebsiella* infection. In contrast to this, however, Audibert *et al.* (1980) observed that some muramyl-peptides, e.g. MurNAc–L-Ala–D-isoGln–L-Lys–D-Ala, held a potent adjuvant activity, but lacked the anti-infectious activity. These findings together may suggest that the antigen-specific and non-specific enhancement of host resistance is mediated by different mechanisms, and consequently by different target cells.

Recent Japanese studies have been aimed at the practical use of MDP derivatives as anti-infectious drugs. Matsumoto *et al.* (1981a,b) compared a number of 6-*O*-acyl derivatives of MDP for their anti-infectious activities against the septic type of *Escherichia coli* infection, and concluded that L18–MDP was the most effective compound among them. L18–MDP augmented the resistance of mice against *Pseudomonas aeruginosa, Staphylococcus aureus* and *Candida albicans* infections, but not against an encapsulated strain of *K. pneumoniae* and *Listeria monocytogenes*, a well-known intracellular parasite (Osada *et al.*, 1982b). They also observed a synergistic effect of L18–MDP and some antibiotics on the protection of mice against *E. coli, P. aeruginosa* and

C. albicans even in aged mice or in mice immunocompromised by treatment with X-irradiation or cyclophosphamide administration (Osada *et al.*, 1982a). L18–MDP also enhanced the resistance against *P. aeruginosa* of guinea pigs whose defence mechanisms were suppressed by treatment with cortisone acetate (Osada *et al.*, 1982d). The increased resistance to microbial infections of animals treated with L18–MDP might be at least partly attributable to the increased antimicrobial activity of PMNL against the pathogens, since various functions of PMNL were shown to be activated by L18–MDP both *in vivo* (Osada *et al.*, 1982a,d) and *in vitro* (Osada *et al.*, 1982c) (see section II. B.3). Recently, Matsumoto *et al.* (1983) compared various derivatives of MDP, having substituted functions in the γ-carboxyl group of their D-isoglutamyl residue, for anti-infectious activities in mice against *E. coli* and other pathogens including *C. albicans*. They found that MDP–Lys(L18) (Figure 1d) was the most active compound, being more effective than L18–MDP. But MDP–Lys(L18) was still scarcely effective against encapsulated *K. pneumoniae* infection.

2. Anti-tumour Activity

Juy and Chedid (1975) showed that MDP could exert anti-tumour activity *in vitro* via macrophage activation, but did not exhibit any anti-tumour activity *in vivo*. Extensive studies by Azuma, Yamamura and their coworkers with a variety of lipophilic derivatives of muramyl-dipeptides are described in review articles (Azuma *et al.*, 1979a; Yamamura and Azuma, 1982; Kotani *et al.*, 1983), of which only mention will be made of the studies with quinonyl–MDP-66, methyl-2-{2-acetamido-2-deoxy-6-*O*-[1O-(2,3-dimethoxy-5-methyl-1,4-benzoquinon-6-yl)-decanoyl] D-glucopyranos-3-*O*-yl}–D-propionyl–L-valyl–D-isoglutaminate (Figure 3), which was arguably the most effective of the MDP derivatives (Azuma *et al.*, 1979b; Saiki *et al.*, 1981). This compound suspended in PBS suppressed the growth of Meth-A tumour in syngeneic BALB/c mice, and regressed line 10 hepatoma in strain 2 guinea pigs when it was injected intralesionally in 10% squalene-treated form (oil-attached form). Saiki *et al.* (1983) showed that quinonyl–MDP-66 restored the impaired immune status in mice bearing Lewis lung carcinoma, in terms of increased induction of allogeneic activity against *L. monocytogenes*.

Recent noteworthy findings would be those of Sone, Fidler and their colleagues. They reported that MDP entrapped within liposomes stimulated alveolar macrophages to exhibit cytocidal effects against syngeneic as well as xenogeneic or allogeneic tumour cells, both *in vitro* (Sone and Fidler, 1980) and *in vivo* (Fidler, 1981). They further showed (Fidler *et al.*, 1981) that repeated intravenous injections of MDP incorporated in multilamellar liposomes into mice, which had been injected into the footpads with melanoma cells and subjected to a midfemoral amputation, markedly reduced the incidence of spontaneous tumour metastases. Comparison of the ability of various liposomes, different in structure and lipid compositions, to deliver MDP to macrophages, led them to conclude that multilamellar vesicles composed of distearoyl-phosphatidylcholine:phosphatidylserine (7:3 mol ratio) were the best vehicle. They further showed that muramyl-tripeptide–phosphatidylethanolamine (MTP–PE) achieved a higher level of macrophage activation in terms of tumouricidal activity than MDP in their *in vitro* assay system (Schroit and Fidler, 1982). Key *et al.* (1982) demonstrated, by immunofluorescence and electron microscopic analyses, that 15% of alveolar macrophages and 5% of metastasis-associated macrophages from mice bearing syngeneic melanoma given by intravenous injection of liposomes (whether with added MTP–PE or none) contained liposomes. In addition, they showed that macrophages from mice given liposomes containing MTP–PE, but not those from mice treated with empty liposomes, were tumouricidal against the target cells *in vitro*. These findings indicate the importance of selecting appropriate vehicles for administration of MDP-related compounds in tumour immunotherapy.

C. Harmful Effects of Muramyl-peptides

In this section, we will describe some known detrimental activities of muramyl-peptides, to which attention should be given in attempts to use MDP and related compounds in clinical or preventive medicine.

1. Induction of Experimental Autoimmune Diseases

Nagai *et al.* (1978b) reported that MDP induced experimental allergic encephalomyelitis (EAE) in guinea pigs when it was administered in a w/o emulsion with a synthetic heptapeptide, which mimicked residues 116–122 of the encephalitogenic basic protein of human myelin. They also showed a correlation between the EAE-provoking and DTH-inducing activities of MDP and its analogues (Nagai *et al.*, 1978a). Attempts to dispense with w/o emulsion have so far been unsuccessful, even with the use of B30–MDP. Maeda *et al.* (1980) confirmed the EAE-inducing activity of MDP in rats.

Adjuvant arthritis in rats whose induction does not require the use of extraneous antigen is another experimental model of autoimmune diseases induced by MDP and related compounds. MDP was once thought to be devoid of this activity unless it was administered together with an appropriate antigen (Koga *et al.*, 1980) or other immunomodulating compounds such as polyriboinosinic acid:polyribocytidylic acid [poly-(I:C)] (Kohashi *et al.*, 1979). However, Nagao and Tanaka (1980) showed the induction of adjuvant arthritis in WKA rats by an intrafootpad injection of MDP in a w/o emulsion prepared with a certain batch of Freund's incomplete adjuvant (Difco). Kohashi *et al.* (1980) confirmed this and showed that the arthritis induced by MDP was composed of a thymus-dependent chronic phase and thymus-independent acute phase, by the use of congenitally athymic nude rats and a spontaneous hypertensive, T-cell deficient rat strain. They also found that MDP in the w/o emulsion did not induce any disease in immunodeficient rats, but consecutive intravenous administrations of an aqueous form of L18–MDP and B30–MDP caused the development of polyarthritis with acute inflammatory reactions with a 100% incidence in both immunologically normal and deficient rats (Kohashi *et al.*, 1981a,b). It should be added, however, that the ability of MDP to induce adjuvant arthritis reported by Japanese investigators has not always been confirmed by French and US workers, although Zidek *et al.* (1982) showed that MDP dissolved in saline induced arthritis in Lewis rats when injected subcutaneously into the neck area daily for 9–32 days at doses of 0.1 to 2.0 mg per rat. Discrepancies among different workers may suggest the existence of unknown secondary factors (either genetic or environmental) which may affect the induction of arthritis by MDP. In this connection, the finding of Hamilton *et al.* (1982) that MDP acted on human monocytes to release factors capable of stimulating the plasminogen activator activity of human synovial fibroblasts is of interest, in view of the fact that this could be responsible for some of the tissue damage and vascular effects associated with rheumatoid arthritis.

MDP was neither immunogenic nor reactogenic by itself as antigen (Audibert *et al.*, 1978) unless it was conjugated to proteins (Reichert *et al.*, 1980) or synthetic carriers (Mozes *et al.*, 1980). As described in section II. B.2, MDP could induce antibodies against self- and altered self-determinants *in vitro* (Löwy *et al.*, 1980a).

Thus it is possible that the ability of MDP to induce autoimmune diseases is mainly mediated by its activity on T-lymphocytes, but is also partially affected by its direct and indirect activities on other cell types.

As other possible detrimental activities of muramyl-peptides, Yamamoto *et al.* (1980) reported that 6-*O*-mycoloyl–MDP produced lung granuloma in mice when it was injected intravenously together with purified, protein derivative (PPD) in a w/o emulsion, and Richerson *et al.* (1982) showed that MDP induced chronic granulomatous pneumonitis in rabbits when it was inhaled together with ovalbumin in an aerosol.

2. Pyrogenicity

Since the report of Kotani *et al.* (1976) that MDP and adjuvant-active analogues caused a febrile response in rabbits after intravenous injection, whilst the adjuvant-inactive analogues were inert, the pyrogenicity of MDP and related compounds has been the subject of many studies (Kotani *et al.*, 1981, 1982; Parant 1979) to elucidate the mechanism of the febrile response and also to develop non-pyrogenic MDP derivatives with useful BRM activities. Two mechanisms seem to be responsible for the pyrogenicity of MDP; one is indirect by the liberation of endogenous pyrogen from leucocytes stimulated by MDP

(Dinarello *et al.*, 1978), and the other is a direct effect of MDP on the thermoregulatory centres (Riveau *et al.*, 1980). The fever response due to the former mechanism can be reduced by indomethacin, while the latter fever could not be inhibited by this agent (Parant *et al.*, 1980b; Riveau *et al.*, 1980). With regard to the indirect mechanisms, Windle *et al.* (1983) recently demonstrated that purified rabbit PMNL did not secrete endogenous pyrogens in response to MDP, while rabbit blood mononuclear cells which spontaneously secreted pyrogens produced more in response to MDP. They concluded that the monocyte-macrophages were the primary source of endogenous pyrogen production by MDP. It may be noted here that MDP and its analogues induced gelation of the amoebocyte lysate of *Tachypleus tridentatus*, although much higher dosages were required than LPS, whereas adjuvant-inactive analogues of MDP were inactive (Kotani *et al.*, 1977b).

There are in the literature a few reports of MDP derivatives which are non-pyrogenic, but which are fully potent with respect to other BRM activities. One such compound is the lipophilic derivative of MDP, in which the 6-*O*-hydroxyl group of the muramic acid residue is replaced by α-branched long-chain fatty acids. Compounds such as B30–MDP are practically non-pyrogenic, although they evoke a distinct febrile response in rabbits following intracisternal injection (Kotani *et al.*, 1981). Another similar compound is murabutide (Figure 2) (Lefrancier *et al.*, 1982), which is devoid of pyrogenicity in both direct and indirect mechanisms (no induction of endogenous pyrogen), and does not induce a febrile response even after the very sensitive intracerebroventricular administration (Chedid *et al.*, 1982; Damais *et al.*, 1982). Nevertheless, this compound retained the ability to enhance both an antigen-specific immune response and non-specific host resistance to infections (Chedid *et al.*, 1982), and to stimulate macrophages to secrete LAF (Damais *et al.*, 1982). In addition, murabutide does not induce leucocytopaenia (decrease of circulating granulocytes, lymphocytes and monocytes) which was observed following the intravenous injection of MDP in rabbits (Chedid *et al.*, 1982). Another approach by Rotta *et al.* (1983) demonstrated that among synthetic compounds mimicking subunits of streptococcal peptidoglycan, a hexapeptide devoid of muramic acid was distinctly pyrogenic. Repeated administration of these pyrogens to rabbits induced tolerance to the pyrogenicity of corresponding materials. Such rabbits showed tolerance to MDP were not tolerant to the pyrogenic hexapeptide. And animals that were tolerant to either MDP or the hexapeptide were not tolerant to peptidoglycan. From these findings they assumed that peptidoglycan contained more than one pyrogenic subunit.

3. Other Harmful Activities

Nagao *et al.* (1982a) observed that necrotic inflammation was provoked by MDP at the site of a previous injection of tubercle bacilli in guinea pigs. In brief, guinea pigs were prepared by an intra-footpad injection of heat-killed tubercle bacilli included in a w/o emulsion. Subsequently, they produced an extensive inflammation with a marked swelling, exudation, haemorrhage, necrosis and ulceration at the pretreated site, 24 h after the provocative injection of aqueous MDP. Sometimes animals died of generalized shock. Susceptibility to this effect was affected by species and strain differences, the phenomenon being clearly observed with guinea pigs of some lines, including outbred Hartley strain, but not with rats (WKA) and rabbits. They further investigated the conditions required for preparation and provocation of this phenomenon in Hartley guinea pigs (Nagao and Tanaka, 1983b). Regarding the preparative activity, myco-bacterial and to a lesser extent nocardial cells were found to be active among several gram-positive bacterial cells. LPS was neither active in preparation nor in provocation. On the other hand, MDP showed preparative activity if it was administered with an appropriate antigen such as ovalbumin in a w/o emulsion, suggesting the participation of DTH-type hypersensitivity in the preparatory process. With regard to the provocative activity, MDP and some of its derivatives [L18–MDP, MDP–Lys, MDP–Lys(L18), GlcNAc–MurNAc-dipeptide, MDP–meso-2,6-diaminopimelic acid (a A_2pm type)] were active, MurNAc(–GlcNAc)-dipeptide and GlcNAc–MurNAc-tripeptide were marginally active, while MurNAc-tetrapeptide (a A_2pm type) and larger peptidoglycan fragments prepared by use of peptidoglycan-degrading enzymes were inactive. B30–MDP was inactive when injected as a suspension in PBS, but was active in provocation as a solution in Nikkol HCO-60, a non-ionic detergent for clinical use. The mechanism of this phenomenon remains to be solved by further study, but seems to be different from those involved in Shwartzman's phenomenon (Shwartzman, 1928).

The recent study of McAdam *et al.* (1983) concerns a possible undesirable activity of muramyl-peptides. A secondary amyloidosis induced in mice by administration of FCA was accompanied by serum amyloid protein (SAA) synthesis. This was induced in cultured hepatocytes by a macrophage-derived interleukin 1. These workers showed that SAA production in mice was markedly elevated after intraperitoneal injection of MDP (100 μg) in saline, but not with an MDP analogue whose L-Ala residue was replaced by D-Ala. Murabutide required a 100-fold greater dosage than MDP for the stimulation of SAA synthesis. Mice that received an intraperitoneal injection of MDP together with amyloid-enhancing factor in FIA produced histologically detectable amyloidosis, but even repeated intraperitoneal injections of MDP in saline did not induce secondary amyloidosis.

Finally, we will briefly refer to a toxicity study of MDP and nor-MDP by Wachsmuth and Dukor (1982). Their data indicated that in mice repeated intravenous or subcutaneous administrations of huge amounts of MDP and nor-MDP were very well tolerated without any detectable adverse effects, whilst in dogs MDP induced substantial inflammatory reactions and activation of the reticuloendothelial system which was manifest even after two injections of 5 mg (per kg per day); nor-MDP also induced similar toxic reactions. They concluded: 'In view of the dramatic species differences in the sensitivity to muramyl-peptides, particular care should be exercised in interpretation of the pharmacological and toxicological data obtained with this class of compounds in experimental animals and in the extrapolation of such findings to man.'

IV. A NEW ASPECT REGARDING MURAMYL-PEPTIDES AS ENDOGENOUS IMMUNOMODULATORS OR VITAMINS

A few years ago, one of us set forth the opinion that, 'Considering that we spend our entire lives together with multitudes of bacteria, present both inside and outside our bodies, it is logical to assume that the biological properties of bacterial wall peptidoglycan must somehow be associated with our (the host) defence mechanisms and other essential physiological phenomena. Therefore, in the future it seems to be significant to evaluate the physiological, pathological, and pharmacological activities of bacterial cell wall, with regard to potential roles in the maturation and maintenance of these functions' (Kotani, 1980; see also Kotani *et al.*, 1981). At that time this statement had not been supported by any experimental evidence, except the finding that the cell walls of bacterial species which undergo no natural interactions with mammals exhibited no or only weak immunopharmacological activities in the majority of *in vivo* and *in vitro* assays (Kotani *et al.*, 1977c,d; Takada *et al.*, 1979b; Ogawa *et al.*, 1982b), in contrast to the walls of bacteria parasitic or indigenous to mammals. It was suggested that this difference was probably determined by the chemical or molecular structure of a peptidoglycan portion (Schleifer and Kandler, 1972). However, experimental data supporting the above speculation have now rapidly accumulated. Krueger *et al.* (1982a) demonstrated that a sleep-promoting principle, Factor S, which was first isolated from brain and cerebrospinal fluid of sleep-deprived animals and then purified from human urine (Krueger *et al.*, 1978, 1980), was a small glycopeptide composed of glutamic acid, alanine, diaminopimelic acid, and muramic acid in molar ratios of 2:2:1:1. Krueger *et al.* (1982b) finally revealed that synthetic MDP and MDP–L-Lys could mimic the sleep-inducing (somnogenic) effects of the natural peptide.

Evidence indicating the physiological role played by muramyl-peptides came from another line of approach, namely studies on the metabolic fate of peptidoglycan fragments including MDP and its derivatives. Parant *et al.* (1979) reported that when [^{14}C]MDP was injected intravenously or subcutaneously into mice, more than 50% of the compound was recovered in urine during the 30 min after the injection, and more than 90% after 2 h without degradation of the molecule. On the other hand, Tomašić *et al.* (1980) revealed that the ^{14}C-labelled peptidoglycan monomer, GlcNAc–MurNAc–L-Ala–D-isoGln–meso-A$_2$pm–D-Ala–D-Ala, was partially degraded *in vivo* into the disaccharide and pentapeptide moieties. This study was confirmed by findings that more than 90% of a peptidoglycan monomer was metabolized *in vitro* after 2 h of incubation with plasma and serum from mouse and man (Ladešić *et al.*, 1981), and that *N*-acetylmuramyl–L-alanine amidase (mucopeptide amidohydrolase) was detected in human, mouse, bovine and sheep sera (Valinger *et al.*, 1982). Yapo *et al.* (1982) also observed that muramyl-pentapeptide (MurNAc–L-Ala–D-isoGln–meso-A_2pm–D-Ala–D-Ala) was digested to meso-A_2pm and D-iso-Gln–meso-A_2pm–D-Ala–D-Ala. Thus, there seem to be several enzymes in mammals that recognize various muramyl-peptides as substrate and may contribute to the regulation of immune status.

The above findings moved Lederer, a pioneer of studies of immunomodulating activities of bacterial cell walls and related synthetic compounds, to propose: 'It is well known that germ-free animals are highly susceptible to infection; their immune systems are practically nonexistent and need stimulation by bacterial (peptidoglycan) products to become fully operative. We are thus led to consider muramyl peptides as a new category of vitamins: trace compounds, derived from the food (or the intestinal flora) and indispensable for the normal health of our organism (Lederer, 1982).

On the other hand, Chedid (1983b) has expressed his opinion that muramyl-peptides can work as possible endogenous immunopharmacological mediators, on the basis of evidence that MDP-activated macrophages produced Factor S as a different entity from both LAF and endogenous pyrogen, and that anti-MDP monoclonal antibody bound to Factor S isolated from human urine or rabbit brain could also specifically inhibit the activity of human monokines. Thus several of the biological activities of the muramyl-peptides could be due to biological mimicry with endogenous products.

REFERENCES

Adam, A., Souvannavong, V., and Lederer, E. (1978). Non-specific MIF-like activity induced by the synthetic immunoadjuvant: *N*-acetylmuramyl–L-alanyl–D-isoglutamine (MDP). *Biochem. Biophys. Res. Commun.*, **85**, 684–690.

Adam, A., Petit, J.-F., Lefrancier, P., and Lederer, E. (1981). Muramyl peptides. Chemical structure, biological activity and mechanism of action. *Mol. Cell. Biochem.*, **41**, 27–47.

Akagawa, K. S., and Tokunaga, T. (1980). Effect of synthetic muramyl dipeptide (MDP) on differentiation of myeloid leukemic cells. *Microbiol. Immunol.*, **24**, 1005–1011.

Arnon, R., Sela, M., Parant, M., and Chedid, L. (1980). Antiviral response elicited by a completely synthetic antigen with built-in adjuvanticity. *Proc. Natl. Acad. Sci. USA*, **77**, 6769–6772.

Audibert, F., and Chedid, L. (1976). Distinctive adjuvanticity of synthetic analogs of mycobacterial water-soluble components. *Cell. Immunol.*, **21**, 243–249.

Audibert, F., and Chedid, L. (1980). Recent advances concerning the use of muramyl dipeptide derivatives as vaccine potentiators. *Prog. Clin. Biol. Res.*, **47**, 325–338.

Audibert, F., and Jolivet, M. (1982). Immunization by a diphtheria toxin oligopeptide and MDP, a model for synthetic vaccines. In *Immunomodulation by Microbial Products and Related Synthetic Compounds* (Eds. Y. Yamamura, S. Kotani, I. Azuma, A. Koda and T. Shiba), pp.241–244. Excerpta Medica, Amsterdam.

Audibert, F., Heymer, B., Gros, C., Schleifer, K. H., Seidl, P. H., and Chedid, L. (1978). Absence of binding of MDP, a synthetic immunoadjuvant, to anti-peptidoglycan antibodies. *J. Immunol.*, **121**, 1219–1222.

Audibert, F., Parant, M., Damais, C., Lefrancier, P., Derrien, M., Choay, J. and Chedid, L. (1980). Dissociation of immunostimulant activities of muramyl dipeptide (MDP) by linking amino-acids or peptides to the glutaminyl residue. *Biochem. Biophys. Res. Commun.*, **96**, 915–923.

Audibert, F., Jolivet, M., Chedid, L., Alouf, J. E., Boquet, P., Rivaille, P., and Siffert, O. (1981). Active antitoxic immunization by a diphtheria toxin synthetic oligopeptide. *Nature*, **289**, 593–594.

Audibert, F., Jolivet, M., and Carelli, C. (1983). Use of MDP with diphtheric or other synthetic oligopeptides as a model for totally synthetic vaccines. *Adv. Immunopharmacol.*, **2**, 429–434.

Azuma, I., Sugimura, K., Taniyama, T., Yamawaki, M., Yamamura, Y., Kusumoto, S., Okada, S., and Shiba, T. (1976). Adjuvant activity of mycobacterial fractions: adjuvant activity of synthetic *N*-acetylmuramyl-dipeptide and the related compounds. *Infect. Immun.*, **14**, 18–27.

Azuma, I., Uemiya, M., Saiki, I., Yamawaki, M., Tanio, Y., Kusumoto, S., Shiba, T., Kusama, T., Tobe, K., Ogawa, H., and Yamamura, Y. (1979a). Synthetic immunoadjuvants. New immunotherapeutic agents. *Dev. Immunol.*, **6**, 311–330.

Azuma, I., Yamawaki, M., Uemiya, M., Saiki, I., Tanio, Y., Kobayashi, S., Fukuda, T., Imada, I., and Yamamura, Y. (1979b). Adjuvant and antitumor activities of quinonyl-*N*-acetylmuramyl-dipeptides. *Gann*, **70**, 847–848.

Binz, H., Tarcsay, L., Wigzell, and Dukor, P. (1981). Specific impaired alloreactivity of mice immunized with syngeneic MLC T-lymphoblasts using muramylpeptides as adjuvant. *Transplant. Proc.*, **13**, 566–573.

Carelli, C., Audibert, F., Gaillard, J., and Chedid, L. (1982). Immunological castration of male mice by a totally synthetic vaccine administered in saline. *Proc. Natl. Acad. Sci. USA*, **79**, 5392–5395.

Chedid, L. (1983a). Adjuvants for vaccines. *Adv. Immunopharmacol.*, **2**, 401–406.

Chedid, L. (1983b). Muramyl peptides as possible endogenous immunopharmacological mediators. *Microbiol. Immunol.*, **27**, 723–732.

Chedid, L., and Audibert, F. (1982). Utilization of muramyl dipeptide derivatives as adjuvants of synthetic vaccines. In *Immunomodulation by Microbial Products and Related Synthetic Compounds* (Eds. Y. Yamamura, S. Kotani, I. Azuma, A. Koda and T. Shiba), pp.48–59. Excerpta Medica, Amsterdam.

Chedid, L., Audibert, F., Lefrancier, P., Choay, J., and Lederer, E. (1976). Modulation of the immune response by a synthetic adjuvant and analogs. *Proc. Natl. Acad. Sci. USA*, **73**, 2472–2475.

Chedid, L., Parant, M., Parant, F., Lefrancier, P., Choay, J., and Lederer, E. (1977). Enhancement of nonspecific immunity to *Klebsiella pneumoniae* infection by a synthetic immunoadjuvant (*N*-acetylmuramyl-L-alanyl-D-isoglutamine) and several analogs. *Proc. Natl. Acad. Sci. USA*, **74**, 2089–2093.

Chedid, L., Audibert, F., and Johnson, A. G. (1978). Biological activities of muramyl dipeptide, a synthetic glycopeptide analogous to bacterial immunoregulating agents. *Prog. Allergy*, **25**, 63–105.

Chedid, L. A., Parant, M. A., Audibert, F. M., Riveau, G. J., Parant, F. J., Lederer, E., Choay, J. P., and Lefrancier, P. L. (1982). Biological activity of a new synthetic muramyl peptide adjuvant devoid of pyrogenicity. *Infect. Immun.*, **35**, 417–424.

Cummings, N. P., Pabst, M. J., and Johnston, R. B., Jr. (1980). Activation of macrophages of enhanced release of superoxide anion and greater killing of *Candida albicans* by injection of muramyl dipeptide. *J. Exp. Med.*, **152**, 1659–1669.

Damais, C., Parant, M., and Chedid, L. (1977). Nonspecific activation of murine spleen cells *in vitro* by a synthetic immunoadjuvant (*N*-acetylmuramyl–L-alanyl–D-isoglutamine). *Cell. Immunol.*, **34**, 49–56.

Damais, C., Parant, M., Chedid, L., Lefrancier, P., and Choay, J. (1978). *In vitro* spleen cell responsiveness to various analogs of MDP (*N*-acetylmuramyl–L-alanyl–D-isoglutamine), a synthetic immunoadjuvant, in MDP high-responder mice. *Cell. Immunol.*, **35**, 173–179.

Damais, C., Riveau, G., Parant, M., Gerota, J., and Chedid, L. (1982). Production of lymphocyte activating factor in the absence of endogenous pyrogen by rabbit or human leukocytes stimulated by a muramyl dipeptide derivative. *Int. J. Immunopharmacol.*, **4**, 451–462.

Dewhirst, F. E. (1982). *N*-acetyl muramyl dipeptide stimulation of bone resorption in tissue culture. *Infect. Immun.*, **35**, 133–137.

Dinarello, C. A., Elin, R. J., Chedid, L., and Wolff, S. M. (1978). The pyrogenicity of the synthetic adjuvant muramyl dipeptide and two structural analogues. *J. Infect. Dis.*, **138**, 760–767.

Dziak, R., Rowe, D. J., Brown, M. J., and Hausmann, E. (1982). Effects of synthetic muramyl dipeptide on bone metabolism in the fetal rat. *Arch. Oral. Biol.*, **27**, 787–791.

Emori, K., and Tanaka, A. (1978). Granuloma formation by synthetic bacterial cell wall fragment: muramyl dipeptide. *Infect. Immun.*, **19**, 613–620.

Fevrier, M., Birrien, J. L., Leclerc, C., Chedid, L., and Liacopoulos, P. (1978). The macrophage, target cell of the synthetic adjuvant muramyl dipeptide. *Eur. J. Immunol.*, **8**, 558–562.

Fidler, I. J. (1981). The *in situ* induction of tumoricidal activity in alveolar macrophages by liposomes containing muramyl dipeptide is a thymus-independent process. *J. Immunol.*, **127**, 1719–1720.

Fidler, I. J., Sone, S., Fogler, W. E., and Barnes, Z. L. (1981). Eradication of spontaneous metastases and activation of alveolar macrophages by intravenous injection of liposomes containing muramyl dipeptide. *Proc. Natl. Acad. Sci. USA*, **78**, 1680–1684.

Fraser-Smith, E. B., Waters, R. V., and Matthews, T. R. (1982). Correlation between *in vivo* anti-*Pseudomonas* and anti-*Candida* activities and clearance of carbon by the reticuloendothelial system for various muramyl dipeptide analogs, using normal and immunosuppressed mice. *Infect. Immun.*, **35**, 105–110.

Fukutomi, Y., Onozaki, K., Hashimoto, T., Nagao, S., and Tanaka, A. (1981). Scanning electron microscopic study of guinea pig macrophages activated by MDP. *Proc. Jpn. Soc. Immunol.*, **11**, 145–146 (in Japanese).

Galelli, A., Garrec, Y. L., Chedid, L., Lefrancier, P., Derrien, M., and Level, M. (1980). Macrophage stimulation *in vitro* by an inactive muramyl dipeptide derivative after conjugation to a multi-poly(DL-alanyl)–poly(L-lysine) carrier. *Infect. Immun.*, **28**, 1–5.

Hadden, J. W. (1978). Effects of isoprinosine, levamisole, muramyl dipeptide, and SM1213 on lymphocyte and macrophage function *in vitro*. *Cancer Treat. Rep.*, **62**, 1981–1985.

Hadden, J. W., England, A., Sadlik, J. R., and Hadden, E. M. (1979). The comparative effects of isoprinosine, levamisole, muramyl dipeptide and SM1213 on lymphocyte and macrophage proliferation and activation *in vitro*. *Int. J. Immunopharmacol.*, **1**, 17–27.

Hamada, S., Narita, T., Kotani, S., and Kato, K. (1971). Studies on cell walls of group A *Streptococcus pyogenes*, type 12. II. Pyrogenic and related biological activities of the higher molecular weight fraction of an enzymatic digest of the cell walls. *Biken J.*, **14**, 217–231.

Hamilton, J. A., Zabriskie, J. B., Lachman, L. B., and Chen, Y. (1982). Streptococcal cell walls and synovial cell activation. Stimulation of synovial fibroblast plasminogen activator activity by monocytes treated with group A streptococcal cell wall sonicates and muramyl dipeptide. *J. Exp. Med.*, **155**, 1702–1718.

Harada, K., Kotani, S., Takada, H., Tsujimoto, M., Hirachi, Y., Kusumoto, S., Shiba, T., Kawata, S., Yokogawa, K., Nishimura, H., Kitaura, T., and Nakajima, T. (1982). Liberation of serotonin from rabbit blood platelets by bacterial cell walls and related compounds. *Infect. Immun.*, **37**, 1181–1190.

Heymer, B., and Rietschel, E. T. (1977). Biological properties of peptidoglycans. In *Microbiology 1977* (Ed. D. Schlessinger), pp.344–349. American Society for Microbiology, Washington, DC.

Homma, Y., Onozaki, K., Hashimoto, T., Miura, K., Nagao, S., and Tanaka, A. (1981). Different effect of (L)-fucose binding lectin on macrophages migration inhibition caused by guinea pig migration inhibitory factor and synthetic muramyl dipeptide. *Int. Arch. Allergy Appl. Immunol.*, **65**, 27–33.

Hotta, H., Hotta, S., Takada, H., and Kotani, S. (1982). Enhancement of dengue virus type 2 replication in mouse macrophage cultures by bacterial cell walls and their components. *Jpn. J. Microbiol.*, **37**, 222 (in Japanese).

Hotta, H., Hotta, S., Takada, H., Kotani, S., Tanaka, S., and Ohki, M. (1983). Enhancement of dengue-2 virus replication in mouse macrophage cultures by bacterial cell walls, peptidoglycans and a polymer of peptidoglycan subunits. *Infect. Immun.*, **41**, 462–469.

Igarashi, T., Okada, M., Azuma, I., and Yamamura, Y. (1977). Adjuvant activity of synthetic *N*-acetylmuramyl–L-alanyl–D-isoglutamine and related compounds on cell-mediated cytotoxicity in syngeneic mice. *Cell. Immunol.*, **34**, 270–278.

Imai, K., and Tanaka, A. (1981). Effect of muramyldipeptide, a synthetic bacterial adjuvant, on enzyme release from cultured mouse macrophages. *Microbiol. Immunol.*, **25**, 51–62.

Imai, K., Tomioka, M., Nagao, S., Kushima, K., and Tanaka, A. (1980). Biochemical evidence for activation of guinea pig macrophages by muramyl dipeptide. *Biomed. Res.*, **1**, 300–307.

Iribe, H., Koga, T., Onoue, K., Kotani, S., Kusumoto, S., and Shiba, T. (1981). Macrophage-stimulating effect of a synthetic muramyl dipeptide and its adjuvant-active and -inactive analogs for the production of T-cell activating monokines. *Cell. Immunol.*, **64**, 73–83.

Iribe, H., Koga, T., and Onoue, K. (1982). Production of T cell-activating monokine of guinea pig macrophages induced by MDP and partial characterization of the monokine. *J. Immunol.*, **129**, 1029–1032.

Iribe, H., Koga, T., Kotani, S., Kusumoto, S., and Shiba, T. (1983). Stimulating effect of MDP and its adjuvant-active analogs on guinea pig fibroblasts for the production of thymocyte-activating factor. *J. Exp. Med.*, **157**, 2190–2195.

Ishihara, Y., Takada, H., Kotani, S., Kusumoto, S., Shiba, T., Kawata, S., and Yokogawa, K. (1982). Stimulation of polymorphonuclear leukocytes by bacterial cell wall components and related synthetic compounds. In *Immunomodulation by Microbial Products and Related Synthetic Compounds* (Eds. Y. Yamamura, S. Kotani, I. Azuma, A. Koda and T. Shiba), pp.217–220. Excerpta Medica, Amsterdam.

Jolivet, M., Sache, E., and Audibert, F. (1981). Biological studies of lipophilic MDP-derivatives incorporated in liposomes. *Immunol. Commun.*, **10**, 511–522.

Juy, D., and Chedid, L. (1975). Comparison between macrophage activation and enhancement of nonspecific resistance to tumors by mycobacterial immunoadjuvants. *Proc. Natl. Acad. Sci. USA*, **72**, 4105–4109.

Kaku, M., Yagawa, K., Nagao, S., and Tanaka, A. (1983). Enhanced superoxide anion release from phagocytes by muramyl dipeptide or lipopolysaccharide. *Infect. Immun.*, **39**, 559–564.

Kato, K., Kotani, S., Kawano, K., Monodane, T., Kitamura, H., Kusumoto, S., and Shiba, T. (1982). Monocytosis-inducing activity of *L. monocytogenes* cell wall and muramyl dipeptide. In *Immunomodulation by Microbial Products and Related Synthetic Compounds* (Eds. Y. Yamamura, S. Kotani, I. Azuma, A, Koda and T. Shiba), pp.181–184. Excerpta Medica, Amsterdam.

Kawasaki, A. (1982). Activation of human complement system by bacterial cell walls, their water-soluble enzymatic digests and related synthetic compounds. *J. Osaka Univ. Dent. Soc.*, **27**, 46–61 (in Japanese with English summary).

Key, M. E., Talmadge, J. E., Fogler, W. E., Bucana, C., and Fidler, I. J. (1982). Isolation of tumoricidal macrophages from lung melanoma metastases of mice treated systemically with liposomes containing a lipophilic derivative of muramyl dipeptide. *J. Natl. Cancer Inst.*, **69**, 1189–1198.

Kishimoto, T., Hirai, Y., Nakanishi, K., Azuma, I., Nagamatsu, A., and Yamamura, Y. (1979). Regulation of antibody response in different immunoglobulin classes. VI. Selective suppression of IgE response by administration of antigen-conjugated muramylpeptides. *J. Immunol.*, **123**, 2709–2715.

Kiyono, H., McGhee, J. R., Kearney, J. F., and Michalek, S. M. (1982). Enhancement of *in vitro* responses of murine Peyer's patch cultures by concanavalin A, muramyl dipeptide and lipopolysaccharide. *Scand. J. Immunol.*, **15**, 329–339.

Koga, T., Sakamoto, S., Onoue, K., Kotani, S., and Sumiyoshi, A. (1980). Efficient induction of collagen arthritis by the use of a synthetic muramyl dipeptide. *Arthritis Rheum.*, **23**, 993–997.

Kohashi, O., Kotani, S., Shiba, T., and Ozawa, A. (1979). Synergistic effect of polyriboinosinic acid:polyribocytidylic acid and either bacterial peptidoglycans or synthetic *N*-acetylmuramyl peptides on production of adjuvant-induced arthritis in rats. *Infect. Immun.*, **26**, 690–687.

Kohashi, O., Tanaka, A., Kotani, S., Shiba, T., Kusumoto, S., Yokogawa, K., Kawata, S., and Ozawa, A. (1980). Arthritis-inducing ability of a synthetic adjuvant, *N*-acetylmuramyl peptides, and bacterial disaccharide peptides related to different oil vehicles and their composition. *Infect. Immun.*, **29**, 70–75.

Kohashi, O., Kohashi, Y., Kotani, S., and Osawa, A. (1981a). A new model of experimental arthritis induced by an aqueous form of synthetic adjuvant in immunodeficient rats (SHR and nude rats). *Ryumachi*, **21** (Suppl.), 149–156.

Kohashi, O., Pearson, C. M., Tamaoki, N., Tanaka, A., Shimamura, K., Ozawa, A., Kotani, S., Saito, M., and Hoiki, K. (1981b). Role of thymus for *N*-acetyl muramyl–L-alanyl–D-isoglutamine-induced polyarthritis and granuloma formation in euthymic and athymic nude rats or in neonatally thymectomized rats. *Infect. Immun.*, **31**, 758–766.

Kotani, S. (1980). Modulation of host defence mechanisms by bacterial cell walls and related synthetic compounds. *Hoechst Immuno-Rev.*, **15** (special number), 38–69 and 95–103.

Kotani, S., Watanabe, Y., Shimono, T., Harada, K., Shiba, T., Kusumoto, S., Yokogawa, K., and Taniguchi, M. (1976). Correlation between the immunoadjuvant activities and pyrogenicities of synthetic *N*-acetylmuramyl-peptides or -amino acids. *Biken J.*, **19**, 9–13.

Kotani, S., Kinoshita, F., Morisaki, I, Shimono, T., Okunaga, T., Takada, H., Tsujimoto, M., Watanabe, Y., Kato, K., Shiba, T., Kusumoto, S., and Okada, S. (1977a). Immunoadjuvant activities of synthetic 6-*O*-acyl-*N*-acetylmuramyl-L-alanyl– D-isoglutamine with special reference to the effect of its administration with liposomes. *Biken J.*, **20**, 95–103.

Kotani, S., Watanabe, Y., Kinoshita, F., Kato, K., Harada, K., Shiba, T., Kusumoto, S., Tarumi, Y., Ikenaka, K., Okada, S., Kawata, S., and Yokogawa, K. (1977b). Gelation of the amoebocyte lysate of *Tachypleus tridentatus* by cell wall digest of several gram-positive bacteria and synthetic peptidoglycan subunits of natural and unnatural configurations. *Biken J.*, **20**, 5–10.

Kotani, S., Watanabe, Y., Kinoshita, F., Kato, K., and Perkins, H. R. (1977c). Immunoadjuvant activities of the enzymatic digests of bacterial cell walls lacking immunoadjuvancy by themselves. *Biken J.*, **20**, 87–90.

Kotani, S., Watanabe, Y., Kinoshita, F., Schleifer, K. H., and Perkins, H. R. (1977d). Inabilities as an immunoadjuvant of cell walls of the group B peptidoglycan types and those of arthrobacters. *Biken J.*, **20**, 1–4.

Kotani, S., Tsujimoto, M., Morisaki, I., Okunaga, T., Kinoshita, F., Takada, H., Kato, K., Shiba, T., Kusumoto, S., Inage, M., Yamamura, Y., and Azuma, I. (1978). Immunoadjuvant activities of mycoloyl and related high-molecular acyl derivatives (synthetic and semisynthetic) of *N*-acetylmuramyl-dipeptides. In *Thirteenth Joint Meeting Tuberculosis Panel. US–Japan Co-operative Medical Science Program*, pp.163–178. Osaka.

Kotani, S., Takada, H., Tsujimoto, M., Ogawa, T., Kato, K., Okunaga, T., Ishihara, Y., Kawasaki, A., Morisaki, I., Kono, N., Shimono, T., Shiba, T., Kusumoto, S., Inage, M., Harada, K., Kitaura, T., Kano, S., Inai, S., Nagaki, K., Matsumoto, M., Kubo, T., Kato, M., Tada, Z., Yokogawa, K., Kawata, S., and Inoue, A. (1981). Immunomodulating and related biological activities of bacterial cell walls and their components, enzymatically prepared or synthesized. In *Immunomodulation by Bacteria and Their Products* (Eds. H. Friedman, T. W. Klein, and S. Szentivanyi), pp.231–273. Plenum Press, New York.

Kotani, S., Takada, H., Tsujimoto, M., Kubo, T., Ogawa, T., Azuma, I., Ogawa, H., Matsumoto, K., Siddiqui, W. A., Tanaka, A., Nagao, S., Kohashi, O., Kanoh, S., Shiba, T., and Kusumoto, S. (1982). Nonspecific and antigen-specific stimulation of host defence mechanisms by lipophilic derivatives of muramyl dipeptides. In *Bacteria and Cancer* (Eds. J. Jeljaszewicz, G. Pulverer and W. Roszkowski), pp.67–107. Academic Press, London.

Kotani, S., Azuma, I., Takada, H., Tsujimoto, M., and Yamamura, Y. (1983). Muramyl dipeptides: Prospect for cancer treatments and immunostimulation. *Adv. Exp. Med. Biol.*, **166**, 117–158.

Kotani, S., Takada, H., Tsujimoto, M., Ogawa, T., Mori, Y., Koga, T., Iribe, H., Tanaka, A., Nagao, S., McGhee, J. R., Michalek, S. M., Morisaki, I., Nishimura, C., Ikeda, S., Kohashi, O., Ogawa, H., Ozawa, S., Hamada, S., Kawata, S., Shiba, T., and Kusumoto, S. (1984). Lipophilic muramyl peptides and synthetic lipid A analogs as immunomodulators, In (Eds. Yamamura, Y., and Tada, T.), Progress in Immunology V; Fifth International Congress of Immunology. p.1359–1377. Academic Press, Tokyo.

Krueger, J. M., Pappenheimer, J. R., and Karnovsky, M. L. (1978). Sleep-promoting factor S: purification and properties. *Proc. Natl. Acad. Sci. USA*, **75**, 5235–5238.

Krueger, J. M., Bacsik, J., and Garcia-Arraras, J. (1980). Sleep-promoting material from human urine and its relation to factor S from brain. *Am. J. Physiol.*, **238**, E116–E123.

Krueger, J. M., Pappenheimer, J. R., and Karnovsky, M. L. (1982a). The composition of sleep-promoting factor isolated from human urine. *J. Biol. Chem.*, **257**, 1644–1669.

Krueger, J. M., Pappenheimer, J. R., and Karnovsky, M. L. (1982b). Sléep-promoting effects of muramyl peptides. *Proc. Natl. Acad. Sci. USA*, **79**, 6102–6106.

Ladešíc, B., Tomašíc, J., Kveder, S., and Hršak, I. (1981). The metabolic fate of ^{14}C-labelled immunoadjuvant peptidoglycan monomer. II. *In vitro* studies. *Biochim. Biophys. Acta*, **678**, 12–17.

Leclerc, C., and Chedid, L. (1982). Macrophage activation by synthetic muramyl peptides. *Lymphokines*, **7**, 1–21.

Leclerc, C., Bourgeois, E., and Chedid, L. (1979). Enhancement by muramyl dipeptide of *in vitro* nude mice responses to a T-dependent antigen. *Immunol. Commun.*, **8**, 55–64.

Leclerc, C., Bourgeois, E., and Chedid, L. (1982). Demonstration of muramyl dipeptide (MDP)-induced T suppressor cells responsible for MDP immunosuppressive activity. *Eur. J. Immunol.*, **12**, 249–252.

Lederer, E. (1982). Immunomodulation by muramyl peptides: recent developments. *Clin. Immunol. Newslett.*, **3**, 83–86.

Lefrancier, P., Derrien, M., Jemet, X., Choay, J., Lederer, E., Audibert, F., Parant, M., Parant, M., and Chedid, L. (1982). Apyrogenic, adjuvant-active *N*-acetylmuramyl-dipeptides. *J. Med. Chem.*, **25**, 87–90.

Löwy, I., Bona, C., and Chedid, L. (1977). Target cells for the activity of a synthetic adjuvant: muramyl dipeptide. *Cell. Immunol.*, **29**, 195–199.

Löwy, I., Leclerc, C., and Chedid, L. (1980a). Induction of antibodies directed against self and altered-self determinants by a synthetic adjuvant, muramyl dipeptide and some of its derivatives. *Immunology*, **39**, 441–450.

Löwy, I., Theze, J., and Chedid, L. (1980b). Stimulàtion of the *in vivo* dinitrophenyl antibody response to the DNP conjugate of L-glutamic acid^{60}–L-alanine^{30}–L-tyrosine^{10} (GAT) polymer by a synthetic adjuvant, muramyl dipeptide (MDP): target cells for adjuvant activity and isotypic pattern of MDP-stimulated response. *J. Immunol.*, **124**, 100–104.

Maeda, K., Koga, T., Sakamoto, S., Onoue, K., Kotani, S., Kusumoto, S., Shiba, T., and Sumiyoshi, A. (1980). Structural requirement of synthetic *N*-acetylmuramyl dipeptides for induction of experimental allergic encephalomyelitis in the rat. *Microbiol. Immunol.*, **24**, 771–776.

Matsumoto, K., Ogawa, H., Kusama, T., Nagase, O., Sawaki, N., Inage, M., Kusumoto, S., Shiba, T., and Azuma, I. (1981a). Stimulation of nonspecific resistance to infection induced by 6-*O*-acyl muramyl dipeptide analogs in mice. *Infect. Immun.*, **32**, 748–758.

Matsumoto, K., Ogawa, H., Nagase, O., Kusama, T., and Azuma, I. (1981b). Stimulation of nonspecific host resistance to infection induced by muramyldipeptides. *Microbiol. Immunol.*, **25**, 1047–1058.

Matsumoto, K., Otani, T., Une, T., Osada, Y., Ogawa, H., and Azuma, I. (1983). Muramyl dipeptide analogs substituted in the γ-carboxyl group and evaluation of N^α-muramyl dipeptide–N^ϵ-stearoyllysine. *Infect. Immun.*, **39**, 1029–1040.

McAdam, K. P. W. J., Foss, N. T., Garcia, C., DeLellis, R., Chedid, L., Rees, R. J., and Wolff, S. M. (1983). Amyloidosis and the serum amyloid response to muramyl dipeptide analogs and different mycobacterial species. *Infect. Immun.*, **39**, 1147–1154.

Michalek, S. M., Morisaki, I., Kotani, S., Hamada, S., and McGhee, J. R. (1983). Oral immunization with antigen in liposomes containing MDP enhances secretory IgA immune responses. In International Symposium on *Immunomodulation by Chemically-Defined Adjuvants*, Program and Abstracts, p.45. Sapporo, Japan.

Misaki, A., Yukawa, S., Tsuchiya, K., and Yamasaki, T. (1966). Studies on cell walls of *Mycobacteria*. I. Chemical and biological properties of the cell walls and the mucopeptide of BCG. *J. Biochem. (Tokyo)*, **59**, 388–396.

Morrison, D. C., and Ryan, J. L. (1979). Bacterial endotoxins and host immune responses. *Adv. Immunol.*, **28**, 293–450.

Mozes, E., Sela, M., and Chedid, L. (1980). Efficient genetically controlled formation of antibody to a synthetic antigen [poly(LTyr,LGlu)–poly(DLAla)–poly(LLys)] covalently bound to a synthetic adjuvant (*N*-acetylmuramyl–L-alanyl–D-isoglutamine). *Proc. Natl. Acad. Sci. USA*, **77**, 4933–4937.

Nagai, Y., Akiyama, K., Kotani, S., Watanabe, Y., Shimono, T., Shiba, T., and Kusumoto, S. (1978a). Structural specificity of synthetic peptide adjuvant for induction of experimental allergic encephalomyelitis. *Cell. Immunol.*, **35**, 168–172.

Nagai, Y., Akiyama, K., Suzuki, K., Kotani, S., Watanabe, Y., Shimono, T., Shiba, T., Kusumoto, S., Ikuta, F., and Takeda, S. (1978b). Minimum structural requirements for encephalitogen and for adjuvant in the induction of experimental allergic encephalomyelitis. *Cell. Immunol.*, **35**, 158–167.

Nagao, S., and Tanaka, A. (1980). Muramyl dipeptide-induced adjuvant arthritis. *Infect. Immun.*, **28**, 624–626.

Nagao, S., and Tanaka, A. (1983a). Inhibition of macrophage DNA synthesis by immunomodulators. I. Suppression of [³H]thymidine incorporation into macrophages by MDP and LPS. *Microbiol. Immunol*, **27**, 377–387.

Nagao, S., and Tanaka, A. (1983b). Extensive necrosis caused by the injection of MDP. *Jpn. J. Bacteriol.*, **38**, 76–77 (in Japanese).

Nagao, S., Tanaka, A., Yamamoto, Y., Koga, T., Onoue, K., Shiba, T., Kusumoto, S., and Kotani, S. (1979). Inhibition of macrophage migration by muramyl peptides. *Infect. Immun.*, **24**, 308–312.

Nagao, S., Miki, T., and Tanaka, A. (1981a). Macrophage activation by muramyl dipeptide (MDP) without lymphocyte participation. *Microbiol. Immunol.*, **25**, 41–50.

Nagao, S., Ota, F., Emori, K., Inoue, K., and Tanaka, A. (1981b). Epithelioid granuloma induced by muramyl dipeptide in immunologically deficient rats. *Infect. Immun.*, **34**, 993–999.

Nagao, S., Iwata, Y., and Tanaka, A. (1982a). Extensive necrosis caused by the injection of MDP. In *Immunomodulation by Microbial Products and Related Synthetic Compounds* (Eds. Y. Yamamura, S. Kotani, I. Azuma, A. Koda and T. Shiba), pp.189–192. Excerpta Medica, Amsterdam.

Nagao, S., Tanaka, A., Onozaki, K., and Hashimoto, T. (1982b). Differences between macrophage migration inhibitions by lymphokines and muramyl dipeptide (MDP) or lipopolysaccharide (LPS): migration enhancement by lymphokines. *Cell. Immunol.*, **71**, 1–11.

Nichols, W. K., and Prosser, F. H. (1980). Induction of ornithine decarboxylase in macrophages by bacterial lipopolysaccharides (LPS) and mycobacterial cell wall material. *Life Sci.*, **27**, 913–920.

Nozawa, R. T., Sekiguchi, R., and Yokota, T. (1980). Stimulation by conditioned medium of L-929 fibroblasts, *E. coli* lipopolysaccharide, and muramyl dipeptide of candidacidal activity of mouse macrophages. *Cell. Immunol.*, **53**, 116–124.

Ogawa, T., Kotani, S., Fukuda, K., Tsukamoto, Y., Mori, M., Kusumoto, S., and Shiba, T. (1982a). Stimulation of migration of human monocytes by bacterial cell walls and muramyl peptides. *Infect. Immun.*, **38**, 817–824.

Ogawa, T., Kotani, S., Tsujimoto, M., Kusumoto, S., Shiba, T., Kawata, S., and Yokogawa, K. (1982b). Contractile effects of bacterial cell walls, their enzymatic digests, and muramyl dipeptides on ileal strips from guinea pigs. *Infect. Immun.*, **35**, 612–619.

Ogawa, T., Takada, H., Kotani, S., Kusumoto, S., Shiba, T., Kawata, S., Yokogawa, K., and Inoue, A. (1982c). 'Basophile leukocyte stimulation' by bacterial cell walls and related compounds. In *Immunomodulation by Microbial Products and Related*

Synthetic Compounds (Eds. Y. Yamamura, S. Kotani, I. Azuma, A. Koda and T. Shiba), pp.221–224. Excerpta Medica, Amsterdam.

Ogawa, T., Kotani, S., Kusumoto, S., and Shiba, T. (1983). Possible chemotaxis of human monocytes by *N*-acetylmuramyl–L-alanyl–D-isoglutamine. *Infect. Immun.*, **39**, 449–451.

Okunaga, T. (1980). Potentiation of immune responses to influenza split virus vaccine by synthetic 6-*O*-acyl-muramylpeptides. *J. Osaka Univ. Dent. Soc.*, **25**, 29–52 (in Japanese with English summary).

Oppenheim, J. J., Togawa, A., Chedid, L., and Mizel, S. (1980). Components of mycobacteria and muramyl dipeptide with adjuvant activity induce lymphocyte activating factor. *Cell. Immunol.*, **50**, 71–81.

Osada, Y., Mitsuyama, M., Matsumoto, K., Une, T., Otani, T., Ogawa, H., and Nomoto, K. (1982a). Stimulation of resistance of immunocompromised mice by a muramyl dipeptide analog. *Infect. Immun.*, **37**, 1285–1288.

Osada, Y., Mitsuyama, M., Une, T., Matsumoto, K., Otani, T., Satoh, M., Ogawa, H., and Nomoto, K. (1982b). Effect of L18–MDP(Ala), a synthetic derivative of muramyl dipeptide, on nonspecific resistance of mice to microbial infections. *Infect. Immun.*, **37**, 292–300.

Osada, Y., Otani, T., Sato, M., Une, T., Matsumoto, K., and Ogawa, H. (1982c). Polymorphonuclear leukocyte activation by a synthetic muramyl dipeptide analog. *Infect. Immun.*, **38**, 848–854.

Osada, Y., Ohtani, T., Une, T., Ogawa, H., and Nomoto, K. (1982d). Enhancement of non-specific resistance to *Pseudomonas pneumonia* by a synthetic derivative of muramyl dipeptide in immunosuppressed guinea pigs. *J. Gen. Microbiol.*, **128**, 2361–2370.

Pabst, M. J., Cummings, N. P., Shiba, T., Kusumoto, S., and Kotani, S. (1980a). Lipophilic derivative of muramyl dipeptide is more active than muramyl dipeptide in priming macrophages to release superoxide anion. *Infect. Immun.*, **29**, 617–622.

Pabst, M. J., and Johnston, R. B., Jr. (1980b). Increased production of superoxide anion by macrophages exposed *in vitro* to muramyl dipeptide or lipopolysaccharde. *J. Exp. Med.*, **151**, 101–114.

Pabst, M. J., Hedegaard, H. B., and Johnston, R. B., Jr. (1982). Cultured human monocytes require exposure to bacterial products to maintain an optimal oxygen radical response. *J. Immunol.*, **128**, 123–128.

Parant, M. (1979). Biologic properties of a new synthetic adjuvant, muramyl dipeptide (MDP), *Springer Semin. Immunopathol.*, **2**, 101–118.

Parant, M., Parant, F., Chedid, L., Yapo, A., Petit, J. F., and Lederer, E. (1979). Fate of the synthetic immunoadjuvant, muramyl dipeptide (^{14}C-labelled) in the mouse. *Int. J. Immunopharmacol.*, **1**, 35–41.

Parant, M. A., Audibert, F. M., Chedid, L., Level, M. R., Lefrancier, P. L., Choay, J. P., and Lederer, E. (1980a). Immunostimulant activities of a lipophilic muramyl dipeptide derivative and of desmuramyl peptidolipid analogs. *Infect. Immun.*, **27**, 826–831.

Parant, M., Riveau, G., Parant, F., Dinarello, C. A., Wolff, S. M., and Chedid, L. (1980b). Effect of indomethacin on increased resistance to bacterial infection and on febrile responses induced by muramyl dipeptide. *J. Infect. Dis.*, **142**, 708–715.

Prunet, J., Birrien, J. L., Panijel, J., and Liacopoulos, P. (1978). On the mechanism of early recovery of specifically depleted lymphoid cell populations by nonspecific activation of T cells. *Cell. Immunol.*, **37**, 151–161.

Raisz, L. G., Alander, C., Eilon, G., Whitehead, S. P., and Nuki, K. (1982). Effects of two bacterial products, muramyl dipeptide and endotoxin, on bone resorption in organ culture. *Calcif. Tissue Int.*, **34**, 365–369.

Reichert, C. M., Carelli, C., Jolivet, M., Audibert, F., Lefrancier, P., and Chedid, L. (1980). Synthesis of conjugates containing *N*-acetylmuramyl-L-alanyl-D-isoglutaminyl (MDP). Their use as hapten-carrier systems. *Mol. Immunol.*, **17**, 357–363.

Richerson, H. B., Suelzer, M. T., Swanson, P. A., Butler, J. E., Kopp, W. C., and Rose, E. F. (1982). Chronic hypersensitivity pneumonitis produced in the rabbit by the adjuvant effect of inhaled muramyl dipeptide (MDP). *Am. J. Pathol.*, **106**, 409–420.

Riveau, G., Mašek, K., Parant, M., and Chedid, L. (1980). Central pyrogenic activity of muramyl dipeptide. *J. Exp. Med.*, **152**, 869–877.

Roch-Arveiller, M., Tissot, M., Moachon, L., and Giroud, J. P. (1982). Effect of immunomodulating agents on leucocyte chemotaxis and cyclic nucleotides. *Agent. Action*, **12**, 353–359.

Rotta, J. (1975). Endotoxin-like properties of the peptidoglycan. *Z. Immunitaetsforsch.*, **149** (Suppl.), 230–244.

Rotta, J., Rýc, M., Mašek, K., and Zaoral, M. (1979). Biological activity of synthetic subunits of *Streptococcus* peptidoglycan. I. Pyrogenic and thrombocytolytic activity. *Exp. Cell. Biol.*, **47**, 258–268.

Rotta, J., Zaoral, M., Rýc, M., Straka, R., and Ježek, J. (1983). Biological activity of synthetic subunits of *Streptococcus* peptidoglycan. II. Relation of peptidoglycan subunits and analogues to fever effect and induction of tolerance. *Exp. Cell. Biol.*, **51**, 29–38.

Rutherford, B., Steffin, K., and Sexton, J. (1982). Activated human mononuclear phagocytes release a substance(s) that induced replication of quiescent human fibroblasts. *J. Reticuloendothel. Soc.*, **31**, 281–293.

Saiki, I., Tanio, Y., Yamawaki, M., Uemiya, M., Kobayashi, S., Fukuda, T., Yukimasa, H., Yamamura, Y., and Azuma, I. (1981). Adjuvant activities of quinonyl–*N*-acetyl muramyl dipeptides in mice and guinea pigs. *Infect. Immun.*, **31**, 114–121.

Saiki, I., Tanio, Y., Yamamoto, K., Yamamura, Y., and Azuma, I. (1983). Effect of quinonyl–*N*-acetyl muramyl dipeptide on immune responses in tumor-bearing mice. *Infect. Immun.*, **39**, 137–141.

Schindler, T. E., Chedid, L. A., and Hadden, J. W. (1982). Stimulatory effects of MDP and its butyl ester derivative on macrophage proliferation and activation *in vitro*. *Int. J. Immunopharmacol.*, **4**, 382.

Schleifer, K. H., and Kandler, O. (1972). Peptidoglycan types of bacterial cells walls and their taxonomic implications. *Bacteriol. Rev.*, **36**, 407–477.

Schroit, A. J., and Fidler, I. J. (1982). Effects of liposome structure and lipid composition on the activation of the tumoricidal properties of macrophages by liposomes containing muramyl dipeptide. *Cancer Res.*, **42**, 161–167.

Schwab, J. H. (1979). Acute and chronic inflammation induced by bacterial cell wall structures. In *Microbiology 1979* (Ed. D. Schlessinger), pp.209–214. American Society for Microbiology, Washington, DC.

Sharma, S. D., Tsai, V., Krahenbuhl, J. L., and Remington, J. S. (1981). Augmentation of mouse natural killer cell activity by muramyl dipeptide and its analogs. *Cell. Immunol.*, **62**, 101–109.

Shwartzman, G. (1928). A new phenomenon of local skin reactivity to *B. typhosus* culture filtrate. *Proc. Soc. Exp. Biol. Med.*, **25**, 560–561.

Siddiqui, W. A. (1982). Synthetic adjuvants and experimental human malaria vaccine. In *Immunomodulation by Microbial Products and Related Synthetic Compounds* (Eds. Y. Yamamura, S. Kotani, I. Azuma, A. Koda and T. Shiba), pp.245–249. Excerpta Medica, Amsterdam.

Siddiqui, W. A., Taylor, D. W., Kan, S.-C., Kramer, K., Richmond-Crum, S. M., Kotani, S., Shiba, T., and Kusumoto, S. (1978). Vaccination of experimental monkeys against *Plasmodium falciparum*: a possible safe adjuvant. *Science*, **201**, 1237–1239.

Sone, S., and Fidler, I. J. (1980). Synergistic activation by lymphokines and muramyl dipeptide of tumoricidal properties in rat alveolar macrophages. *J. Immunol.*, **125**, 2454–2460.

Souvannavong, V., Rimsky, L., and Adam, A. (1983). *In vitro* immune response to sheep erythrocytes in macrophage depleted cultures. Restoration with interleukin 1 or a monokine from resident macrophages and stimulation by *N*-acetyl-muramyl–L-alanyl–D-isoglutamine (MDP). *Biochem. Biophys. Res. Commun.*, **114**, 721–728.

Specter, S., Friedman, H., and Chedid, L. (1977). Dissociation between the adjuvant vs mitogenic activity of a synthetic muramyl dipeptide for murine splenocytes. *Proc. Soc. Exp. Biol. Med.*, **155**, 349–352.

Specter, S., Cimprich, R., Friedman, H., and Chedid, L. (1978). Stimulation of an enhanced *in vitro* immune response by a synthetic adjuvant, muramyl dipeptide. *J. Immunol.*, **120**, 487–491.

Staber, F. G., Gisler, R. H., Schumann, G., Tarcsay, L., Schläfli, E., and Dukor, P. (1978). Modulation of myelopoiesis by different bacterial cell–wall components: Induction of colony-stimulating activity (by pure preparations, low-molecular-weight degradation products, and a synthetic low-molecular analog of bacterial cell-wall components) *in vitro*. *Cell. Immunol.*, **37**, 174–187.

Stewart, J., Jones, D. G., and Kay, A. B. (1979). Metabolic studies on the uptake of [^{14}C]-histidine and [^{14}C]-histamine and histamine synthesis by guinea-pig basophils, *in vitro*. *Immunology*, **36**, 539–548.

Stewart-Tull, D. E. S. (1980). The immunological activities of bacterial peptidoglycans. *Annu. Rev. Microbiol.*, **34**, 311–340.

Sugimoto, M., Germain, P. N., Chedid, L., and Benacerraf, B. (1978). Enhancement of carrier-specific helper T cell function by the synthetic adjuvant, *N*-acetylmuramyl–L-alanyl–D-isoglutamine (MDP). *J. Immunol.*, **120**, 980–982.

Sugimura, K., Uemiya, M., Saiki, I., Azuma, I., and Yamamura, Y. (1979). The adjuvant activity of synthetic *N*-acetylmuramyl-dipeptide: evidence of initial target cells for the adjuvant activity. *Cell. Immunol.*, **43**, 137–149.

Takada, H., Kotani, S., Kusumoto, S., Tarumi, Y., Ikenaka, K., and Shiba, T. (1977). Mitogenic activity of adjuvant-active *N*-acetylmuramyl–L-alanyl–D-isoglutamine and its analogues. *Biken J.*, **20**, 81–85.

Takada, H., Tsujimoto, M., Kato, K., Kotani, S., Kusumoto, S., Inage, M., Shiba, T., Yano, I., Kawata, S., and Yokogawa, K. (1979a). Macrophage activation by bacterial cell walls and related synthetic compounds. *Infect. Immun.*, **25**, 48–53.

Takada, H., Tsujimoto, M., Kotani, S., Kusumoto, S., Inage, M., Shiba, T., Nagao, S., Yano, I., Kawata, S., and Yokogawa, K. (1979b). Mitogenic effects of bacterial cell walls, their fragments, and related synthetic compounds on thymocytes and splenocytes of guinea pigs. *Infect. Immun.*, **25**, 645–652.

Takada, H., Nagao, S., Kotani, S., Kawata, S., Yokogawa, K., Kusumoto, S., Shiba, T, and Yano, I. (1980). Mitogenic effects of bacterial cell walls and their components on murine splenocytes. *Biken J.*, **23**, 61–68.

Takada, H., Ishihara, Y., Kawasaki, A., Ogawa, T., Kotani, S., Kusumoto, S., Shiba, T., Kawata, S., and Yokogawa, K. (1982). Macrophage activation by bacterial cell walls and related synthetic compounds. 2. Surface phagocytosis enhancing activity. *Jpn. J. Bacteriol.*, **37**, 314 (in Japanese).

Tanaka, A. (1982). Macrophage activation by muramyl dipeptide (MDP). In *Immunomodulation by Microbial Products and Related Synthetic Compounds* (Eds. Y. Yamamura, S. Kotani, I. Azuma, A. Koda and T. Shiba), pp.72–83. Excerpta Medica, Amsterdam.

Tanaka, A., and Emori, K. (1980). Epithelioid granuloma formation by a synthetic bacterial cell wall component, muramyl dipeptide (MDP). *Am. J. Pathol.*, **98**, 733–742.

Tanaka, A., Nagao, S. Saito, R., Kotani, S., Kusumoto, S., and Shiba, T. (1977). Correlation of stereochemically specific structure in muramyl dipeptide between macrophage activation and adjuvant activity. *Biochem. Biophys. Res. Commun.*, **77**, 621–627.

Tanaka, A., Nagao, S., Nagao, R., Kotani, S., Shiba, T., and Kusumoto, S. (1979). Stimulation of the reticuloendothelial system of mice by muramyl dipeptide. *Infect. Immun.*, **24**, 302–307.

Tanaka, A., Nagao, S., Imai, K., and Mori, R. (1980). Macrophage activation by muramyl dipeptide as measured by macrophage spreading and attachment. *Microbiol. Immunol.*, **24**, 547–557.

Tanaka, A., Emori, K., Nagao, S., Kushima, K., Kohashi, O., Saito, M., and Kataoka, T. (1982a). Epithelioid granuloma formation requiring no T-cell function. *Am. J. Pathol.*, **106**, 165–170.

Tanaka, A., Nagao, S., Ikegami, S., Shiba, T., and Kotani, S. (1982b). The suppression of macrophage DNA synthesis by MDP, a probable correlate of macrophage activation. In *Immunomodulation by Microbial Products and Related Synthetic Compounds* (Eds. Y. Yamamura, S. Kotani, I. Azuma, A. Koda and T. Shiba), pp.201–204. Excerpta Medica, Amsterdam.

Taniyama, T., and Holden, H. T. (1979). Direct augmentation of cytolytic activity of tumor-derived macrophages and macrophage cell lines by muramyl dipeptide. *Cell. Immunol.*, **48**, 369–374.

Tenu, J.-P., Lederer, E., and Petit, J.-F. (1980). Stimulation of thymocyte mitogenic protein secretion and of cytostatic activity of mouse peritoneal macrophages by trehalose dimycolate and muramyl-dipeptide. *Eur. J. Immunol.*, **10**, 647–653.

Tomašić, J., Ladešić, B., Valinger, Z., and Hršak, I. (1980). The metabolic fate of ^{14}C-labeled peptidoglycan monomer in mice. I. Identification of the monomer and the corresponding pentapeptide in urine. *Biochim. Biophys. Acta*, **629**, 77–82.

Tsukamoto, Y., Helsel, W. E., and Wahl, S. M. (1981). Macrophage production of fibronectin, a chemoattractant for fibroblasts. *J. Immunol.*, **127**, 673–678.

Valinger, Z., Ladešić, B., and Tomašić, J. (1982). Partial purification and characterization of *N*-acetylmuramyl-L-alanine amidase from human and mouse serum. *Biochim. Biophys. Acta*, **701**, 63–71.

Wachsmuth, E. D., and Dukor, P. (1982). Immunopathology of muramyl-peptides. In *Immunomodulation by Microbial Products and Related Synthetic Compounds* (Eds. Y. Yamamura, S. Kotani, I. Azuma, A. Koda and T. Shiba), pp.60–71. Excerpta Medica, Amsterdam.

Wahl, S. M., Wahl, L. M., McCarthy, J. B., Chedid, L., and Mergenhagen, S. E. (1979). Macrophage activation by mycobacterial water soluble compounds and synthetic muramyl dipeptide. *J. Immunol.*, **122**, 2226–2231.

Waters, R. V., and Ferraresi, R. W. (1980). Muramyl dipeptide stimulation of particle clearance in several animal species. *J. Reticulonendothel. Soc.*, **28**, 457–471.

Watson, J., and Whitlock, C. (1978). Effect of a synthetic adjuvant on the induction of primary immune responses in T cell-depleted spleen cultures. *J. Immunol.*, **121**, 383–389.

Wilson, C. B., Bohnsack, J., and Weaver, W. M. (1982). Effects of muramyl dipeptide on superoxide anion release and on anti-microbial activity of human macrophages. *Clin. Exp. Immunol.*, **49**, 371–376.

Windle, B. E., Murphy, P. A., and Cooperman, S. (1983). Rabbit polymorphonuclear leukocytes do not secrete endogenous pyrogens or interleukin 1 when stimulated by endotoxin, polyinosine:polycytosine, or muramyl dipeptide. *Infect. Immun.*, **39**, 1142–1146.

Wood, D. D., and Staruch, M. J. (1981). Control of the mitogenicity of muramyl dipeptide. *Int. J. Immunopharmacol.*, **3**, 31–44.

Wuest, B., and Wachsmuth, E. D. (1982). Stimulatory effect of *N*-acetyl muramyl dipeptide *in vivo*: proliferation of bone marrow progenitor cells in mice. *Infect. Immun.*, **37**, 452–462.

Yamamoto, K., Kakinuma, M., Kato, K., Okuyama, H., and Azuma, I. (1980). Relationship of anti-tuberculous protection in lung granuloma produced by intravenous injection of synthetic 6-*O*-mycoloyl–*N*-acetylmuramyl–L-alanyl–D-isoglutamine with or without specific antigens. *Immunology*, **40**, 557–564.

Yamamoto, Y., Nagao, S., Tanaka, A., Koga, T., and Onoue, K. (1978). Inhibition of macrophage migration by synthetic muramyl dipeptide. *Biochem. Biophys. Res. Commun.*, **80**, 923–928.

Yamamura, Y., and Azuma, I. (1982). Cancer immunotherapy with cell-wall skeletons of BCG and *Nocardia rubra* and related synthetic compounds. In *Immunomodulation by Microbial Products and Related Synthetic Compounds* (Eds. Y. Yamamura, S. Kotani, I. Azuma, A. Koda and T. Shiba), pp.17–36. Excerpta Medica, Amsterdam.

Yapo, A., Petit, J. F., and Lederer, E. (1982). Fate of two ^{14}C labelled muramyl peptides: Ac-Mur–L-Ala–γ-D-Glu–meso-A$_2$pm and Ac-Mur–L-Ala–γ-D-Glu–meso-A$_2$pm–D-Ala–D-Ala. Evaluation of their ability to increase non specific resistance to *Klebsiella* infection. *Int. J. Immunopharmacol.*, **4**, 143–149.

Zídek, Z., Mašek, K., and Jiřička, Z. (1982). Arthritogenic activity of a synthetic immunoadjuvant, muramyl dipeptide. *Infect. Immun.*, **35**, 674–679.

Immunology of the Bacterial Cell Envelope
Edited by D. E. S. Stewart-Tull and M. Davies
© 1985 John Wiley & Sons Ltd.

CHAPTER 6

The Impact of Teichoic Acids upon the Immunological System

Frank W. Chorpenning
Department of Microbiology,
The Ohio State University, Columbus, OH 43210, USA

I. INTRODUCTION

A variety of relatively stable microbial products are released into the environment which are capable of producing important biological effects in animals, including man (Chorpenning, 1982). These substances include lipopolysaccharide (LPS), dextran (DX), peptidoglycan (PG), and teichoic acid (TA). The mechanisms by which the latter substance affects the immunological system are the subject of this review.

The phenomena to be discussed involve specific humoral and cellular responses to TA, relationship to disease including possible protection, non-specific activation of lymphocytes, immunomodulation, mitogenicity, cytotoxicity, cellular involvement, and possible relationships between these mechanisms. Other phenomena such as the sequence in development of 'natural' specific responses, cross-reactions, cycling of the response, factors governing immunogenicity, T-independence, and membrane binding will also be discussed. It will be shown by experimental demonstration *in vivo* and *in vitro* that glycerol teichoic acid (GTA) not only induces the expected specific responses of both 'natural' (environmental) and 'immune' varieties, but that it also regulates responses to unrelated antigens. Furthermore, direct evidence is presented to show that environmental GTA present in the food is capable of suppressing unrelated responses *in vivo*.

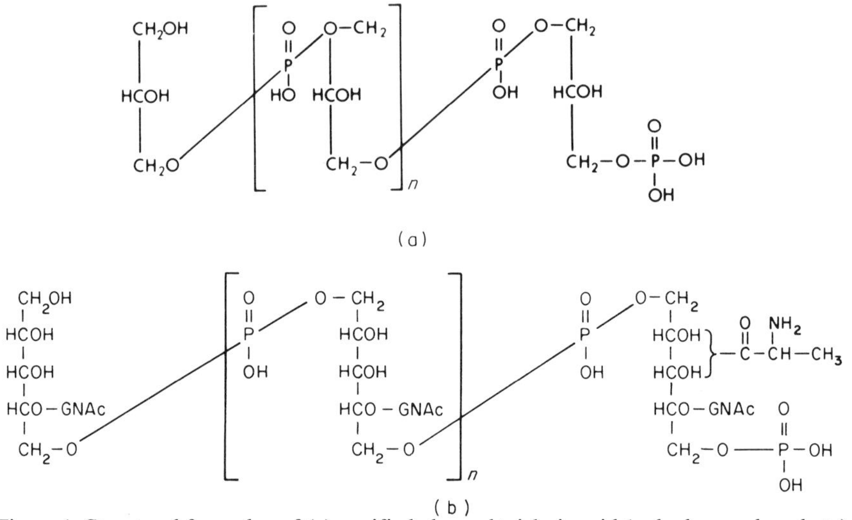

(a)

(b)

Figure 1. Structural formulae of (a) purified glycerol teichoic acid (polyglycerophosphate), and (b) teichoic acid in *Staphylococcus aureus* (polyribitol phosphate)

The teichoic acids are found in most gram-positive bacteria, occurring either in the cell wall or associated with the cell membrane. They are basically stable polymers which usually consist of a glycerophosphate or ribitol phosphate backbone upon which glycosyl or D-alanyl groups may be substituted (Figure 1). However, there are exceptions where saccharide units occur in the basic chain (Button et al., 1966). The glycerol variety may contain fatty acids (Wicken and Knox, 1975); however, it has been isolated from bacilli and the cell walls of *Streptococcus mutans* in a form free of covalently bound lipid (Cooper *et al.*, 1978). The question of whether fatty acids or other esters had been removed during purification was not addressed during the Cooper study. Chain lengths of the GTA polymer may vary depending upon the source (Dziarski, 1976) and probably upon extraction procedures (Cooper *et al.*, 1978). The material extracted from *Bacillus* sp. ATCC 29726 in the latter investigation averaged 19 glyceryl residues in length. The ribitol teichoic acids are found only in certain bacterial cell walls and usually contain D-alanine and saccharide substituents. They do not contain fatty acids.

In the bacterial cell wall, teichoic acids are covalently bound to the peptidoglycan complex (Button *et al.*, 1966), unassociated with lipid.

Lipoteichoic acids (LTA), on the other hand, appear to be associated with the membrane surface (Van Driel *et al.*, 1973). Teichoic acids dissociate readily from bacterial cells in the culture medium and by washing cells with saline solutions. GTA appears to be widespread in the environment due to its stability and multiple sources in gram-positive bacteria. It is present in amounts as high as 8 mg kg^{-1} in laboratory rat chow (Rozmiarek *et al.* 1977), presumably derived from gram-positive bacteria in feed sources.

II. SPECIFIC RESPONSES TO GLYCEROL TEICHOIC ACID

GTA as a component of bacterial cells is immunogenic in rabbits (McCarty, 1959), as are crude phenol extracts (Knox *et al.*, 1970), or complexes of purified GTA (Burger, 1966, Chorpenning and Stamper, 1973; Fiedel and Jackson, 1976), but rabbits are unresponsive to purified GTA. However, the rabbit is notoriously unresponsive to purified bacterial polysaccharides and we have shown that both rats and guinea pigs are responsive to a highly purified, protein-free GTA (Chorpenning *et al.*, 1979b).

An important determinant of GTA is the polyglycerophosphate backbone (PGP), which accounts for many of the cross-reactions observed (Chorpenning *et al.*, 1975; McCarty, 1959; Decker *et al.*, 1972). It is true that TA cross-reactions of other specificities also exist which are related to glycosyl substituents. For example, antibodies to TA containing α-D-glucosyl substituents cross-react with dextran from *Leuconostoc mesenteroides* (Knox and Wicken, 1972).

Antibodies of the PGP specificity arise naturally in human beings and animals (Decker *et al.*, 1972; Bolton and Chorpenning, 1974; Russell and Beighton, 1982), including germ-free (GF) guinea pigs (Frederick and Chorpenning, 1973) and rats (Rozmiarek *et al.*, 1977; Chorpenning *et al.*, 1979a). Cell-mediated immunity also has been demonstrated (Frederick *et al.*, 1972; Bolton and Chorpenning, 1974). The rather unusual occurrence of responses in GF animals was explained by the demonstration that ample GTA for stimulation was present in autoclaved rat chow and that a GTA-free diet abolished antibody production (Rozmiarck *et al.*, 1977). It was shown further that the presence of gram-positive bacteria in the intestinal flora did not stimulate production of the PGP antibodies and that removal of GTA from the diet eliminated these 'natural' antibodies. On the other hand, addition of heat-killed bacilli to the food or water of GTA-deprived rats resulted in antibody production. Similar results were obtained later by Oldfather and Chorpenning (1981), who showed that feeding of purified soluble GTA to deprived rats also restored antibody production. In fact, passive haemolysin titres and splenic plaque-forming cells rose to considerably higher levels than those resulting from oral bacillary or environmental stimulation. This model strongly suggests that 'natural' anti-PGP antibodies arise due to GTA present in the environment.

The characteristics of the naturally occurring anti-PGP antibodies have been studied in human beings, guinea pigs, rabbits, and rats (Frederick and

Chorpenning, 1974). Adult human beings and guinea pigs had antibodies of both IgM and IgG classes, while rabbits possessed only IgM antibodies. Some rats had antibodies in both classes while in others they occurred only in the IgM class. In guinea pigs, the IgG serum fraction was further fractionated on Sephadex DEAE A-50 to separate the IgG_1 and IgG_2. Anti-PGP activity was limited to the IgG_1 subclass. The average affinity of these antibodies for PGP was determined by equilibrium dialysis to range from 10^5 to 10^6 litres mole^{-1}, which is low for a secondary response (assuming repeated exposure to antigen) but is consistent with affinities of other 'natural' antibodies and with some primary responses. This situation may be explained by the occurrence of specific immunosuppression, to be discussed later. In this connection, when guinea pigs (Frederick and Chorpenning, 1973) or rats (Chorpenning *et al.*, 1979b) were injected with large doses of purified GTA, an anamnestic response occurred indicating that any existing suppression had been overcome.

Another interesting aspect of environmental elicitation of antibodies to PGP is their cyclic occurrence in Sprague-Dawley rats (Bolton *et al.*, 1977). In uninjected animals the cycles were asynchronous between individuals and varied in period, but when rats were injected simultaneously with GTA-bearing bacilli the cycles became synchronized. Cycling was evident also in the plaque-forming cells (PFC) of the spleen, mesenteric lymph nodes, and bone marrow. It was present for both direct and indirect PFC in spleen and lymph nodes but for only indirect PFC in the marrow. Recently Bolton (1978) reported that cycling of anti-PGP antibodies and PFC occurred in the peripheral blood of rabbits after the injection of heat-killed bacilli. These observations suggest that a regulatory mechanism is suppressing the level of response.

In rats and guinea pigs the ability to respond to environmental teichoic acid is frequently present at birth or shortly thereafter since IgM antibodies to PGP were produced and PFC observed (Chorpenning *et al.*, 1979a). However, IgG antibodies and indirect PFC do not appear until later in development, the antibodies reaching a frequency of 40% by the twentieth week with the PFC appearing somewhat earlier. It is interesting that cell-mediated immunity (CMI) of PGP specificity as measured by macrophage migration inhibition (MIF) and skin tests also appeared to be delayed in rats and guinea pigs until about 20 weeks of age (Chorpenning *et al.*, 1979a). Since the critical age for the onset of IgG and CMI responsiveness to injected GTA was prior to 12 weeks, it appears that both maturation of the immunologic system and another factor related to the type of stimulation (route, dosage, etc.) are involved in the delay. Furthermore, it appears that development or interaction of T-dependent mechanisms are involved in ways which influence both IgG and CMI responses.

As with a number of bacterial polysaccharides (see Chorpenning, 1982), GTA responses occur in the absence of T-lymphocytes (Oldfather and Chorpenning, 1980). When adult inbred Fisher 344 rats were thymectomized, X-irradiated (600 R), and reconstituted with bone marrow, mitogenic responses to concanavalin A or phytohaemagglutinin and antibody responses to sheep red blood cells (SRBC) were essentially eliminated, but PFC responses to 400 μg GTA were equal to those of control rats. The ability of B-lymphocytes alone to respond to purified GTA was confirmed later by Young and Chorpenning (1982a). BALB/c mouse splenocytes were separated into their component populations and examined for PFC responses to GTA *in vitro*. Purified B-cells exposed to GTA produced specific PFC in the absence of any detectable macrophages (MØ) or T-cells. However, the addition of MØ-T-cell mixtures increased GTA-specific PFC significantly. A further finding of considerable interest was that when GTA-responding B-cells were killed with 10^{-5} M 5-bromodeoxyuridine (BUdR) and light (Zoscke and Bach, 1971), the remaining viable B-cells could respond to GTA, but only if MØ and helper (Ly 1.2) T-cells were added to the culture (Young, 1982). Thus, it appears that the B-cells involved in the T-independent response to GTA are a separate subpopulation from those involved in the T-dependent (augmented) response.

III. RESPONSES TO RIBITOL TEICHOIC ACID

Although fewer studies have been made of 'natural' responses to ribitol teichoic acid (RTA) than of those to GTA, RTA is immunogenic in the complex form (Brock and Rieter, 1971) and 'natural' responses have been observed. The specificity of the reaction has usually been for *N*-acetylglucosamine. Torii *et al.* (1964) showed many years ago that normal human sera contained precipitating antibodies which reacted with RTA from *Staphylococcus aureus*. Specificities for both α- and β-*N*-acetylglucosamine were present. Daugharty *et al.* (1967) also demonstrated antibodies to RTA in normal sera. However, the origin (stimulus) of these antibodies has not been ascertained and the determinants are found in non-TA polysaccharides (Grov. 1969; Karakawa *et al.*, 1971; Cooper *et al.*, 1975). They are also substituents of some GTA antigens (Knox and Wicken, 1973). Apparently, fortuitous cross-reactions between the ribitol and glycerol backbones do not occur and antibodies to RTA usually are not specific for the backbone but rather for glycosyl substituents (Knox and Wicken, 1972). I am unaware of any reports of 'natural' antibodies specific for the RTA backbone.

It was reported earlier (Martin *et al.*, 1966) that RTA produced hypersensitivity in man. However, later investigators demonstrated that delayed-type hypersensitivity (DTH) experimentally induced in mice was due to peptidoglycan not RTA (Easmon and Glynn, 1978; Bolen and Tribble, 1979) and it has been suggested that the Martin RTA preparation contained peptidoglycan (Knox and Wicken, 1973). Thus, it appears that solid evidence for the involvement of RTA in induction of DTH, such as that demonstrated for GTA (Frederick *et al.*, 1972; Bolton and Chorpenning, 1974; Chorpenning *et al.*, 1979a), has not been forthcoming.

IV. INVOLVEMENT OF TEICHOIC ACIDS IN
DISEASE AND DIAGNOSIS

The foregoing observations have considerable significance and it is obvious that any relationship to disease deserves prompt attention. A major consideration is the possible involvement of TA determinants as protective antigens. Immunization of mice against staphylococcal infection by vaccination with whole *S. aureus* organisms or fractions was demonstrated a number of years ago (Ekstedt, 1963a, b) and it was suggested later that the protective antigen was teichoic acid (Ekstedt, 1966; Yoshida and Ekstedt, 1968). The antibody was associated with the IgM fraction (Yoshida and Ekstedt, 1968). Mudd *et al.* (1963) reported that absorption with RTA removed the phagocytosis-promoting factor from serum, reducing the killing of *S. aureus*. However, Shayegani *et al.* (1970) later presented evidence that it was the 'intact mucopeptide' rather than RTA which was the active agent in reducing phagocytosis. It appears that the question still remains open since Warner *et al.* (1966) have published data suggesting that more than one protective-antibody specificity for *S. aureus* exists in human sera and, therefore, different protective mechanisms may have been observed by the two groups of investigators.

A brief preliminary study has been carried out to examine directly the possible protective effects of antibodies to the PGP specificity of GTA (H. B. Stamper and F. W. Chorpenning, unpublished result; reviewed in Chorpenning and Young, 1982). Natural anti-GTA antibodies fractionated on Sephadex G-200 from pooled guinea pig serum and injected into mice protected them against a $1.5 \, LD_{50}$ dose of viable bacteria bearing surface GTA antigen. Also, Bolton (1981a) has shown that less dental caries activity is present in human subjects with higher levels of IgA antibodies for GTA than in those with lower levels of antibody. Russell and Beighton (1982) have suggested reservations regarding this association. These reports indicate the need for further study, and any conclusions should be deferred until confirmatory studies have been reported.

Although it is clearly established that 'natural antibodies' to both GTA and RTA occur, it has been reported also that levels of RTA antibodies rise during certain infections. A comparatively large number of studies have dealt with the use of these antibodies diagnostically. They have involved endocarditis (Crowder and White, 1972; Tuason and Sheagren, 1976; Larinkari *et al.*, 1977; Bayer *et al.*, 1980; Tenenbaun and Archer, 1980), bacteraemia (Tuason and Sheagren, 1976; Larinkari *et al.*, 1977; Curtin *et al.*, 1978; Tenenbaum and Archer, 1980), abscesses (Curtin *et al.*, 1978), osteomyelitis (Larinkari, 1982), and other infections (Flandrois *et al.*, 1979). It was found generally that anti-RTA titres were elevated in patients with *S. aureus* infections but the prognostic value of RTA tests, especially with regard to development of endocarditis, has been disputed (Tenenbaum and Archer, 1980). There has been considerable variability in test results as reported and it has been suggested (Sheagren *et al.*, 1981) that this may be due to differences in antigen preparation, agar for counterimmuno-electrophoresis and gel diffusion, and other technical variations. Little attention has been paid to the specificity of the antigenic determinants involved and it may be that some investigations have dealt with different specificities than others. For example, some studies appear to have employed antigen which contained peptidoglycan. Few studies of the possible use of anti-GTA antibodies in clinical diagnosis have been carried out. One investigation found elevated titres in rheumatic heart disease (Klesius *et al.*, 1974). It is doubtful in view of the extensive cross-reactions which occur that such tests show any great promise.

In view of the well-known pathologic effects of LPS (Berry, 1977) and peptidoglycan (Stewart-Tull, 1980), considerable interest has been shown in possible adverse effects of GTA. With fairly large doses, no pyrogenicity or other adverse effects were seen in experimental animals (Knox and Wicken, 1973; Miller and Jackson, 1973) although DTH was induced (Bolton and Chorpenning, 1974). However, cytotoxicity has been demonstrated at the cellular level in cultures of murine splenocytes when large amounts of purified GTA were employed (Chorpenning *et al.*, 1979c; Dziarski *et al.*, 1980). The amounts of GTA used were considerably greater than required for induction of immunological activities. In addition, LTA has been shown to be toxic for human kidney cells (DeVuono and Panos, 1978).

Other adverse effects induced by TA have been demonstrated experimentally. These include arthritis (Ne'eman and Ginsberg, 1972), renal pathology (Fiedel and Jackson, 1974; Waltersdorff *et al.*, 1977), and, probably, a bacteriogenic transfusion reaction (Chorpenning and Dodd, 1965). In the latter case, a haemolytic transfusion reaction unrelated to isoagglutinin incompatibility was proven by pathological examination. Reactivity of the patients' erythrocytes was altered, and they were destroyed by 'natural' antibody. An experimental model of the mechanism was established *in vitro* and the mechanism was shown later to involve GTA-coated red cells and anti-GTA antibody (Chorpenning and Stamper, 1972). Although the involvement of complement was not proven in the above case, heating removed the haemolytic effect of sera. Therefore, it is likely that the observed haemolysis *in vivo* was complement-mediated. Activation of complement (C) by TA may be involved in other pathologic processs such as those reviewed by Nelson (1974). It has been shown that RTA activates the classical C pathway in normal human serum (Verbrugh *et al.*, 1979) and, perhaps, the alternative pathway, although both are in dispute (Winkelstein and Tomasz, 1978; Wilkinson *et al.*, 1981). Silvestri *et al.* (1979) demonstrated that LTA was anticomplementary and that LTA-coated SRBC were resistant to immune lysis by anti-SRBC; however, we have shown that GTA-coated SRBC are lysed by anti-GTA and C (Bolton *et al.*, 1977). Also, C appeared to be involved in GTA-induced renal dysfunction in rabbits (Fiedel and Jackson, 1974) since it was demonstrated that $\beta_1 C$ was deposited in the glomeruli and a dose-related depletion of serum C correlated with the severity of disease.

Another pathologic phenomenon in which TA may be involved is bacterial adherence to mammalian cells, an important mechanism of virulence. Although binding of purified GTA to erythrocytes has been known for quite a few years (Chorpenning and Stamper, 1973) and the mediation of LTA in streptococcal binding has been reported (Beachey and Ofek, 1976), there was some dispute of this in the case of *Streptococcus mutans* adherence (Hamada and Slade, 1976). It does appear that in the adherence of group A streptococci to human oral epithelial cells LTA is of major importance (Alkan *et al.*, 1977). Inhibition of *Staphylococcus aureus* adherence to nasal epithelial cells by both LTA and RTA was also observed (Aly *et al.*, 1980). Using radiolabelled bacteria, Bolton (1980a) has reported that anti-GTA antibody inhibited the adherence of S. *mutans*, S. *sanguis*, and a *Bacillus* sp. to hydroxyapatite *in vitro* and that neutralization of the antibody by pure GTA reduced the inhibitory effect. These results suggest that GTA is involved in adherence of oral bacteria to tooth surfaces.

Considerably more research needs to be conducted before any definite conclusions regarding the pathologic effects of teichoic acid may be made.

V. POLYCLONAL ACTIVATION OF B LYMPHOCYTES

Of course, polyclonal B-cell activation (PBA) by LPS (Anderson *et al.*, 1972; Coutinho and Moller, 1973) and PG (Dziarski and Dziarski, 1979) has been known for some time and mitogenic activity by GTA had been reported earlier (Oldfather *et al.*, 1977; Beachey *et al.*, 1979). Therefore, the possibility of a PBA effect was anticipated. The phenomenon was demonstrated first in Sprague-Dawley rats (Oldfather and Chorpenning, 1980) which when injected with 100 μg of purified GTA produced significant numbers of PFC for sheep (SRBC), human (HRBC), chicken (CRBC), and 1-fluoro-2,4-dinitrobenzene-treated erythrocytes (DNP cells), as well as for GTA-coated cells. The PBA effect could not be demonstrated in normal Fisher (F344) inbred rats, although they did yield specific responses. However, when these rats were thymectomized, irradiated, and the bone marrow was reconstituted, PBA was easily shown. Thus, it appears that the PBA response is regulated by T-cells in the F344 rat but is not so fully regulated in the Sprague-Dawley rat. A similar observation was made by Nakano *et al.* (1980) in athymic nude mice, using *Staph. aureus* as the inducer.

The PBA phenomenon induced by GTA was confirmed *in vitro* using splenocyte cultures from BALB/c mice (Young and Chorpenning, 1980a). It was shown that PFC for SRBC, CRBC, and HRBC were induced by addition of 3 μg of purified lipid-free GTA to the cultures (10^7 cells). The number of SRBC plaques was increased 5-6-fold above background. Although such a comparison has little meaning if different cell subsets are involved, as suggested by Coutinho *et al.* (1976), it does serve to emphasize the existence of a significant difference in numbers of PFC over controls. Lower doses yielded better specific

GTA responses with lesser PBA responses and a time–dose relationship was demonstrated, the kinetics being speeded up at higher dosage. Although GTA activated *isolated* B-cells to secrete aspecific antibodies, the influence of other cells also was examined in BALB/c mice (Chorpenning and Young, 1982; Young, 1982). With the Protein A assay, it was shown that the PBA response of B-cells to GTA was suppressed significantly when MØ were introduced into the cultures, a finding similar to that of Lemke *et al.* (1975) for LPS. Mitogenesis and the specific response also were suppressed as first reported by Folch *et al.* (1973). Suppression of specific and non-specific responses also occurred via the MØ-T-cell (Ly 2) circuit. Contrary to the findings of Goodman and Weigle (1981) with LPS, helper (Ly 1) T-cells did not appear to be involved in the PBA effect, although they were shown to enhance the specific anti-GTA response in the presence of MØ. Thus specific GTA responses are both T-dependent and T-independent. Interestingly, GTA was also mitogenic for both Ly 1 and Ly 2 T-cells in the presence of MØ, furnishing supporting evidence for their activation in the systems under observation.

The relationship between specific responses to T-independent antigens and their PBA effects have been of considerable interest and some dispute (Bretscher and Cohn, 1970; Moller *et al.*, 1976; Cohn, 1976). One aspect of the argument deals with the number and kinds of cell receptors involved, some investigators favouring a two-signal theory and others (Moller *et al.*, 1976) a one-signal mechanism. In the former theory, there is argument regarding the need of separate signals for proliferation and differentiation. In the latter theory, the Ig receptor would be involved only in antigen concentration on the B-cell and a non-specific signal would trigger antibody secretion. Thus, both specific and PBA responses would be triggered via a non-specific receptor. In either case, a non-specific receptor(s) is invoked for T-independent responses. Our work indicates that there are multiple non-specific receptors and a variety of B-cell subpopulations. *In vitro* experiments (Young *et al.*, 1982) with isolated BALB/c mouse B-cells that were stimulated with *Escherichia coli* LPS, PG, or GTA, separately, exhibited both mitogenesis ($[_3H]$-thymidine uptake) and the PBA effect in each. The amounts of each inducer required for optimal effects were the same for PBA and mitogenesis but considerably different between the three substances. Furthermore, selective killing of proliferating, GTA-stimulated B-cells with BUdR and light (Zoscke and Bach, 1971) abrogated both PBA and mitogenic effects, suggesting that the same subset of B-cells was responsible for both. This treatment also killed some of the cells responsive to LPS but not those responsive to PG. Exposure of GTA–BUdR-treated cells to either LPS or PG indicated that B-cells remained which were responsive to both agents but unresponsive to GTA. Similar treatment with PG eliminated most of the proliferating cells but only 10% of antibody-secreting cells. While treatment with LPS killed proliferating cells and part of the antibody-secreting cells. These data imply that subsets at different stages of maturation were involved.

On the other hand, killing of LPS-treated cells by BUdR practically eliminated cells responding to GTA, while killing of PG-stimulated cells had no effect on GTA responses. From these data it is apparent that several different cell subsets are involved in non-specific responses and that none of these are responsive only to GTA. Thus, it would seem likely that multiple receptors are involved.

The PBA effect induced by 1 μg of GTA per 10^5 B-cells was greatest at the second day after treatment and was more than twice that induced by 25 μg of LPS. Employment of intact spleen cell populations suppressed the response (as observed earlier) but did not alter the general shape of the kinetic curve. However, proliferation increased (Young *et al.*, 1982).

The relationship between specific and PBA responses to GTA was studied in parallel dosage–kinetics experiments (Young, 1982) and in isolated B-cell cultures using BUdR–light treatment (Young, 1982). The overall effect of dosage agreed with the theory of Coutinho and Moller (1975), in that low doses of GTA favoured the specific response while higher doses favoured a PBA effect. At an optimal dose, both mitogenic and PBA responses peaked at about 2 days, while the anti-GTA response peaked at five days. However, when MØ and T-cells were eliminated, the anti-GTA peak occurred at three days, suggesting that the specific T-independent response follows the same mechanism as the polyclonal one. Elimination of the responding B-cells by BUdR–light treatment abrogated this early response along with the PBA effect and such treated cultures could no longer respond to GTA unless MØ-T-cell mixtures were added. This parallelism also suggests that the T-independent GTA mechanism is the same as that of PBA responses, while the T-dependent GTA response obviously follows the classical mechanism (Jerne, 1974; Benacerraf and Germain, 1979; Cantor and Gershon, 1979).

Based upon our work and that of others cited above, it appears that considerable differences exist between the mechanisms of various PBA substances. For example, Wong and Herscowitz (1979) reported that there was no MØ effect on activation of B-cells by TNP–LPS and dextran, while Boswell *et al.* (1980) found them to be necessary for activation by TNP–Ficoll. Lee *et al.* (1980) also reported that MØ were essential. In this connection, Martinez-Alonso *et al.* (1980) reported that MØ were not required for the PBA effect of TNP–LPS but that they were needed for the specific response. In contrast, our findings (above) show that MØ may suppress non-specific activation of B-cells by GTA but that no T-cell help was involved. However, both helper (T_H) and suppressor (T_S) T-cell circuits, as well as MØ, affect the specific response (Chorpenning and Young, 1982).

Recent work by us with three PBA substances of bacterial origin (reviewed above) has furnished further emphasis for the idea that multiple mechanisms exist and that polyclonal activators induce a variety of mechanisms (Young *et al.*, 1982). In these experiments, the patterns of mitosis and polyclonal antibody synthesis in BALB/c B-cell cultures varied considerably when induced by each of the activators, LPS, PD, or GTA. LPS activated two subpopulations of B-cells, a non-proliferating one which secreted polyclonal antibodies and one which proliferated and then secreted antibodies. PG also activated a secreting population and a proliferating one, but the latter did not secrete antibodies. On the other hand, GTA activated only a single population of B-cells which proliferated and secreted polyclonal antibodies. When these differences are considered along with the discrepancies reported in experiments on MØ and T-cell involvement, it becomes apparent that there exist major differences in mechanisms and, probably, in receptors. It indicates also that separate cells or receptors are required for differentiation and proliferation. This may involve two separate signals as suggested by Falkoff *et al.* (1982), who reported a T-cell requirement for antibody secretion but not for proliferation in B-cells stimulated by *Staph. aureus*. It is not clear what molecular agent was used in their study, although it appears to have been assumed to be protein A. Since RTA is also present in *Staph. aureus*, the question of its involvement could arise. Whether RTA can induce PBA effects is not clear, since Räsänen and Arvilommi (1982) reported that it activated both B- and T-cells, but Dziarski (1982) reported that it was not active as a PBA and was not mitogenic for mouse, rat, and human lymphocytes (Dziarski *et al.*, 1980).

Certain aspects of the polyclonal activation phenomenon may be of significance in disease. It has been suggested that lymphocyte and MØ activation by bacterial products may furnish a non-specific first line of defence (Petit and Unanue, 1974; Clagett and Engel, 1978) which could operate via protective antibodies, lymphokines, and MØ activation. Undoubtedly cytolytic antibodies are produced (Chorpenning, 1982) but these have not been correlated with protection. Räsänen *et al.* (1978) have shown that all of nine bacterial strains tested stimulate human B lymphocytes from cord blood to produce leucocyte migration inhibitory factor and suggest that this represents polyclonal triggering. There is no doubt that antibodies of many specificities are secreted as a result of B-cell stimulation by a variety of bacterial substances. This, in itself, has made it difficult to associate the separate events with protection and the number of attempts appear to have been few. Nevertheless, the potential for protection is there.

On the other hand, evidence has been presented that PBA mechanisms may induce pathological changes (Shenker *et al.*, 1980). Thus, the familiar dichotomy of tissue damage occurring as a result of protective mechanisms may exist. Ortiz-Ortiz *et al.* (1980) have shown that *Trypanosoma cruzi* induces PBA in infected mice, secreting IgM antibodies to unrelated antigens which they believe could account for the Ig abnormalities reported in patients with Chaga's disease. This may suggest a role in the aetiology of autoimmune disease which frequently follows parasitic infection. However, another work indicates that even though the high serum IgM level in NZB mice is due to increased polyclonal activation, the appearance of 'natural' thymocytotropic autoantibody is not correlated with

PBA (Hirose *et al.*, 1980). Of course, neither of these findings is exclusive nor conclusive.

Horton *et al.* (1972) isolated a new osteoclast-activating lymphokine from cultures of peripheral blood leucocytes stimulated with phytohaemagglutinin or by dental plaque which has been assumed by some to be of polyclonal origin, but Mackler *et al.* (1974) found that cells from normal adult individuals were not stimulated by plaque. Cord blood leucocytes also were not stimulated by dental plaque (Baker *et al.*, 1976). These findings suggest that antigenic responses, rather than PBA, were being observed. On the other hand, gram-negative bacteria isolated from periodontally diseased sites have been reported recently to induce PBA in normal human peripheral blood lymphocytes (Bick *et al.*, 1981) which seems to reopen the question. Still, no direct cause and effect mechanisms have been demonstrated.

It does seem likely if a cause and effect relationship can be shown between polyclonal B-cell activators and either/or protection and tissue damage that bacterial substances which persist in the environment are important inducers of the phenomena (Chorpenning, 1982; Shenker *et al.*, 1980).

VI. IMMUNOMODULATION BY GLYCEROL TEICHOIC ACID

The non-specific influence of certain substances on unrelated immune responses has been known for quite some time (see Chorpenning, 1982). Early observations dealt with the adjuvant effect which required injection of the adjuvant simultaneously with the antigen. However, injection of a modulatory substance two or more days before the antigen also can produce enhancement of the response, and timing influences the relative level of IgM and IgG antibodies (Battisto and Pappas, 1973). Cell-mediated responses also may be modulated by bacterial agents (Chorpenning and Young, 1982) but this effect has not been shown with GTA and will not be covered in this review.

The evidence that GTA could act as an immunomodulator was first presented by Miller and Jackson (1973; Miller *et al.*, 1976) and other studies *in vivo* showed that differences in route, mouse strain, or species influenced the occurrence of immunomodulation (Lynch *et al.*, 1978). Furthermore, the effect was confirmed with C3H/HeJ and BDF$_1$ mouse splenocytes *in vitro* (Marbrook cultures) and it was shown that the dosage influenced the direction of modulation. Low doses of GTA (0.1–2 μg) enhanced the SRBC-PFC response and higher doses (6–10 μg) suppressed it (Lynch and Chorpenning, 1978; Young and Chorpenning, 1980b). The kinetic curve followed a continuous dose-related gradient from peak enhancement to suppression (reviewed in Chorpenning and Young, 1982). The immunomodulation observed in these experiments was shown to result from stimulation by lipid-free, protein-free GTA (Chorpenning *et al.*, 1979c). In fact, the substance was a simple glycerophosphate chain of 19 glycerol units (average) with no esteryl or glycosyl substituents.

More searching investigation of the mechanism by which GTA influences unrelated responses included study of the involvement of specific antibodies (Bolton, 1980b). It was shown that immunosuppression of the SRBC response was induced in normal Sprague-Dawley rats by intraperitoneal injection of 0.32 μg of GTA per g body weight 24 h before immunization, while GTA-deprived rats (Rozmiarek *et al.*, 1977) exhibited no apparent suppression. Both serum antibody to SRBC and splenic PFC showed 80% suppression in the normal GTA-treated rats which possessed natural anti-GTA antibodies, while the GTA-deprived antibody-free rats showed no suppression. However, when GTA–anti-GTA complexes were injected into the antibody-free rats, suppression of the anti-SRBC response occurred. Bolton (1980b) interpreted these results to imply suppression by antigen–antibody complexes and probably to indicate the action of suppressor T-cells. A similar conclusion could be suggested by earlier unpublished work in our laboratory (Oldfather *et al.*, 1978) showing that GTA induced enhancement of SRBC responses in animals having no natural antibodies (mice) while those having antibodies (rats) exhibited suppression when treated with equal amounts per body weight (2.7 μg per 25 g). In preliminary experiments, increased levels of GTA–anti-GTA complexes favoured suppression.

Other studies of the mechanism(s) involved cell cultures and stimulation of isolated cell populations *in vitro* in an effort to determine which cells were affected by GTA. In one such study, dose-related enhancement of the response to SRBC *in vitro* was significantly (four times) greater when glass-adherent cells were removed from C3H/HeJ splenocyte cultures (Lynch and Chorpenning, 1979). When adherent peritoneal exudate cells were substituted, the suppression observed at higher doses of GTA was abrogated but returned on the addition of splenic adherent cells. Involvement of adherent cells in suppression has been reported also in Wistar rats (Mattingly *et al.*, 1979). Specific responses to GTA also were suppressed by adherent cells (Chorpenning and Young, 1982). In C3H/HeJ mice, neither serum haemolysin nor PFC to GTA were observed in either uninjected or GTA-injected animals. Splenocyte cultures also were unresponsive but yielded good PFC responses when adherent cells were removed. Replacement of adherent cells resulted in return of specific suppression.

Bolton (1981b) has presented an interesting report which indicates the broad influence of GTA modulation on the immunological system. Using cultures of C57BL/6 mouse splenocytes, he showed that the mitogenesis ([^{3}H]-thymidine uptake) induced by concanavalin A (T-cell mitogen) was suppressed by GTA while that induced by LPS (B-cell mitogen) was enhanced. At a relatively high dosage, GTA activates suppressor circuits (below) and also acts as a strong B-cell mitogen. Thus, it could increase the B-cell effect, overshadowing suppressor activity, while having only a suppressive effect on T-cell mitogenesis.

In experiments with BALB/c mouse splenocytes stimulated *in vitro* with SRBC, two approaches were used to study cellular involvement (Chorpenning and Young, 1982). In the first group of experiments, cultures of isolated B-cells were treated with cytotoxic anti-Thy 1.2 antiserum to kill any residual T-cells, the B-cells were stimulated with GTA, and were treated with BUdR–light (Zoscke and Bach, 1971). Thus, the B-cell subpopulation reacting mitogenically (and in PBA) to GTA was killed. The remaining viable B-cells were then cultured with T-cells and MØ in the presence of GTA and SRBC. Control cultures with the intact (untreated) B-cell population yielded the highest PFC response to SRBC, while cultures without GTA yielded the lowest number of PFC and the non-mitotic B-cell subpopulation yielded an intermediate response. Therefore, it appears that enhancement of the SRBC response by GTA has two components, one involving B-cell proliferation, probably associated with PBA, and one involving stimulation or activation of other cells.

In the second series of experiments, separated cell populations were pretreated with GTA, washed, and added to intact splenocyte cultures. Pretreated (1 μg GTA per 10^6 cells) MØ or MØ–T-cell mixtures suppressed SRBC responses when added to intact splenocyte cultures. When T_S-cells were depleted with anti-Lyt 2.2 cytotoxic antiserum, suppression was abrogated and enhancement occurred. Pretreatment of MØ–Lyt 1.2 cell mixtures with 0.3 μg of GTA induced enhanced SRBC responses in spleen cell cultures, while pretreatment of either cell population alone failed to induce enhancement. Thus, it appears that GTA acts via the MØ to induce antithetical dose-related events in either T_S- or T_H-cells. Similar results obtained with LPS led Uchiyama and Jacobs (1978) to suggest that LPS modulation of antibody synthesis also was dependent upon helper and suppressor cell populations. Adherent cells are known to be involved in such regulatory circuits (Altman, 1980; Villeneuve *et al.*, 1980; Anderson *et al.*, 1981). Pretreatment of B-cells with a high dose of GTA before addition to splenocyte cultures resulted in suppression of the SRBC response while pretreatment with a low dose (0.3 μg) produced enhancement. Whether or not these effects involve lymphokines (Cohen, 1982) or monokines was not determined by the present experiments. The results with pretreated B-cells are interesting in this connection, since pretreated *heat-killed* B-cells produced no effect. Therefore, transfer of GTA does not appear to be involved and lymphokine release or direct cell action is indicated. It is particularly interesting that B-cells can act as a target for GTA totally apart from its mitogenic action and then can modulate other immune responses in a dose-related manner.

The question of receptor involvement in cell activation by GTA has been touched upon only with regard to binding experiments. Ofek *et al.* (1975) suggested that a lipid moiety of GTA was involved in binding to erythrocytes and, presumably, to other cells, but Cooper *et al.* (1978) and Chorpenning *et al.* (1979c) reported that binding and immunomodulation could occur in the absence of fatty acids. A possible explanation for these disparate findings was presented by Chorpenning and Young (1982), who suggested that loss of binding capacity after ammonolysis was due to shortening of the chain rather than to deacylation.

Both B- and T-cells were shown to possess binding sites for LTA but it was reported to be mitogenic only for T-lymphocytes (Beachey *et al.*, 1979). GTA undoubtedly binds to B-cells and is highly mitogenic for them (Young *et al.*, 1982). It is moderately mitogenic for both T_S- and T_H-cell subsets via the MØ (Young, 1982). Proliferation appears to be highly significant in the immunomodulatory mechanisms of GTA and probably contributes to non-specific responses via the PBA mechanism, MØ activation, and activation of both T_S- and T_H-lymphocytes.

Based upon the investigations reviewed above, it appears that GTA is capable of modulating unrelated responses by multiple pathways involving all major cell populations of the immunological system. B lymphocytes are directly activated polyclonally and secrete antibodies which exhibit specific reactivity, enhancing the specific response. In the presence of MØ, T_H-lymphocytes or T_S-lymphocytes are activated, depending upon the dosage, and may enhance or suppress non-specifically. MØ are directly activated by GTA, resulting in non-specific suppression, partially via T-cell circuits. B-cells also can cause either enhancement or suppression of unrelated responses, but whether this is due to lymphokines has not been determined. It seems that experimental immunomodulation by GTA may follow two circuits other than those of the classical regulatory system. In T-cell activity induced by GTA, the MØ appears to be the target cell for inducing T_H or T_S effector cell action while either the MØ or B-cell may be the target for suppression without the aid of T-cells.

Perhaps the most significant observation regarding immunomodulation by bacterial substances was that an immunomodulator from environmental sources could induce significant long-term suppression in animals (Oldfather and Chorpenning, 1981). Sprague-Dawley rats were fed a GTA-free diet (Rozmiarek *et al.*, 1977) and their splenocytes were examined for IgM responses (PFC) to injection of foreign erythrocytes. Responses (haemolytic plaque assay) were four-fold higher in GTA-deprived animals than in rats eating the usual diet, but when the rats were fed purified GTA (200 μg per week) for five weeks they again exhibited suppressed responses. The degree of suppression was dose-related and feeding of either gram-positive bacteria or the conventional diet also restored suppression. Since the conventional diet contained about 8 mg GTA per kg and average consumption per rat approached 100 g per week, it was not surprising that feeding of 200 μg GTA per week to rats which had been deprived of GTA since weaning (at age three weeks) resulted in suppression similar to that seen in conventional rats. In view of the previously indicated need for anti-GTA antibody in induction of suppression, it should be noted that there was ample time for that response.

From the foregoing, it is clear that dietary GTA induces suppression of responses to foreign erythrocytes in the rat. If we accept red blood cells as a surrogate for bacterial cells, bactericidal action and perhaps other protective mechanisms could be suppressed. It is interesting that specific anti-GTA responses also are suppressed, as previously mentioned, since GTA is a major antigen in many gram-positive bacteria. Specific suppression undoubtedly accounts for the very low IgM anti-GTA antibody levels in some species and the absence of detectable circulating antibody in Swiss and C3H/HeJ mice.

Although no direct demonstration of immunomodulation by environmental bacterial products had been reported prior to our study, modulation by intestinal bacteria has been observed using germ-free (GF) rats (Wells and Balish, 1980). In these experiments GF rats colonized with *Fusobacterium necrophorum* yielded enhanced responses to the mitogens concanavalin A and phytohaemagglutinin over that of GF animals. Mattingly *et al.* (1979) also observed suppression of SRBC responses in conventional Wistar rats which was not present in GF rats. They attributed this suppression to activation of 'suppressor' MØ by microbial products in the normal flora of the rats. In view of our findings, this mechanism may indeed be *one* of those involved in immunosuppression and any or several microbial substances such as LPS, PG, GTA, or dextran (Chorpenning, 1982) may be the active agent. However, it is important to remember that there are differences in the cell populations acted upon by these agents (Young *et al.*, 1982) and in their dosages and mechanisms. Under a given set of circumstances, they could easily induce antithetical effects. The modulatory effects by intestinal flora as opposed to those of ingested bacterial products also comes into question and has considerable influence on the outcome. For example, in the two investigations cited above (Wells and Balish, 1980; Mattingly *et al.*, 1979) intestinal flora seem to be responsible for immunomodulation, yet in our study the intestinal flora of the rats was essentially the same in conventional or GTA-free groups (Rozmiarek *et al.*, 1977) and ample GTA must have been present in the gram-positive flora to produce an effect if properly presented. However, on a GTA-free diet neither circulating antibody nor PFC of GTA specificity appeared, while GF rats (no intestinal flora) fed a sterile conventional diet produced anti-GTA responses, and GF rats fed a GTA-free diet did not. No discriminating experiments have been done regarding environmental GTA modulation in GF animals, but in view of the need for introduction via the upper gastrointestinal tract or parenterally for immunization, it is doubtful whether any difference in modulation between GF and conventional rats could be demonstrated.

It is apparent that immunomodulation by environmental GTA is an important factor in immune responses of the rat and some other species. Both specific and non-specific modulation are involved and multiple regulatory circuits appear to operate. Most likely, the antibody cycling observed (reviewed in Chorpenning and Young, 1982) is a result of the operation of such regulation, as is unresponsiveness in mice. A major part of GTA modulation is induced via the MØ, acting either through T-cell circuits or more directly. Dosage has a major influence on whether enhancement or suppression of responses will occur, but route, species, and timing also are important factors. Direct activation of the

B-lymphocyte also may be important, not only because of the PBA contribution to antibody responses, but because GTA-activated B-cells may release lymphokines with either suppressive or enhancing activities. Thus, all major cell populations of the immunological system are involved in modulation by GTA. Whether or not all of these cells and circuits are involved when modulation is due to natural environmental exposure has not been determined. It may be assumed, however, that in the restricted situation of the rat experiments route, dosage, and species dictated that suppression would result.

VII. COMMENTS

It is readily apparent from the observations reviewed above that GTA has an extensive impact on the immunological system of several laboratory animals. This impact is highly significant when occurring under natural conditions as a result of environmental stimulation. Effects which are involved include induction of specific natural humoral and cellular immunity, possible protection, polyclonal activation, and immunomodulation. It is likely that the PBA effect of GTA contributes to a non-specific first line of defence against infection, and stimulation of other cells by GTA may result in activated MØ and release of lymphokines. In the natural situation, there is no evidence that immunomodulation has an enhancing effect on responses. Thus, the beneficial effects of modulation are purely speculative. It may be possible to employ GTA in clinical immunopotentiation or suppression, but such experiments as yet have not been carried out in animals.

In view of the natural immune responses to GTA demonstrated in humans, it may be suspected that the other immunological phenomena demonstrated in animals may occur as well.

The other side of the coin concerns possible adverse effects of GTA. Although no naturally occurring pathological changes have been observed or any associated with DTH, there were instances (above) of experimentally induced disease. Also, it is clear that high concentrations of GTA are toxic for some mammalian cells *in vitro*. Yet, neither immunogenic nor immunomodulating doses appear to be toxic *in vivo*. The suppression of immune responses observed under natural conditions *in vivo* may, of course, be considered to be an adverse effect.

ACKNOWLEDGEMENTS

I am pleased to acknowledge the valuable contributions by Drs. Hugh B. Stamper, Jr., Ronald W. Bolton, Harold R. Cooper, Gene P. Decker, G. Thomas Frederick, John J. Lynch, Jr., John W. Oldfather, Harry Rozmiarek, and Deborah A. Young to the work from my laboratory which is reviewed herein. I also wish to thank Dr. Robert M. Pfister for the support which made this project possible and Pat Titus for preparation of the manuscript.

REFERENCES

Alkan, M. L., Ofek, I., and Beachey, E. H. (1977). Adherence of pharyngeal and skin strains of group A streptococci to human skin and oral epithelial cells. *Infect. Immun.*, **18**, 555–557.

Altman, A. (1980). Immunoregulatory networks. *Immunol. Today*, **1**, 73–74.

Aly, R., Shinefield, H. R., Litz, C., and Maibach H. I. (1980). Role of teichoic acid in the binding of *Staphylococcus aureus* to nasal epithelial cells. *J. Infect. Dis.*, **141**, 163–165.

Anderson, J., Sjöberg, O., and Moller, G. (1972). Induction of immunoglobulin and antibody syntheses *in vitro* by lipoplysaccharides. *Eur. J. Immunol.*, **2**, 349–353.

Anderson, S. A., Isakson, P. C., Pure, E., Muirhead, M., Uhr, J. W., and Vitetta, E. S. (1981). Immunosuppression in a murine B cell leukemia (BCL$_1$): role of an adherent cell in the suppression of primary *in vitro* antibody responses. *J. Immunol.*, **126**, 1603–1607.

Baker, J. J., Chan, S. P., Socransky, S. S., Oppenheim, J. J., and Mergenhagen, S. E. (1976). Importance of *Actinomyces* and certain gram-negative anaerobic organisms in the transformation of lymphocytes from patients with periodontal disease. *Infect. Immun.*, **13**, 1363–1368.

Battisto, J. R., and Pappas, F. (1973). Regulation of immunoglobulin synthesis by dextran. *J. Exp. Med.*, **138**, 176–193.

Bayer, A. S., Tillman, D. B., Concepcion, N., and Guze, L. B. (1980). Clinical value of teichoic acid antibody titers in the diagnosis and management of the staphylococcemias. *Western J. Med.*, **132**, 294–300.

Beachey, E. H., and Ofek, I. (1976). Epithelial cell binding of group A streptococci by lipoteichoic acid on fimbriae denuded of M protein. *J. Exp. Med.*, **143**, 759–771.

Beachey, E. H., Dale, J. B., Grebe, S., Ahmed, A., Simpson, W. A., and Ofek, I. (1979). Lymphocyte binding and T cell mitogenic properties of group A streptococcal lipoteichoic acid. *J. Immunol.*, **122**, 189–195.

Benacerraf, B., and Germain, R. N. (1979). Specific suppressor responses to antigen under I region control. *Fed. Proc.*, **38**, 2053–2057.

Berry, L. J. (1977). Bacterial toxins. *Crit. Rev. Toxicol.*, **5**, 239–318.

Bick, P. H., Carpenter, A. B., Holdeman, L. V., Miller, G. A., Ranney, R. R., Palcanis, K. G., and Tew, J. G. (1981). Polyclonal B-cell activation induced by extracts of gram-negative bacteria isolated from periodontally diseased sites. *Infect. Immun.*, **34**, 43–49.

Bolen, J. B., and Tribble, J. L. (1979). Delayed hypersensitivity to *Staphylococcus aureus* in mice: *In vivo* responses to isolated staphylococcal antigens. *Immunology*, **38**, 809–817.

Bolton, R. W. (1978). Cyclic appearance of antibody-producing cells in the peripheral blood in response to a chemically-defined polyglycerophosphate antigen. *Immunol. Commun.*, **7**, 383–392.

Bolton, R. W. (1980a). Adherence of oral streptococci to hydroxyapatite *in vitro* via glycerol-teichoic acid. *Arch. Oral Biol.*, **25**, 111–114.

Bolton, R. W. (1980b). Immunosuppression of anti-sheep erythrocyte responses by glycerol teichoic acid immune complexes. *Infect. Immun.*, **30**, 723–727.

Bolton, R. W. (1981a). Naturally-occurring IgA antibodies to glycerol-teichoic acid in human saliva. Correlation with caries activity. *J. Dent. Res.*, **60**, 878–882.

Bolton, R. W. (1981b). Modulation of murine lymphocyte mitogen responses by glycerol-teichoic acid. *Immunol. Commun.*, **10**, 631–640.

Bolton, R. W., and Chorpenning, F. W. (1974). Naturally occurrng cellular and humoral immunity to teichoic acid in rats. *Immunology*, **27**, 517–523.

Bolton, R. W., Rozmiarek, H., and Chorpenning, F. W. (1977). Cyclic antibody formation to polyglycerophosphate in normal and injected rats. *J. Immunol.*, **118**, 1154–1158.

Boswell, H. S., Sharrow, S. O., and Singer, A. (1980). Role of accessory cells in B cell activation. I. Macrophage presentation of TNP–Ficoll: evidence for macrophage-B cell interaction. *J. Immunol.*, **124**, 989–996.

Bretscher, P. A., and Cohn, M. (1970). A theory of self–nonself discrimination. *Science*, **169**, 1042–1049.

Brock, J. H., and Reiter, B. (1971). Sensitisation of sheep erythrocytes by cell wall teichoic acid of *Staphylococcus aureus*. *Immunochemistry*, **8**, 933–938.

Burger, M. M. (1966). Teichoic acids: antigenic determinants, chain separation, and their location in the cell wall. *Proc. Natl. Acad. Sci. USA*, **56**, 910–917.

Button, D., Archibald, A. R., and Baddiley, J. (1966). The linkage between teichoic acid and glycosaminopeptide in the walls of a strain of *Staphylococcus lactis*. *Biochem. J.*, **99**, 11–14.

Cantor, H., and Gershon, R. K. (1979). Immunological circuits: cellular composition. *Fed. Proc.*, **38**, 2058–2064.

Chorpenning, F. W. (1982). Immunologic effects of teichoic acid in the environment: a review. *Ohio J. Sci.*, **82**, 31–37.

Chorpenning, F. W., and Dodd, M. C. (1965). Polyagglutinable erythrocytes associated with bacteriogenic transfusion reactions. *Vox Sang.*, **10**, 460–471.

Chorpenning, F. W., and Stamper, H. B., Jr. (1972). The mechanism of erythrocyte alteration associated with certain transfusion reactions. *Proc. AABB–ISBT Transfusion Congress*, p.68. American Association of Blood Banks, Washington, DC.

Chorpenning, F. W., and Stamper, H. B. (1973). Spontaneous absorption of teichoic acid to erythrocytes. *Immunochemistry*, **10**, 15–20.

Chorpenning, F. W., and Young, D. A. (1982). Immunomodulatory and cyclic effects of glycerol teichoic acid. In *Regulatory Implications of Oscillatory Dynamics in the Immune Response*. Vol. II (Eds. C. DeLisi and J. Hierraux), pp.89–126. CRC Press, Boca Raton, FL.

Chorpenning, F. W., Cooper, H. R., and Rosen, S. (1975). Cross-reactions of *Streptococcus mutans* due to cell wall teichoic acid. *Infect. Immun.*, **12**, 586–591.

Chorpenning, F. W., Bolton, R. W., Frederick, G. T., and Rozmiarek, H. (1979a). Development of cellular and humoral responses to teichoic acid. *Dev. Comp. Immunol.*, **3**, 709–724.

Chorpenning, F. W., Cooper, H. R., Oldfather, J. W., and Lynch, J. J., Jr. (1979b). Immunogenicity of soluble versus cellular glycerol teichoic acid. *Infect. Immun.*, **26**, 211.

Chorpenning, F. W., Lynch, J. J., Jr., Cooper, H. R., and Oldfather, J. W. (1979c). Modulation of the immune response to sheep erythrocytes by lipid-free glycerol teichoic acid. *Infect. Immun.*, **26**, 262–269.

Clagett, J. A., and Engel, D. (1978). Polyclonal activation: a form of primative immunity and its possible role in pathogenesis of inflammatory diseases. *Dev. Comp. Immunol.*, **2**, 235–242.

Cohen, S. (1982). Lymphokines and immune regulation. I. Introduction and summary. *Fed. Proc.*, **41**, 2478–2479.

Cohn, M. (1976). Summary discussion of directions of immunobiology. In *Mitogens in Immunobiology* (Eds. J. J. Oppenheim, and O. L. Rosenstreich), pp.663–702. Academic Press, New York.

Cooper, H. R., Chorpenning, F. W., and Rosen, S. (1975). Preparation and chemical composition of the cell walls of *Streptococcus mutans*. *Infect. Immun.*, **11**, 823–828.

Cooper, H. R., Chorpenning, F. W., and Rosen, S. (1978). Lipid-free glycerol teichoic acids with potent membrane-binding activity. *Infect. Immun.*, **19**, 462–469.

Coutinho, A., and Moller, G. (1973). B cell mitogenic properties of thymus-independent antigens. *Nature*, **245**, 12–14.

Coutinho, A., and Moller, A. (1975). Thymus-independent B cell induction and paralysis. *Adv. Immunol.*, **21**, 113–236.

Coutinho, A., Gronowicz, E., Moller, G., and Lemke, H. (1976). Polyclonal B cell activators (PBA). In *Mitogens in Immunobiology* (Eds. J. J. Oppenheim, and D. L. Rosenstreich), pp.173–190. Academic Press, New York.

Crowder, J. G., and White, A. (1972). Teichoic acid antibodies in staphylococcal and nonstaphylococcal endocarditis. *Ann. Intern. Med.*, **77**, 87–90.

Curtin, J. A., Choa, M. S., Marcus, D., Sheagren, J. N., and Tuazon, C. U. (1978). *Staphylococcus aureus* bacteremia. Relationship between formation of antibodies to teichoic acid and development of metastatic abscesses. *J. Infect. Dis.*, **137**, 57–63.

Daugharty, H., Martin, R. R., and White, A. (1967). Antibodies against staphylococcal teichoic acids and type-specific antigens in man. *J. Immunol.*, **98**, 1123–1129.

Decker, G. P., Chorpenning, F. W., and Frederick, G. T. (1972). Naturally-occurring antibodies to bacillary teichoic acids. *J. Immunol.*, **108**, 214–222.

DeVuono, H., and Panos, C. (1978). Effect of L-form *Streptococcus pyogenes* and of lipoteichoic acid on human cells in tissue culture. *Infect. Immun.*, **22**, 255–265.

Dziarski, R. (1976). Teichoic acids. *Curr. Top. Microbiol. Immunol.*, **74**, 113–135.

Dziarski, R. (1982). Studies on the mechanism of peptidoglycan- and lipoplysaccharide-induced polyclonal activation. *Infect. Immun.*, **35**, 507–514.

Dziarski, R., and Dziarski, A. (1979). Mitogenic activity of staphlococcal peptidoglycan. *Infect. Immun.*, **23**, 706–710.

Dziarski, R., Dziarski, A., and Levinson, A. I. (1980). Mitogenic responsiveness of mouse, rat, and human lymphocytes to *Staphlococcus aureus* cell wall, teichoic acid, and peptidoglycan. *Int. Arch. Allergy Appl. Immunol.*, **63**, 383–395.

Easmon, C. S. F., and Glynn, A. A. (1978). Role of *Staphylococcus aureus* cell wall antigens in the stimulation of delayed hypersensitivity after staphylococcal infection. *Infect. Immun.*, **19**, 341–342.

Ekstedt, R. D. (1963a). Studies on immunity to staphylococcal infection in mice. I. Effect of dosage, viability, and interval between immunization and challenge on resistance to infection following injection of whole cell vaccines. *J. Infect. Dis.*, **112**, 143–151.

Ekstedt, R. D. (1963b). Studies on immunity to staphylococcal infection in mice. II. Effect of immunization with fractions of *Staphylococcus aureus* prepared by physical and chemical methods. *J. Infect. Dis.*, **112**, 152–157.

Ekstedt, R. D. (1966). Studies on immunity to staphylococcal infection in mice. IV. The role of specific and nonspecific immunity. *J. Infect. Dis.*, **116**, 514–522.

Falkoff, R. J. M., Zhu, L. P., and Fauci, A. S. (1982). Separate signals for B cell proliferation and differentiation in response to *Staphylococcus aureus*. Evidence for a two-signal model of B cell activation. *J. Immunol.*, **129**, 97–102.

Fiedel, B. A., and Jackson, R. S. (1974). Implications of a strep-lipoteichoic acid in renal dysfunction in hyperimmunized rabbits. *Abstr. Ann. Meeting—ASM*, (M364), 126.

Fiedel, B. A., and Jackson, R. W. (1976). Immunogenicity of a purified and carrier-complexed streptococcal lipoteichoic acid. *Infect. Immun.*, **13**, 1585–1590.

Flandrois, J. P., Reverdy, M. E., Fleurette, J., Jullien, P., Veysseyre, C., Modjadedy, A., and Gery, C. (1979). Diagnostic serologique des infections a *Staphylococcus aureus* par dosage des anticorps anti-acids teichoique AB. *Pathol. Biol.*, **27**, 281–284.

Folch, H., Yoshinaga, M., and Waksman, B. H. (1973). Regulation of lymphocyte responses *in vitro*. III. Inhibition by adherent cells of the T-lymphocyte response to phytohemagglutinin. *J. Immunol.*, **110**, 835–839.

Frederick, G. T., and Chorpenning, F. W. (1973). Comparisons of natural and immune antibodies to teichoic acids in germfree and conventional guinea pigs. In *Germfree Research: Biological Effect of Gnotobiotic Environments* (Ed. J. B. Heneghan), pp.517–524, Academic Press, New York.

Frederick, G. T., and Chorpenning, F. W. (1974). Characterization of antibodies specific for polyglycerophosphate. *J. Immunol.*, **113**, 489–493.

Frederick, G. T., Holmes, R. A., and Chorpenning, F. W. (1972). Naturally occurring cell-mediated immunity to purified glycerol-teichoic acid antigen in guinea pigs. *J. Immunol.*, **109**, 1399–1401.

Goodman, M. G., and Weigle, W. O. (1981). T cell regulation of polyclonal B cell responsiveness. III. Overt T helper and latent T suppressor activities from distinct subpopulations of unstimulated splenic T cells. *J. Exp. Med.*, **153**, 844–856.

Grov, A. (1969). Studies on antigen preparations from *Staphylococcus aureus*. 7. The component of polysaccharide A sensitizing tanned erythrocytes. *Acta Pathol. Microbiol. Scand.*, **76**, 621–628.

Hamada, S., and Slade, H. D. (1976). Adherence of serotype e *Streptococcus mutans* and the inhibitory effect of Lancefield Group E and S. Mutans type e antiserum. *J. Dent. Res.*, **55**, 65–74.

Hirose, S., Maruyama, N., Ohta, K., and Shirai, T. (1980). Polyclonal B cell activation and autoimmunity in New Zealand mice. I. Natural thymocytotoxic autoantibody (NTA). *J. Immunol.*, **125**, 610–615.

Horton, J. E., Raisz, L. G., and Oppenheim, J. J. (1972). Bone resorbing activity in supernatant fluid from cultured human peripheral blood leukocytes. *Science*, **177**, 793–795.

Jerne, N. K. (1974). Towards a network theory of the immune response. *Ann. Immunol. (Inst. Pasteur)*, **125**C, 373–389.

Karakawa, W. W., Wagner, J. E., and Pazur, J. H. (1971). Immunochemistry of the cell wall carbohydrate of group L hemolytic streptococci. *J. Immunol.*, **107**, pp. 554–562.

Klesius, P. H., Zimmerman, R. A., Mathews, J. H., and Auernheime, A. H. (1974). Human antibody response to group A streptococcal teichoic acid. *Can. J. Microbiol.*, **20**, 853–859.

Knox, K. W., and Wicken, A. J. (1972). Serological studies on the teichoic acids of *Lactobacillus plantarum*. *Infect. Immun.*, **6**, 43–49.

Knox, K. W., and Wicken, A. J. (1973). Immunological properties of teichoic acids. *Bact. Rev.*, **37**, 215–257.

Knox, K. W., Hewett, M. J., and Wicken, A. J. (1970). Studies on the group F antigen of lactobacilli: Antigenicity and serological specificity of teichoic acid preparations. *J. Gen. Microbiol.*, **60**, 303–313.

Larinkari, U. M. (1982). Assay of teichoic acid antibodies and anti-staphylolysin in the diagnosis of staphylococcal osteomyelitis. *Scand. J. Infect. Dis.*, **14**, 123–128.

Larinkari, U. M., Valtonen, M. V., Sarvas, M., and Valtonen, V. V. (1977). Teichoic acid antibody test. Its use in patients with coagulase-positive staphylococcal bacteremia. *Arch. Intern. Med.*, **137**, 1522–1525.

Lee, K. C., Shiozawa, C., Shaw, A., and Diener, E. (1980). Requirement for accessory cells in the antibody response to T cell independent antigens *in vitro*. *Eur. J. Immunol.*, **6**, 63–69.

Lemke, H., Coutinho, A., Opitz, H.-G., and Gronowicz, E. (1975). Macrophages suppress direct B cell activation by lipoplysaccharide. *Scand. J. Immunol.*, **4**, 707–713.

Lynch, J. J., Jr., and Chorpenning, F. W. (1978). Effects of dosage on modulation of sheep red cell responses by teichoic acid. *Fed. Proc.*, **37**, 1489.

Lynch, J. J., Jr., and Chorpenning, F. W. (1979). Adherent cell mediated modulation of the response to sheep erythrocytes induced by teichoic acid. *Fed. Proc.*, **38**, 190.

Lynch, J. J., Jr., Chorpenning, F. W., and Oldfather, J. W. (1978). Route, strain, and species difference in modulation of SRBC response by teichoic acid. *Abstr. Ann. Meeting — ASM*, No. E170.

Mackler, B. F, Altman, L. C., Wahl, S., Rosenstreich, D. L., Oppenheim, J. J., and Mergenhagen, S. E. (1974). Blastogenesis and lymphokine synthesis by T and B lymphocytes from patients with periodontal disease. *Infect. Immun.*, **10**, 844–850.

Martin, R. R., Daugharty, H., and White, A. (1966). Staphylococcal antibodies and hypersensitivity to teichoic acids in man. In *Antimicrobial Agents and Chemotherapy — 1965* (Ed. G. L. Hobby), pp.91–96. American Society for Microbiology, Washington, USA.

Martinez-Alonso, C., Bernabe, R. R., and Diaz-Espada, F. (1980). Different macrophage requirement in the specific and polyclonal responses induced by TNP–LPS and LPS. *Scand. J. Immunol.*, **12**, 453–457.

Mattingly, J. A., Eardley, D. D., Kemp, J. D., and Gershon, R. K. (1979). Induction of suppressor cells in rat spleen: Influence of microbial stimulation. *J. Immunol.*, **122**, 787–790.

McCarty, M. (1959). The occurrence of polyglycerophosphate as an antigenic component of various gram-positive bacterial species. *J. Exp. Med.*, **109**, 361–378.

Miller, G. A., and Jackson, R. W. (1973). The effect of *Streptococcus pyogenes* teichoic acid on the immune response of mice. *J. Immunol.*, **110**, 148–156.

Miller, G. A., Urban, J., and Jackson, R. W. (1976). Effects of a streptococcal lipoteichoic acid on host responses in mice. *Infect. Immun.*, **13**, 1408–1417.

Moller, G., Coutinho, A., and Gronowicz, E. (1976). Role of mitogenic components of thymus-independent antigens. In *Mitogens in Immunobiology* (Eds. J. J. Oppenheim, and D. L. Rosenstreich), pp.291–311. Academic Press, New York.

Mudd, S. A., Yoshida, I. W. Li, and Lenhart, N. A. (1963). Identification of a somatic antigen of *Staphylococcus aureus* critical for phagocytosis by human blood. *Nature*, **199**, 1200–1201.

Nakano, M., Toyoda, H., Tanabe, M. J., Matsumoto, T., and Masuda, S. (1980). Polyclonal antibody production in murine spleen cells induced by staphylococcus. *Microb. Immunol.*, **24**, 981–994.

Ne'eman, N., and Ginsburg, I. (1972). Cell sensitizing antigen of group a streptococci. II. Immunological and immunopathological properties. *Isr. J. Med. Sci.*, **8**, 1807–1816.

Nelson, A. (1974). The complement system. In *The Inflammatory Process*, Vol. III, 2nd edn. Academic Press, San Francisco.

Ofek, I., Beachey, E. H., Jefferson, W., and Campbell, G. L. (1975). Cell membrane-binding properties of group A streptococcal lipoteichoic acid. *J. Exp. Med.*, **141**, 990–1003.

Oldfather, J. W., and Chorpenning, F. W. (1980). Role of T-lymphocytes in antibody responses to glycerol teichoic acid. *Ohio J. Sci.*, **80** (Suppl.), 45.

Oldfather, J. W., and Chorpenning, F. W. (1981). Suppression of the primary IgM response by environmental teichoic acid. *Eur. J. Immunol.*, **11**, 437–440.

Oldfather, J. W., Cooper, H. R., and Chorpenning, F. W. (1977). Investigation of possible mitogenic activity by glycerol teichoic acid. *Abstr. Ann. Meeting — ASM*, (E201).

Oldfather, J. W., Chorpenning, F. W., Lynch, J. J., Jr., and Rozmiarek, H. (1978). Influence of responsiveness to teichoic acid on its immunomodulatory effects. *Abstr. Ann. Meeting — ASM*, (E168).

Ortiz-Ortiz, L., Parks, D. E., Rodriguez, M., and Weigle, W. O. (1980). Polyclonal B lymphocyte activation during *Trypanosoma cruzi* infection. *J. Immunol.*, **124**, 121–124.

Petit, J.-C., and Unanue. (1974). Effects of bacterial products on lymphocytes and macrophages: Their possible role in natural resistance to *Listeria* infection in mice. *J. Immunol.*, **113**, 984–992.

Räsänen, L., and Arvilommi, H. (1982). Cell walls, peptidoglycans, and teichoic acids of gram-positive bacteria as polyclonal inducers and immunomodulators of proliferative and lymphokine responses of human B and T lymphocytes. *Infect. Immun.*, **35**, 523–527.

Räsänen, L., Karhumaki, E., and Arvilommi, H. (1978). Bacteria induce lymphokine synthesis polyclonally in human B lymphocytes. *J. Immunol.*, **121**, 418–420.

Rozmiarek, H., Bolton, R. W., and Chorpenning, F. W. (1977). Environmental origin of natural antibodies to teichoic acid. *Infect. Immun.*, **16**, 505–509.

Russell, R. R. B., and Beighton, D. (1982). Specificity of natural antibodies reactive with *Streptococcus mutans* in monkey. *Infect. Immun.*, **35**, 741–748.

Shayegani, M., Hisatsune, K., and Mudd, S. (1970). Cell wall component which affects the ability of serum to promote phagocytosis and killing of *Staphylococcus aureusn*. *Infect. Immun.*, **2**, 750–756.

Sheagren, J. N., Menes, B. L., Han, D. P., Sanders, J. L., and Sheagren, M. A. (1981). Technical aspects of the *Staphylococcus aureus* teichoic acid antibody assay: gel diffusion and counter immunoelectrophoretic assays, antigen preparation, antigen selection, concentration effects, and cross-reactions with other organisms. *J. Clin. Microbiol.*, **13**, 293–300.

Shenker, B. J., Mann, T. N., and Willoughby, W. F. (1980). Role of polyclonal cell activation in the initiation of immune complex-mediated pulmonary injury following antigen inhalation. *Environ. Health Perspect.*, **35**, 43–54.

Silvestri, L. J., Knox, K. W., Wicken, A. J., and Hoffman, E. M. (1979). Inhibition of complement-mediated lysis of sheep erythrocytes by cell-free preparation from *Streptococcus mutans* BHT. *J. Immunol.*, **122**, 54–60.

Stewart-Tull, D. E. S. (1980). The immunological activities of bacterial peptidoglycans. *Annu. Rev. Microbiol.*, **34**, 311–340.

Tenenbaum, M. J., and Archer, G. L. (1980). Prognostic value of teichoic acid antibodies in *Staphylococcus aureus* bacteremia: A reassessment. *South. Med. J.*, **73**, 140–143.

Torii, M., Kabat, E. A., and Bezer, A. E. (1964). Separation of teichoic acid of *Staphylococcus aureus* into two immunologically distinct specific polysaccharides with α- and β-*N*acetylglucosaminyl linkages respectively. *J. Exp. Med.*, **120**, 13–29.

Tribble, J. L., and Bolen, J. B. (1979). Delayed hypersensitivity to *Staphylococcus aureus* in mice: *in vitro* responses to isolated staphylococcal antigens. *Immunology*, **38**, 819–825.

Tuason, C. U., and Sheagren, J. N. (1976). Teichoic acid antibodies in the diagnosis of serious infections with *Staphylococcus aureus*. *Ann. Intern. Med.*, **84**, 543–546.

Uchiyama, T., and Jacobs, D. M. (1978). Modulation of immune responses by bacterial lipopolysaccharide (LPS): Cellular basis of stimulatory and inhibitory effects of LPS on the *in vitro* IgM antibody response to a T-dependent antigens. *J. Immunol.*, **121**, 2347–2351.

Van Driel, D., Wicken, A. J., Dickson, M. R. and Knox, K. W. (1973). Cellular location of the teichoic acids of *Lactobacillus casei* NCTC 6375. *J. Ultrastruct. Res.*, **43**, 483–497.

Verbrugh, H. A., Van Dijk, W. C., Peters, R., Van Der Tol, M. E., and Verhoef, J. (1979). The role of *Staphylococcus aureus* cell-wall peptidoglycan teichoic acid and protein A in the processes of complement activation and opsonization. *Immunology*, **37**, 615–621.

Villeneuve, L., Brousseau, P., Chaput, J., and Elie, R. (1980). Role of adherent cells in graft-versus-host induced suppression of the humoral immune response. *Scand. J. Immunol.*, **12**, 321–330.

Waltersdorff, R. L., Fiedel, B. A., and Jackson, R. W. (1977). Induction of nephrocalcinosis in rabbit kidneys after long-term exposure to a streptococcal teichoic acid. *Infect. Immun.*, **17**, 665–667.

Warner, P., Slipetz, W. K., and Kroeker, J. (1966). Mouse-protective antibodies in human sera against the Smith strain of *Staphylococcus aureus*. *Can. J. Microbiol.*, **12**, 949–955.

Wells, C. L., and Balish, E. (1980). Modulation of the rat's immune status by monoassociation with anaerobic bacteria. *Can. J. Microbiol.*, **26**, 1192–1198.

Wicken, A. J., and Knox, K. W. (1975). Lipoteichoic acids: A new class of bacterial antigen. *Science*, **87**, 1161–1167.

Wilkinson, B. J., Kim, Y., and Peterson, P. K. (1981). Factors affecting complement activation by *Staphylococcus aureus* cell walls. *Infect. Immun.*, **32**, 216–224.

Winkelstein, J. A., and Tomasz, A. (1978). Activation of the alternative complement pathway by pneumococcal cell wall teichoic acid. *J. Immunol.*, **120**, 174–178.

Wong, D. M., and Herscowitz, H. B. (1979). Immune activation by T-independent antigens: Lack of effect of macrophage depletion on the immune response to TNP-LPS, PVP, and dextran. *Immunology*, **37**, 765–769.

Yoshida, K., and Ekstedt, R. D. (1968). Antibody response to *Staphylococcus aureus* in rabbits: Sequence of immunoglobulin synthesis and its correlation with passive protection in mice. *J. Bacteriol.*, **96**, 1540–1545.

Young, D. A., and Chorpenning, F. W. (1980a). Specificity of splenocyte activation by glycerol teichoic acid (GTA). *Abstr. Ann. Meeting—ASM*, (E45).

Young, D. A., and Chorpenning, F. W. (1980b). Kinetics of immunomodulation by glycerol teichoic acid in BALB/c mice. *Ohio J. Sci.*, **80**, Prog. Abstr. p.44.

Young, D. A. (1982). A comparative study of the responses elicited by lipopolysaccharide, peptidoglycan, and glycerol teichoic acid in immunocompetent murine spleen cell populations. PhD Dissertation, The Ohio State Univ., Columbus, Ohio.

Young, D. A., Cline, D. J., and Chorpenning, F. W. (1982). Polyclonal and mitogenic responses of splenic BALB/c cells to three different bacterial products. *Fed. Proc.*, **41**, 420.

Zoscke, D. C., and Bach, F. H. (1971). *In vitro* elimination of specific immunoreactive cells with 5-bromodeoxyuridine. *J. Immunol. Methods*, **1**, 55.

Immunology of the Bacterial Cell Envelope
Edited by D. E. S. Stewart-Tull and M. Davies
© 1985 John Wiley & Sons Ltd.

CHAPTER 7

Immunology of Outer Membrane Proteins of Gram-Negative Bacteria

Cyril J. Smyth

Department of Microbiology, Moyne Institute, Trinity College, Dublin 2, Ireland

I. INTRODUCTION

Gram-negative bacteria possess a complex cell envelope comprising at least three distinguishable layers, namely, the inner or cytoplasmic membrane, the

177

peptidoglycan layer and associated periplasmic space, and the outer membrane, which acts as a selective barrier on the exterior surface of the cell (Inouye, 1979; Nikaido and Nakae, 1979; Lugtenberg, 1981). The development of methods for the preparation of sphaeroplasts of gram-negative bacterial cells, for the fractionation of bacterial envelopes and for the separation of inner and outer membranes, thereby allowing the isolation of outer membrane with or without peptidoglycan, has played no small role in the probing of structural and functional details of outer membranes (Miura and Mizushima, 1969; Schnaitman, 1970; Osborn and Munson, 1974; Owen *et al.* 1982; Lugtenberg and Van Alphen, 1983). A review of some aspect of the biology of outer membranes has almost become an annual occurrence, so rapid have the advances in knowledge of their structure, assembly, genetics, antigenicity and topography been (Salton, 1971; Braun and Hantke, 1974; Costerton *et al.*, 1974; Inouye, 1975, 1979; Salton and Owen, 1976; DiRienzo *et al.*, 1978; Braun, 1978; Osborn and Wu, 1980; Hall and Silhavy, 1981; Owen, 1981, 1983a,b; Lugtenberg, 1981; Lugtenberg and Van Alphen, 1983). What these reviews also attest to is the plethora of techniques applied to the analysis of the constituents of outer membranes and the topographical disposition of components within them.

Although originally developed for the separation of the membranes of *Escherichia coli* and *Salmonella typhimurium*, the same procedures with slight modification have been applied successfully to a variety of gram-negative bacteria within and without the family *Enterobacteriaceae* (Owen *et al.*, 1982; Lugtenberg and Van Alphen, 1983). These studies have shown that outer membranes have an essentially similar composition, namely that they contain lipopolysaccharide (LPS), phospholipid and protein as major constituents. The quantitative proportions of these major constituents vary from investigation to investigation. Reasons for this have been discussed in detail by Lugtenberg and Van Alphen (1983). In addition to the above-mentioned components, minor constituents may be present such as the enterobacterial common antigen shared by most members of the *Enterobacteriaceae* (Mäkelä and Mayer, 1976; Mayer and Schmidt, 1979).

Other contributions to this book deal with the immunology of the lipopolysaccharide of outer membranes. The focus of this chapter is restricted to the immunology of outer membrane proteins of gram-negative bacteria. However, some general aspects of isolation and characterization of outer membranes are relevant for an understanding of studies on the antigenicity and immunogenicity of outer membrane proteins.

II. ISOLATION AND CHARACTERIZATION OF OUTER MEMBRANES

A. Isolation of Outer Membranes

Owen *et al.* (1982) have reviewed procedures for the separation of inner and outer membranes from 18 species of gram-negative bacteria. Examples for an additional ten species were cited by Lugtenberg and Van Alphen (1983). Suffice to say, that procedures originally developed for the isolation of inner and outer membranes of *E. coli* and *S. typhimurium* have been applied successfully to other gram-negative bacteria. The modifications for particular organisms usually lie in the method of cell lysis, while fractionation of the envelope membranes is based in most cases on isopycnic centrifugation on sucrose gradients based on the original description of Miura and Mizushima (1969).

Outer membranes can be isolated without peptidoglycan after sphaeroplast lysis or as outer membrane–peptidoglycan complexes following disruption of cells in a French pressure cell (Lugtenberg and Van Alphen, 1983). Outer membrane fragments which slough off the bacterial cell surface during growth in broth can also be harvested from cell-free culture supernatant fluid and from heat-treated and sonicated cells (see Owen *et al.*, 1982, for references).

Another strategy adopted by some investigators is based on the belief that certain detergents solubilize the cytoplasmic membrane of isolated envelopes in a selective manner leaving the outer membrane intact as an insoluble residue. Triton X-100 and sodium lauryl sarcosinate (sarkosyl) have been studied in detail (Schnaitman, 1971a,b; Filip *et al.*, 1973). However, there is a lack of solid quantitative data on the fate of outer membrane components using these methods and some outer membrane proteins may be solubilized under these conditions (Chopra and Shales, 1980). Moreover, the residues obtained by ultracentrifugation of detergent-treated cell envelopes or sphaeroplast envelopes are not true outer membranes but rather delipidated aggregates of outer membrane proteins, possibly also having lost considerable amounts of LPS.

Criteria for the purity of outer membranes of gram-negative bacteria and the distribution of molecular markers between the inner and outer membranes have been reviewed in detail (Owen *et al.*, 1982).

B. Analysis of Outer Membrane Proteins

The outer membrane of gram-negative bacteria accounts for some 9–12% of cellular protein. In contrast to the inner membrane, the outer membrane contains few enzymes. Those reported in various gram-negative species include phospholipase A_1, lysophospholipase, lysophosphatidic acid phosphatase, tetramethylphenylenediamine oxidase, β-lactamase, proteolytic activities including signal peptidase, UDP–glucose hydrolase, monoacylglycerophosphoethanolamine acylase, pullanase and *N*-acetylmuramyl–L-alanine amidase (Owen *et al.*, 1982; Lugtenberg and Van Alphen, 1983). Some of these are also present in inner membranes.

Two techniques, because of their high resolution, have been of particular value for the examination of outer membrane protein profiles of gram-negative bacteria, namely, sodium dodecyl sulphate–polyacrylamide gel electrophoresis (SDS–PAGE) (see Owen *et al.*, 1982, and Lugtenberg and Van Alphen, 1983, for review of procedures) and electroimmunochemical methods (Owen and Smyth, 1977; Owen, 1981; Bjerrum, 1983; Axelsen, 1983).

1. SDS–PAGE

Electrophoretic separation of SDS-solubilized outer membrane proteins on slab gels of polyacrylamide or linear gradient polyacrylamide gels followed by staining or autoradiography or fluorography, when the bacteria are grown in the presence of a radio-labelled substrate, has revealed that gram-negative bacterial outer membranes have highly distinctive polypeptide profiles (e.g. Overbeeke and Lugtenberg, 1980; Tsai *et al.*, 1981; Achtman *et al.*, 1983). This technique allows identification of outer membrane proteins based on their apparent molecular weights relative to known standard proteins and on their altered electrophoretic mobilities following treatment with SDS at temperatures below 60°C as opposed to boiling. This property of so-called heat modifiability of proteins results from incomplete unfolding which gives rise to decreased binding of SDS (Osborn and Wu, 1980; Lugtenberg and Van Alphen, 1983). The most widely used techniques are those of Laemmli (1970) and Lugtenberg *et al.* (1975), the latter method being particularly suitable for resolution of outer membrane proteins in the 30 000 to 40 000 molecular weight range. Electrophoretic homogeneity by SDS–PAGE is also a useful criterion for the purity of so-called purified proteins.

2. Immunoprecipitation-in-gel Techniques

Alternative high-resolution techniques which allow analysis of membrane proteins as discrete antigens or antigen complexes are electroimmunochemical methods. In particular, crossed immunoelectrophoresis (CIE) has been of particular value (Owen, 1981; Bjerrum, 1983; Axelsen, 1983). The method has the advantage over SDS–PAGE that it permits resolution with retention of intrinsic biological properties or activities. Membrane proteins, solubilized and dissociated usually by non-ionic detergents, are electrophoresed in agarose gel in one dimension and then at 90° to the first dimension into a similar gel containing immunoglobulins. Each membrane antigen or complex is displayed as a rocket- or arc-shaped immunoprecipitate. The final pattern is a complex two-dimensional array of immunoprecipitates (Owen and Smyth, 1977; Owen, 1981, 1983a,b). In addition, the method is quantitative, the area enclosed by the immunoprecipitate being proportional to the concentration of antigen and inversely proportional to the concentration of immunoglobulins. To date, the technique has been applied most extensively to *Escherichia coli* strains K-12 and ML308–225 (Smyth *et al.*, 1978; Owen, 1981, 1983b) (Figure 1), although the method has been used successfully with *Neisseria gonorrhoeae* (Smyth *et al.*, 1976; Collins and Salton, 1980) and *Neisseria meningitidis* (Hoff and Frasch, 1979). Moreover, the antigenic components giving rise to immunoprecipitates can be identified in terms of polypeptides resolved using SDS–PAGE after

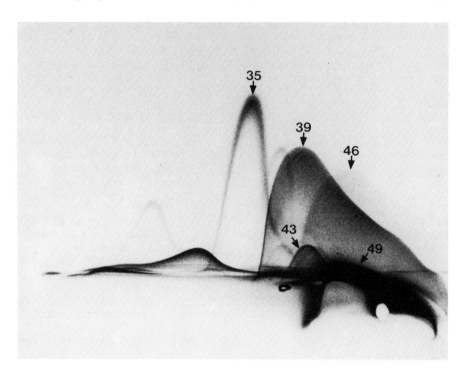

Figure 1. Crossed immunoelectrophoresis of isolated ^{35}S-labelled outer membranes from *Escherichia coli* ML308-225. Some of the salient immunoprecipitates have been numbered according to the scheme of Owen (1983b) and correspond to the following antigens mentioned in the text: 35, antigen No. 35; 39, OmpF/C proteins; 43, antigen No. 43; 46, OmpA protein; 49, Lpp protein (Braun's lipoprotein). Anode is to the left and top of the autoradiogram. (Figure kindly supplied by Peter Owen from unpublished data)

precipitate excision, solubilization in SDS and electrophoresis (Owen, 1983a,b). CIE and its variant techniques provide possibilities for stringent monitoring of the purity of outer membrane proteins with the use of suitable monospecific and polyvalent antisera. Furthermore, the topological distribution of proteins within a membrane and their surface expression on cells can be investigated (Owen, 1981, 1983a,b).

III. NOMENCLATURE OF OUTER MEMBRANE PROTEINS

The outer membrane proteins of *E. coli* have been divided into major and minor proteins. Using different SDS–PAGE systems, several groups of researchers in the 1970s resolved a characteristic set of polypeptide bands termed major outer membrane proteins, so-called because of their prominence in outer membrane protein profiles in SDS–PAGE, thereby leading to different

Table 1   Outer membrane proteins of *E. coli* lacking enzymic activity[*]

Protein	Relative molecular weight	No. of molecules per cell	Peptidoglycan associated	Proposed or established function
OmpF	37 205	$\sim 10^5$	+	General porin
OmpC	36 000	$\sim 10^5$	+	General porin
OmpA	35 159	$\sim 10^5$		Stabilization of mating
PhoE	36 782	$\sim 5 \times 10^4$	+	Porin for anions
Tsx	26 000	$\sim 10^4$		Porin for nucleosides, deoxyribonucleosides
LamB	47 392	$\sim 10^5$	+	Porin for maltose and maltodextrins
BtuB	60 000	~ 250		Uptake of vitamin B_{12}
Cir	74 000	?		Uptake of Fe^{3+}
FhuA	78 000	$\sim 10^3$		Uptake of ferrichrome
Fec	80 500	?		Uptake of Fe^{3+}-citrate
FepA	81 000	?		Uptake of Fe^{3+}-enterochelin
83K	83 000	?		Uptake of Fe^{3+}
TraT	25 000	?	+	Surface exclusion
K	40 000	?		Unknown
Lc	36 000	?	+	General porin replacing OmpC protein
NmpC	36 000	?		General porin in strains lacking OmpC/F
31K	31 000	?		Attachment of DNA
O-13	31 000	$\sim 1.6 \times 10^4$	+	Unknown
PAL	21 000	$\sim 10^4$	+	Unknown
III	18 000	$\sim 10^4$		Unknown
Lipoprotein	7 200	$\sim 7.5 \times 10^5$	+	Anchors outer membrane to peptidoglycan
LPS-binding	15 000	?		Structural

*Compiled from Lugtenberg (1981), Lugtenberg and Van Alphen (1983) and Arbuthnott *et al.* (1983).

nomenclature systems which have been compared in a number of reviews (Osborn and Wu, 1980; Bachmann and Brooks Low, 1980; Lugtenberg and Van Alphen, 1983). A uniform nomenclature system has been agreed for *E. coli* and *S. typhimurium* whereby each protein is named after its structural gene (Osborn and Wu, 1980). For example, the OmpF protein is encoded by the *ompF* structural gene. Some ten outer membrane proteins have been described which comprise 80% of the outer membrane protein content. These proteins may be present in 100 000 copies per cell (Osborn and Wu, 1980). Approximately 10–20 minor protein components have been described which are implicated in vitamin B_{12} uptake, iron transport, nucleoside transport, maltose uptake, phage receptors, and blocking or stabilization of mating aggregates, or to which as yet no function has been ascribed. The properties of constitutive and inducible outer membrane proteins of *E. coli* are shown in Table 1 [for fuller descriptions of the properties of these proteins, see Arbuthnott *et al.* (1983), Lugtenberg (1981) and Lugtenberg and Van Alphen (1983)]. The lipoprotein of the outer membrane is by far the most abundant protein of the gram-negative bacterial cell.

In general, the outer membranes of other gram-negative bacteria have not been characterized to anywhere near the extent of those of *E. coli* K-12, in particular. However, proteins with apparently analogous functions in *Pseudomonas aeruginosa, N. gonorrhoeae* and *N. meningitidis* have been described for the LamB, PhoE, OmpF, OmpC, OmpA, and PAL proteins and murein lipoprotein of *E. coli* in one or more of these bacteria (Arbuthnott *et al.*, 1983). Unfortunately, no uniform nomenclature has yet been established. Moreover, it has not proved possible to establish the presence of some proteins in certain gram-negative bacteria, e.g. of a murein lipoprotein in *N. gonorrhoeae* (Hebeler *et al.*, 1978).

IV. PURIFICATION AND PURITY OF OUTER MEMBRANE PROTEINS

Several of the outer membrane proteins of *E. coli* have been purified using ionic and non-ionic detergents and even obtained on a preparative scale, e.g. lipoprotein, OmpF, and protein III (synonyms: a, 3b or O-11) (see Braun, 1978, and Lugtenberg and Van Alphen, 1983, for references). This progress in the field of characterization of outer membrane proteins has permitted greater understanding of structural and functional relationships within this membrane. These proteins are integral proteins and bind strongly to each other, to LPS, to phospholipids and in some cases to peptidoglycan.

Extraction and purification of such proteins raises several questions which are pertinent to studies of their biological properties including antigenicity, immunogenicity and mitogenicity. For example, to what extent is the native conformation or configuration changed and how different is the conformation in the 'renatured' state from that *in situ* in the outer membrane? How free are purified outer membrane proteins from LPS given its manifest biological properties? How does the immunogenicity of an outer membrane protein in its integrated state in the membrane differ from its immunogenicity as an isolated delipidated, possibly aggregated protein?

For example, purification of the OmpF protein and other pore proteins (porins) by the method of Rosenbusch (1974) or minor modifications thereof, results in high yields of highly purified, even chemically pure, denatured monomers. However, the biologically active porin is trimeric. To obtain this, the trimers can be removed from peptidoglycan using high salt concentrations (Nakamura and Mizushima, 1976) or isolated using deoxycholate or octylglucosides (see Lugtenberg and Van Alphen, 1983, for references).

Purity of isolated outer membrane proteins has been monitored by SDS–PAGE, CIE and by chemical analysis. However, although several methods are available for the estimation of LPS because of its several unique chemical components, the limits of sensitivity of such procedures should be borne in mind in relation to the amounts of LPS required to elicit its biological effects. Moreover, the absence of heptose and ketodeoxyoctonate (KDO) in the lipopolysaccharide and of β-hydroxymyristic acid on the lipid A of *Bacteroides fragilis* and *B. melaninogenicus* presents particular problems with respect to the purification of outer membrane proteins of these organisms (Hofstad and Sveen, 1979; Mansheim *et al.*, 1979).

Thus, despite the advances in methodology and legerdemain in purifying outer membrane proteins, the difficulties involved in obtaining them undenatured and free from contaminating LPS or Braun's lipoprotein should not be understated. Antisera raised to purified outer membrane proteins have been shown to contain precipitating antibodies against minor protein contaminants and LPS or to be strongly reactive with denatured antigen, because denatured hydrophobic proteins present in such preparations may possibly be more immunogenic than the 'native' molecules or because antigenic determinants are exposed which are not normally recognized *in vivo* because of strong association with phospholipids or LPS.

V. ANTIGENIC CROSS-REACTIVITIES OF OUTER MEMBRANE PROTEINS

Immunoprecipitation-in-gel techniques have been extensively used by Høiby and coworkers to investigate cross-reactivities between antigens present in supernatant fractions of lysates of gram-negative bacteria, but the nature of these antigens is by and large unknown (reviewed by Owen and Smyth, 1977; Owen, 1981; Høiby, 1977). Other investigators have examined the immunological relatedness of outer membrane proteins of a limited spectrum of gram-negative bacteria.

Two approaches have proved to be of particular use in such studies, namely, crossed, tandem-crossed and SDS–PAGE-crossed immunoelectrophoresis (Van Tol *et al.*, 1979; Axelsen, 1983), or SDS–PAGE coupled with antibody-labelling of separated components (Van Raamsdonk *et al.*, 1977; Overbeeke and Lugtenberg, 1980). In the latter instance, after SDS–PAGE, the slab gel is sliced, washed, incubated with specific antibody and then either with ^{125}I-labelled staphylococcal protein A or anti-immunoglobulin conjugated with horseradish peroxidase. The band pattern of labelled polypeptides is developed by autoradiography and enzyme staining with a peroxidase substrate, respectively. Preimmunization sera are used as controls.

A. Enterobacteriaceae

The possibility that outer membrane proteins might act as common immunogens among several genera of gram-negative bacteria received stimulus with the report that Braun's lipoprotein (Braun, 1975) was a common antigen within the family *Enterobacteriaceae* (Braun *et al.*, 1976). Using passive haemagglutination and immune haemolysis for titration, antibodies against lipoprotein were detected in rabbit antisera prepared against whole cell vaccines of encapsulated and non-capsulated strains of *E. coli* of various serotypes, *Shigella* spp., *Salmonella minnesota*, mutants of these latter strains with complete or incomplete R-LPS, and *Citrobacter* S and R forms. Using CIE, co-CIE and tandem CIE, Owen and Kaback (1979) showed full antigenic identity between the Braun's lipoproteins of *E. coli* and *S. typhimurium*. By the latter methods, the lipoproteins can be examined in a non-denatured state by solubilization with the non-ionic detergent Triton X-100.

Using interfacial precipitin tests with SDS-solubilized outer membrane proteins followed by SDS–PAGE of the immunoprecipitates, Dankert and Hofstra (1978) subsequently showed that rabbit antisera to whole cell vaccines of *E. coli* O26:K60 contained antibodies to the spectrum of outer membrane proteins present in SDS extracts of outer membranes. Moreover, these same antibodies were reactive in interfacial precipitin tests with solubilized outer membrane proteins of other *E. coli* serotypes and of strains of other genera of the *Enterobacteriaceae* (Hofstra and Dankert, 1979).

The cross-reactivities of the OmpA, OmpC and OmpF proteins have been studied by SDS–PAGE-crossed immunoelectrophoresis and by the SDS–PAGE immunoperoxidase and SDS–PAGE ^{125}I-labelled protein A techniques (Van Tol *et al.*, 1979; Beher *et al.*, 1980; Hofstra and Dankert, 1980a,b; Overbeeke and Lugtenberg, 1980; Hofstra *et al.*, 1980; Overbeeke *et al.*, 1980).

Despite differences in the electrophoretic mobilities of the non-peptidoglycan-bound, heat-modifiable OmpA-like proteins of *E. coli* strains of different origin and serotype, all reacted with antibodies raised to OmpA, purified from either *E. coli* K-12 or *E. coli* O26:K60 by SDS extraction of outer membranes followed by column chromatography and acetone precipitation (Hofstra and Dankert, 1980b; Overbeeke and Lugtenberg, 1980). In *Proteus* species, except *Proteus morganii*, and *Providencia stuartii*, the heat-modifiable, non-peptidoglycan-bound, i.e. OmpA-like, proteins that were cross-reactive were of a higher molecular weight than usually associated with OmpA proteins in the *Enterobacteriaceae*, namely 38 000 to 40 000 as opposed to 33 000 to 36 000 in *E. coli* and other species (Hofstra and Dankert, 1980b). Moreover, in SDS–PAGE-CIE and in quantitative double immunodiffusion, the OmpA proteins in *Proteus* species reacted less strongly with antisera than did the corresponding proteins in the outer membranes of the other enterobacterial species tested (Hofstra *et al.*, 1980; Beher *et al.*, 1980). Both the unmodified and the heat-modified forms of these OmpA proteins reacted with the antisera (Hofstra *et al.*, 1980; Beher *et al.* 1980; Hofstra and Dankert, 1980b). Antisera to the OmpF and OmpC proteins of *E. coli* K-12 did not react with the OmpA protein (Overbeeke *et al.*, 1980).

The OmpC and OmpF proteins, both of which are peptidoglycan-bound, form aqueous pores through the outer membrane and have thus been termed general porins. Although these porins have very similar total amino acid compositions and amino terminal sequences, considerable differences have been found in their peptide map patterns after cleavage with cyanogen bromide and proteolytic enzymes (Lugtenberg and Van Alphen, 1983). In all *E. coli* investigated, except strain B/r which only produces the OmpF protein, both OmpC and OmpF are present, the relative amounts of the two proteins being dependent on such factors as the composition of the growth medium and its osmolarity such that the sum of these proteins is quantitatively constant (Lugtenberg *et al.*, 1976; Nakamura and Mizushima, 1976).

In the investigations of Hofstra and Dankert (1980a,b,c) it is not possible to distinguish cross-reactions between the OmpC and OmpF proteins in *E. coli* and between these *E. coli* proteins and OmpC- and OmpF-like proteins in other test species because the antiserum almost certainly contained antibodies to both OmpC and OmpF on account of the nature of the purified immunogen. Moreover, the OmpC and OmpF proteins, whether from *E. coli* K-12 or *E. coli* O26:K60, which have been used to raise antisera for most of the cross-reactivity studies had been SDS- and heat-treated. Thus, each of the peptidoglycan-bound proteins in all *E. coli* strains reacted with the antiserum, whether the strain had one or two porin bands. In the analysis of outer membrane preparations of other enterobacteria, the peptidoglycan-bound proteins corresponding to OmpC/OmpF reacted with the *E. coli* antiserum, although in the cases of *Proteus vulgaris, Proteus mirabilis* and *Providencia stuartii*, reactions were considerably less strong in the SDS–PAGE-CIE experiments (Hofstra *et al.*, 1980). The OmpC/OmpF equivalents in these three species had lower apparent molecular weights than those of the heat-modified forms of the OmpA cross-reactive proteins (cf. *E. coli* in Table 1).

In contrast, Overbeeke and Lugtenberg (1980) used antisera raised to individually purified outer membrane proteins. They showed that in all of 45 faecal, urine and blood isolates of *E. coli*, the major peptidoglycan-associated proteins reacted with antibodies against OmpC or OmpF or both proteins of *E. coli* K-12. However, the affinities of these antisera differed for these two outer membrane proteins. The anti-OmpF serum had a greater affinity for polypeptide bands corresponding to OmpF and protein III of strain K-12, whereas the anti-OmpC serum had a higher affinity for the polypeptide bands corresponding to the OmpC protein of strain K-12.

The immunological relationship between several outer membrane proteins was further investigated semiquantitatively using haemagglutination inhibition tests. The three general porins, the OmpF, OmpC and PhoE proteins, were cross-reactive although the amounts of purified proteins required for haemagglutination inhibition by heterologous proteins were significantly higher. Antigenic relationships between *E. coli* K-12 porins and functionally and biochemically similar proteins in other enterobacteria were also investigated. Good cross-reactivity to strong relationships were shown between the three *E. coli* porins and those of *S. typhimurium* and *Klebsiella aerogenes* and between the porin preparation of *Enterobacter cloacae* and the OmpC and OmpF proteins of *E. coli* K-12, whereas the reactions between *Proteus mirabilis* porins and *E. coli* porins were much weaker, in line with the SDS–PAGE findings (*vide supra*).

In contrast, haemagglutination inhibition findings indicated that the OmpA-equivalent outer membrane proteins of the species tested were not related immunologically to the OmpA protein of *E. coli* K-12. These semiquantitative findings agree with those of Beher *et al.* (1980) who used immunodiffusion, and with some of the qualitative findings of Hofstra and Dankert (1980b) and Hofstra *et al.* (1980).

A LPS-binding protein from *Re* mutants of *Salmonella minnesota* has also been shown to cross-react serologically with antigens expressed on the surface of strains of *S. typhimurium*, *E. coli*, *Klebsiella* serovars, *Shigella dysenteriae* and *Shigella boydii* on the basis of antiserum absorption studies with specific antiserum to purified LPS-binding protein (Geyer *et al.*, 1979). The authors proposed that this protein may be a common surface antigen within the Enterobacteriaceae.

A novel outer membrane antigen, No. 35 in the standard CIE pattern of immunoprecipitates obtained for Triton X-100 extracts of membrane vesicles of *E. coli* strain ML308–225 (Owen, 1981, 1983b), has been shown to consist of at least three polypeptides of 94 000 (α), 40 500 (β) and 26 400 (γ) molecular weight. Using specific antiserum raised to immunoprecipitates excised from CIE immunoplates, antigen No. 35 has been detected by CIE methods in the envelopes of other *E. coli* strains examined. Partially identical antigens have also been identified in *S. typhimurium*, *Shigella flexneri*, *Klebsiella aerogenes*, *Enterobacter cloacae*, *Serratia marcescens* and *Erwinia carotovora*, but not in *Proteus vulgaris* or *Proteus mirabilis* using CIE and tandem CIE (Owen, 1983b). In further studies using SDS–PAGE followed by electrophoretic transfer of polypeptides to nitrocellulose and immunological detection using specific antibody and peroxidase-labelled anti-immunoglobulin or radioiodinated staphylococcal protein A, so-called Western blotting (Burnette, 1981; Towbin *et al.*, 1979), antibodies to the 94 000 subunit revealed equivalent polypeptides in the SDS–PAGE profiles of other enterobacterial envelopes in which a cross-reactive antigen was present, as indicated by CIE methods (Dr. P. Owen, personal communication). Although the antigen No. 35-specific antiserum contained antibodies to all three subunits (Owen, 1983b), methodological problems have occurred in trying unequivocally to demonstrate cross-reactivity due to anti-α and anti-β antibodies (Dr. P. Owen, personal communication).

B. Gram-negative Bacteria other than Enterobacteriaceae

Despite the demonstration of biochemically and/or functionally similar proteins in a number of other gram-negative bacteria (Lugtenberg and Van Alphen, 1983; Arbuthnott *et al.*, 1983), there have been few reports that the immunological cross-reactivity observed in the *Enterobacteriaceae* extends outside this family. Proteins functionally or apparently equivalent to Braun's lipoprotein have been described in *Aeromonas hydrophila, Pseudomonas aeruginosa* and *Rhodopseudomonas sphaeroides*, but not in *Neisseria gonorrhoeae* (Lugtenberg and Van Alphen, 1983). Another class of lipoproteins, peptidoglycan-associated lipoproteins (PAL), have been found in the outer membranes of a number of gram-negative bacteria, as well as several new lipoproteins in *E. coli* (see Lugtenberg and Van Alphen, 1983, for review). None of these was cross-reactive with Braun's lipoprotein from *E. coli*. Non-enterobacterial inter-species cross-reactivity has not yet been reported.

A protein cross-reactive with the OmpA protein of *E. coli* has been detected in *Aeromonas salmonicida* and *Haemophilus influenzae* (unpublished data cited by Lugtenberg and Van Alphen, 1983), although such a reaction was not detected by Beher *et al.* (1980) in extracts of the latter species. Negative findings have been recorded for *Pseudomonas aeruginosa, P. fluorescens, Acinetobacter calcoaceticus* var. *anitratus, Moraxella* sp. and *Neisseria gonorrhoeae* (Beher *et al.*, 1980; Hofstra and Dankert, 1980b). *Aeromonas hydrophila* and *Alcaligenes faecalis* lacked non-peptidoglycan-associated outer membrane proteins (Hofstra and Dankert, 1980b).

Analogous proteins cross-reactive with *E. coli* OmpF and/or OmpC proteins were not found in *Pseudomonas aeruginosa, P. fluorescens, Aeromonas hydrophila, Alcaligenes faecalis* and *Acinetobacter calcoaceticus* var. *anitratus* (Hofstra and Dankert, 1980b).

To date inter-generic or inter-familial cross-reactivity investigations have not been carried out with antisera to purified outer membrane proteins from bacteria outwith the family *Enterobacteriaceae*.

C. Immunological Characterization of Native and Heat-dissociated Forms of *E. coli* Porins

Hofstra and Dankert (1980c) observed during the preparation and quantitation of antibodies to outer membrane proteins that antibodies against a purified OmpC/OmpF porin mixture, prepared as described by Rosenbusch (1974), were hardly absorbed at all by outer membrane preparations. Accordingly, antisera raised in rabbits by immunization with purified porin trimers (Nakamura and Mizushima, 1976) and porin monomers (Rosenbusch, 1974) were compared with respect to their specificity and affinity for the homologous and heterologous antigens (Hofstra and Dankert, 1981). Antibodies to native porin oligomers reacted strongly quantitatively and qualitatively with the homologous antigen as detected by SDS–PAGE immunoperoxidase analysis, enzyme-linked immunosorbent assay (ELISA) and immunodiffusion, but showed no significant reaction with SDS- and heat-denatured porin monomers. Moreover, they were completely absorbed out by outer membrane preparations. Taken together these observations pinpoint that cross-reactivities among OmpF/OmpC proteins detected with antisera raised to denatured porins may not reflect cross-reactivities of these proteins in their native configurations. These findings are also of relevance to the potential use of purified outer membrane proteins in vaccines or as carriers of haptens for immunization (*vide infra*).

Thus, although the antigenicity of outer membrane proteins has received considerable attention, there is a need to adapt strategies that have been used commonly to date, namely SDS–PAGE-linked procedures using antisera raised to outer membrane proteins that have almost certainly been altered antigenically by the extraction procedures adopted. The use of non-ionic detergents for extraction and of CIE-related techniques to permit excision of immunoprecipitates for raising specific sera without the need to purify outer membrane proteins offers one approach (Harboe and Closs, 1983). Such reagents could be used with the high resolution of CIE to identify undenatured outer membrane proteins and to permit unequivocal assessment of inter- and intra-generic antigenic relationships between gram-negative bacteria.

VI. TYPING OF BACTERIAL SEROVARS BASED ON OUTER MEMBRANE PROTEINS

A. *Neisseria meningitidis*

Serogrouping of *N. meningitidis* into eight serogroups is based on the antigenic heterogeneity and immunological specificity of the capsular polysaccharides, namely serogroups A, B, C, X, Y, Z, 29E ($ = Z'$) and W-135. These serogroups have been subdivided into a number of serovars based on immunologically distinct LPS and major outer membrane proteins. Epidemiologically there is an association of certain meningococcal serogroups and serovars with disease (reviewed by Frasch, 1979; Poolman *et al.*, 1982).

Serogroups B, C, Y and W-135 have been divided into serovars by antigenic differences among the major outer membrane proteins. Within serogroup B, 15 serovars have been distinguished, of which serovars 3 and 7 cross-react with serovars 8 and 2, respectively (Frasch, 1979). Polypeptide band profiles of outer membranes of these different serovars in SDS–PAGE revealed characteristic sets of major outer membrane proteins in the 25 000 to 46 000 molecular weight range (Tsai *et al.*, 1981; Mocca and Frasch, 1982; Poolman *et al.*, 1980a). Serogroups B and C shared many of these serovars. Serovar 2 occurs with particularly high prevalence among patients with serogroup B, C, Y or W-135

Table 2   Molecular basis of designating serovars based on major outer membrane
proteins in *Neisseria meningitidis*

Class containing serovar-specific immunodeterminants*	Molecular weight range $(\times 10^{-3})^\S$	Heat-modifiable	Major outer membrane protein serovar§
1	43–46	–	2a, 6, 9, 12, 14, 15, 16
2[†]	35–42	$\pm$ ¶	1, 2a, 2b, 2c, 11
3[‡]	35–42	$\pm$	
4	34–36	–	None yet detected
5	25–32	+	2a, 2b, 9, 12, 13

*Nomenclature of Tsai *et al.* (1981).
[†]Analogous in function to OmpF/C proteins of *E. coli.*
[‡]Analogous in function to OmpA protein of *E. coli.*
§Data of Poolman *et al.* (1982).
¶Heat-modifiable in some strains; no strain has both heat-modifiable and non-modifiable proteins.

meningococcal disease and is rarely isolated from healthy carriers (Frasch, 1979, 1983; Poolman *et al.* 1982). Serovar 2 has also been subdivided into serovars 2a, 2b and 2c based on variations in serovar-specific immunodeterminants on major outer membrane proteins in the 34 000 to 42 000 molecular weight range (Poolman *et al.*, 1980a) and most of the group B isolates are presently of serovar 2b.

The major outer membrane proteins of *N. meningitidis* can be characterized by molecular weight, heat-modifiability and variability in expression both quantitatively and qualitatively (Poolman *et al.*, 1980a,b; Tsai *et al.*, 1981). The molecular basis of variability is unknown. Many of the serovar-specific immuno-determinants have been characterized with respect to particular major outer membrane proteins (Table 2). In addition, strains belonging to certain serovars may carry additional serovar-specific immunodeterminants on other outer membrane proteins, further complicating typing mosaics. Moreover, many minor outer membrane proteins may be important in designating serovars (Poolman *et al.*, 1982).

B. *Neisseria gonorrhoeae*

The polypeptide profiles of the outer membranes of gonococci on SDS–PAGE show considerable variations even within a single strain. However, the major proteins can be classified into three types (Watt and Heckels, 1983). Protein I (equivalent to OmpF/C of *E. coli*) is present in all gonococcal phenotypes and has a subunit molecular weight in the range 32 000 to 40 000. Protein II is produced by strains with an opaque colonial phenotype. This heat-modifiable protein is analogous to the OmpA protein of *E. coli* and has a molecular weight in the range 24 000 to 30 000. A single strain may produce as many as six such proteins. Protein III with a molecular weight of 31 000 is present in many strains and may replace single subunits in the porin trimer of protein I.

Gonococci have been divided into serovars on the basis of immunological differences in their protein I, formerly called the major or principal outer membrane protein (Johnston, 1977, 1978). Sixteen serologically different protein I serovars were identified among strains obtained from various places all over the world. Variations in the molecular weights of the protein in outer membranes appeared to be related to the antigenic differences. Using a reduced protein I typing scheme, Buchanan and Hildebrandt (1981) assigned almost all strains from disseminated gonococcal infections to serovars 1 and 2 by ELISA.

VII. OUTER MEMBRANE PROTEIN VACCINES

Interest in the use of outer membrane proteins as candidate immunogens has emerged for two reasons: the non-immunogenicity of certain purified capsular polysaccharides of gram-negative bacteria, and the toxicity of whole cell vaccines of gram-negative bacteria due to the lipid A of the lipopolysaccharide. Since outer membrane proteins are major components of the gram-negative bacterial surface, the potential development of immunochemically defined vaccines based on outer membrane proteins has provided new impetus and hope for immunoprophylaxis of certain infections, e.g. group B meningococcal disease.

A. *Neisseria meningitidis*

Bactericidal antibodies play a critical role in immunity to meningococcal disease (Frasch, 1983). The chemically defined, purified capsular polysaccharide vaccines developed by Gotschlich and coworkers represented a major breakthrough in immunization against *N. meningitidis* (reviewed by Peltola, 1983; Frasch, 1983). However, purified group B polysaccharide, an $\alpha(2\rightarrow8)$-linked polymer of *N*-acetylneuraminic acid immunochemically identical to *E. coli* K1 polysaccharide, is non-immunogenic, despite the fact that in group B meningococcal disease a significant antibody response to this polysaccharide occurs (Frasch, 1983). As a model for the usefulness of outer membrane protein vaccines, a non-encapsulated variant of a group B, serovar 2 strain was chosen for the preparation of outer membrane proteins on account of the high prevalence of this serovar among patients with meningococcal disease. Initial studies showed that a purified class 2 outer membrane protein (41 000 molecular weight) possessing serovar 2 immunodeterminants (Table 2) and a particulate protein vaccine comprising primarily the 41 000 molecular weight protein both stimulated high levels of bactericidal antibodies in experimental animals (reviewed by Frasch, 1983). Unfortunately, although the particulate vaccine proved to be safe in all age groups tested in clinical trials, it was poorly immunogenic, a fact at variance with the animal studies. It has been proposed that the surprisingly poor results were due to partial protein denaturation which may be related to labile antigenic determinants.

Accordingly, attempts were made to develop soluble protein vaccines (Frasch, 1983). Addition of group B meningococcal polysaccharide to outer membrane protein preparations rendered the latter 'soluble'. Highly purified group B polysaccharide was combined with purified serovar 2 outer membrane protein of class 2 or LPS-depleted outer membrane vesicles, to yield non-covalent complexes which were colloidal suspensions rather than free solutions. None of the polysaccharide became protein-bound. The studies of Gotschlich *et al.* (1981) strongly indicated that most likely polysaccharide molecules with terminal phosphoglycerides were responsible for the group B polysaccharide–protein interaction. These soluble vaccines were more immunogenic in animals than the particulate vaccine and provided greater protection. In clinical trials, the combination soluble vaccines were shown to elicit bactericidal antibodies without serious side-effects.

Significantly, when non-covalently complexed with the serovar 2 outer membrane protein the group B polysaccharide was immunogenic. The ratio of polysaccharide to outer membrane protein for optimal antibody responses to both components was investigated. A polysaccharide:protein ratio of 1:3 was that most effective in eliciting group B polysaccharide antibodies (largely IgM) whereas the 1:1 complex appeared optimal for inducing anti-outer-membrane-protein antibodies (Frasch, 1983). The efficacy of a combined outer membrane protein–polysaccharide A, B, C, Y and W-135 vaccine in preventing meningococcal disease remains to be established.

B. *Haemophilus influenzae*

H. influenzae Pittman type **b** is the most common cause of endemic bacterial meningitis in infants and young children. There is a considerable body of experimental evidence indicating that the phosphoribose ribosyl phosphate capsule plays a critical role in the pathogenesis of *H. influenzae* infections (Moxon and Vaughn, 1981). The failure of this capsular antigen to induce production of protective antibodies in infants less than 14 months of age has stimulated the search for alternative surface antigens eliciting bactericidal antibodies as potential vaccine candidates (Hill, 1983).

The polypeptide composition of isolated outer membranes of *H. influenzae* type **b** was investigated by Loeb *et al.* (1981). They defined six prominent bands which had the following molecular weights: **a**, 46 000; **b**, 38 000; **c**, 37 000; **d**, 34 000; **e**, 28 000; and **f**, 26 000. Proteins **a** and **d** were heat-modifiable and protein **f** has since been shown to be the non-heat-modified form of protein **d** (Van Alphen *et al.*, 1983). Twenty-two subtypes of *H. influenzae* type **b** have been described on the basis of major outer membrane protein patterns (Granhoff *et al.*, 1982; Van Alphen *et al.*, 1983). In addition, several other higher and lower molecular weight minor polypeptide bands were usually present. Studies at the University of Rochester, New York, using an SDS–PAGE radio-immunoassay, showed that sera from adult patients had, on average, antibodies to 12 individual proteins, while even sera from convalescing infants had on average antibodies against eight outer membrane proteins (cited by Hill, 1983). All the patients' sera had antibodies to the major outer membrane protein **d/f**, 83% to protein **e** (which seemed to be common to all strains) and 70% to protein **a**.

In a series of investigations, Hansen and coworkers demonstrated that acute and convalescent phase sera from patients with *H. influenzae* meningitis and from experimental infant and adult rats convalescing from *H. influenzae* type **b** infection contained antibodies directed against cell-surface exposed outer membrane proteins, in particular to a 39 000 molecular weight protein (Hansen *et al.*, 1981a,b; Gulig *et al.*, 1982). Monoclonal antibodies to this outer membrane protein, which probably corresponds to protein **b** or protein **c** or a mixture of both proteins, only passively immunized rats to systemic *H. influenzae* type **b** infection with strains possessing the 39 000 outer membrane protein possessing an antigenic determinant recognized by the monoclonal antibodies (Hansen *et al.*, 1982). These observations indicate that antigenic differences exist between strains and that cross-reactive outer membrane proteins (Gulig *et al.*, 1983) or pools of antigenic subtypes may be required for a vaccine preparation. Antibodies against a 37 000 protein termed P2 (possibly protein C) have also been shown by another group to protect infant rats against challenge with the donor strain but not against strains of a heterologous outer membrane protein subtype (Hill, 1983).

In contrast, Van Alphen *et al.* (1983) demonstrated that the antibodies in the sera of patients with meningitis were directed predominantly against the heat-modifiable major outer membrane protein **a**. Antibodies to purified protein **a** were not bactericidal in tests with human complement against capsulated *H. influenzae* type **b** *in vitro*.

In addition to these outer membrane proteins, Gulig *et al.* (1982) reported that convalescent infant sera contained antibodies to minor high-molecular-weight outer membrane proteins ($\geqslant 100\,000$) which were exposed on the cell surface and possessed antigenic determinants accessible to antibodies. Within one outer membrane protein subtype, inter-strain differences in several of these minor proteins were noted (Van Alphen *et al.*, 1983). Neither the degree of protection conferred by antibodies to these cell-surface components nor the bactericidal efficacy of such antibodies has been investigated.

Although the research on the potential for outer membrane protein vaccines against *H. influenzae* type **b** has been encouraging, much still requires to be done if an effective vaccine against the single most important cause of endemic bacterial meningitis in infants is to be achieved. Given the apparent diversity of antibodies to outer membrane proteins in patients' sera, LPS-depleted outer membrane vesicles may prove to be more effective as a vaccine than was the case for *N. meningitidis* (Frasch, 1983).

C. *Salmonella*

The currently recognized *Salmonella* vaccines comprise whole killed bacteria. Their protective value is controversial. These vaccines (referred to as TAB vaccines for *S. typhi, S. paratyphi* A and B) are pyrogenic and toxic and appear to confer incomplete protection of short duration. Accordingly, efforts have been made to develop vaccines based on defined non-toxic surface components. For testing their potential efficacy, infections in mice have been used as a model system with *S. typhimurium* because they bear a close resemblance pathologically and the symptoms are similar to human enteric fever (Kuusi *et al.*, 1979; Svenson *et al.* 1979).

The porin complex of *S. typhimurium*, comprising outer membrane proteins of 34 000, 35 000 and 36 000 molecular weight (Lugtenberg and Van Alphen, 1983), was chosen as a candidate vaccine because such properties as bacteriophage reception suggested that these porins were surface-exposed and might be reached by anti-porin antibodies. The method used for purification of the porin complex from a rough (Rb_2) strain was so mild that the isolated porins retained their ability to inactivate phage (Nurminen, 1978). Moreover, they were not exposed to SDS treatment (see section V.C). Passive administration of antibodies raised to porins (absorbed to remove antibodies to rough LPS) and vaccination with purified porins conferred highly significant protection against experimental infections in mice (Kuusi *et al.*, 1979; Svenson *et al.*, 1979). Moreover, the antigenic specificities of the *Salmonella* porin preparations appeared to be universal for the genus rather than species-specific (Svenson *et al.*, 1979). Furthermore, artificial *Salmonella* vaccines comprising an O-antigenic octasaccharide chain of *S. typhimurium* covalently linked to purified porins induced better protection against experimental infection in mice than that obtained by vaccination with octasaccharide or porin vaccines separately (Svenson *et al.*, 1979). In follow-up studies using other conjugates, these artificial vaccines have been shown to elicit opsonizing antibodies that enhance phagocytosis (Jörbeck *et al.*, 1981). However, antisera raised to crude LPS-free porins of *S. typhimurium* lacked a protective capacity in passive immunization experiments, while sera raised to porins reconstituted with rough LPS were protective (Kuusi *et al.*, 1981). The rough LPS probably acted as an adjuvant and may also have stabilized the trimeric configuration of the porins, whereas the LPS-free purified porin, although still trimeric, had probably lost its native conformation. Thus, pyrogen-free porins would require to be manipulated *in vitro* to reconstitute protective preparations.

In the future it may prove possible to combine pyrogen-free porins with chemically pure Vi antigen, the microcapsular, highly acidic polysaccharide composed of $\alpha(1\rightarrow4)$-linked *O*- and *N*-acetylated galactosaminouronic acid units, which has long been assumed to be important in protective immunity to typhoid in man (Johnson *et al.*, 1982), in much the same way as group B polysaccharide has been complexed with purified outer membrane proteins of *N. meningitidis*. Alternatively, the oligosaccharide–porin conjugate approach to a multispecific *Salmonella* vaccine appears to hold promise for an effective, non-toxic immunogen for salmonellosis.

VIII. FUTURE PERSPECTIVES

The past decade has seen substantial advances in techniques and procedures for the analysis and purification of outer membrane proteins. Candidate antigens for vaccine development can be identified by SDS–PAGE Western blotting or direct immunolabelling methods using patients' sera to elucidate immune responses during natural infection. The use of conjugated vaccines or complexed vaccines comprising chemically and antigenically defined components seems the way forward at present. However, one must not lose sight of the need to investigate also pathogenic mechanisms to aid in the identification of virulence functions which may be blocked by bactericidal or opsonizing antibodies. Much more effort has been put into rational strategies for vaccine development in recent years and it seems that such approaches are paying dividends.

Given the potential role of biotechnology in vaccine development, genetic engineering in particular has brought new prospects for viral vaccines. To date, cloning of the genes encoding bacterial antigens such as outer membrane structural proteins into readily manipulated hosts to enhance production of candidate immunogens is still in its infancy. Epidemiological control of gonococcal infection may also eventually be possible by vaccination. Pathogenic mechanisms, immune responses and gonococcal surface antigens have been intensively studied yet immunization against gonococcal infection is still elusive (Watt and Heckels, 1983). Antigenic heterogeneity is a major problem, e.g. of outer membrane proteins. With monoclonal antibodies it may be possible to recognize immunodominant peptides in outer membrane proteins (Gabay and Schwartz, 1982; Robertson *et al.*, 1982). Cloning of the DNA sequences for these may allow the development of chemically defined conjugate vaccines (Wilson, 1984).

ACKNOWLEDGEMENTS

I thank P. Owen, R. J. Russell and J. P. Arbuthnott for helpful discussions during the preparation of this chapter and Gillian Johnston for excellent secretarial service.

REFERENCES

Achtman, M., Mercer, A., Kusecek, B., Pohl, A., Heuzenroeder, M., Aaronson, W., Sutton, A., and Silver, R. P. (1983). Six widespread bacterial clones among *Escherichia coli* K1 isolates. *Infect. Immun.*, **39**, 315–335.

Arbuthnott, J. P., Owen, P., and Russell, R. J. (1983). Bacterial antigens. In *Topley and Wilson's Principles of Bacteriology, Virology and Immunity*, 7th edn., Vol. 1 (Eds. G. Wilson, A. Miles and M. T. Parker), pp.337–373. Edward Arnold, London.

Axelsen, N. H. (1983). *Handbook of Immunoprecipitation-in-Gel Techniques*. Blackwell Scientific Publications, Oxford.

Bachmann, B. J., and Brooks Low, K. (1980). Linkage map of *Escherichia coli* K12, edition 6. *Microbiol. Rev.*, **44**, 1–56.

Beher, M. G., Schnaitman, C. A., and Pugsley, A. P. (1980). Major heat-modifiable outer membrane protein in Gram-negative bacteria: comparison with the OmpA protein of *Escherichia coli*. *J. Bacteriol.*, **143**, 906–913.

Bjerrum, O. J. (1983). *Electroimmunochemical Analysis of Membrane Proteins*. Elsevier, Amsterdam.

Braun, V. (1975). Covalent lipoprotein from the outer membrane of *Escherichia coli*. *Biochim. Biophys. Acta*, **415**, 335–377.

Braun, V. (1978). Structure–function relationships of the Gram-negative bacterial cell envelope. In *Relation between Structure and Function in the Prokaryotic Cell* (*Society for General Microbiology Symposium* 28), (Eds. R. Y. Stanier, H. J. Rogers and J. B. Ward), pp.111–138. Cambridge University Press, Cambridge.

Braun, V., and Hantke, K. (1974). Biochemistry of bacterial cell envelopes. *Annu. Rev. Biochem.*, **43**, 89–121.

Braun, V., Bosch, V., Klumpp, E. R., Neff, I., Mayer, H., and Schlecht, S. (1976). Antigenic determinants of murein lipoprotein and its exposure at the surface of Enterobacteriaceae. *Eur. J. Biochem.*, **62**, 555–566.

Buchanan, T. H., and Hildebrandt, J. F. (1981). Antigen-specific serotyping of *Neisseria gonorrhoeae*: characterization based on principal outer membrane protein. *Infect. Immun.*, **32**, 985–994.

Burnette, W. N. (1981). Western blotting: electrophoretic transfer of proteins from sodium dodecyl sulfate–polyacrylamide gels to unmodified nitrocellulose and radiographic detection with antibody and radioiodinated protein A. *Anal. Biochem.*, **112**, 195–203.

Chopra, I., and Shales, S. W. (1980). Comparison of the polypeptide composition of *Escherichia coli* outer membranes prepared by two methods. *J. Bacteriol.*, **114**, 425–427.

Collins, M. L. P., and Salton, M. R. J. (1980). Preparation and crossed immuno-electrophoretic analysis of cytoplasmic and outer membrane fractions from *Neisseria gonorrhoeae*. *Infect. Immun.*, **30**, 281–288.

Costerton, J. W., Ingram, J. M., and Cheng, K.-J. (1974). Structure and function of the cell envelope of Gram-negative bacteria. *Bacteriol. Rev.*, **38**, 87–110.

Dankert, J., and Hofstra, J. (1978). Antibodies against outer membrane proteins in rabbit antisera prepared against *Escherichia coli* O26K60. *J. Gen. Microbiol.*, **104**, 311–320.

DiRienzo, J. M., Nakamura, K., and Inouye, M. (1978). The outer membrane proteins of Gram-negative bacteria: biosynthesis, assembly and functions. *Annu. Rev. Biochem.*, **47**, 481–532.

Filip, C., Fletcher, G., Wulff, J. L., and Earhart, C. F. (1973). Solubilization of the cytoplasmic membrane of *Escherichia coli* by the ionic detergent sodium-lauryl sarcosinate. *J. Bacteriol.*, **115**, 717–722.

Frasch, C. E. (1979). Noncapsular surface antigens of *Neisseria meningitidis*. In *Seminars in Infectious Disease*, Vol. 2 (Eds. L. Weinstein and B. N. Fields), pp.304–337. Stratton Intercontinental Medical Book Corporation, New York.

Frasch, C. E. (1983). Immunization against *Neisseria meningitidis*. In *Immunization Against Bacterial Disease* (*Medical Microbiology*, Vol. 2), (Eds. C. S. F. Easmon and J. Jeljaszewicz), pp.115–144. Academic Press, London.

Gabay, J., and Schwartz, M. (1982). Monoclonal antibody as a probe for structure and function of an *Escherichia coli* outer membrane protein. *J. Biol. Chem.*, **257**, 6627–6630.

Geyer, R., Galanos, C., Westphal, O., and Golecki, J. R. (1979). A lipopolysaccharide-binding cell-surface protein from *Salmonella minnesota*. *Eur. J. Biochem.*, **98**, 27–38.

Gotschlich, E. C., Fraser, B. A., Nishimura, O., Robbins, J. B., and Liu, T.-Y. (1981). Lipid on capsular polysaccharides of Gram-negative bacteria. *J. Biol. Chem.*, **256**, 8915–8921.

Granhoff, D. M., Barenchamp, S. J., and Munson, R. S., Jr. (1982). Outer membrane protein subtypes for epidemiological investigation of *Haemophilus influenzae* type b disease. In *Haemophilus influenzae* (Eds. S. H. Sell and P. F. Wright), pp.43–54. Elsevier/North-Holland, New York.

Gulig, P. A., McCracken, G. H., Jr., Frisch, C. F., Johnston, K. H., and Hansen, E. J. (1982). Antibody response of infants to cell surface-exposed outer membrane proteins of *Haemophilus influenzae* type b after systemic *Haemophilus* disease. *Infect. Immun.*, **37**, 82–88.

Gulig, P. A., Frisch, C. F., and Hansen, E. J. (1983). A set of two monoclonal antibodies specific for the cell surface-exposed 39K major outer membrane protein of *Haemophilus influenzae* type b defines all strains of this pathogen. *Infect. Immun.*, **42**, 516–524.

Hall, M. N., and Silhavy, T. J. (1981). Genetic analysis of the major outer membrane proteins of *Escherichia coli*. *Annu. Rev. Genet.*, **15**, 91–142.

Hansen, E. J., Frisch, C. F., and Johnston, K. H. (1981a). Detection of antibody-accessible proteins on the cell surface of *Haemophilus influenzae* type b. *Infect. Immun.*, **33**, 950–953.

Hansen, E. J., Frisch, C. F., McDade, R. L., Jr., and Johnston, K. H. (1981b). Identification of immunogenic outer membrane proteins of *Haemophilus influenzae* type b in the infant rat model system. *Infect. Immun.*, **32**, 1084–1092.

Hansen, E. J., Robertson, S. M., Gulig, P. A., Frisch, C. F., and Haanes, E. J. (1982). Immunoprotection of rats against *Haemophilus influenzae* type b disease mediated by monoclonal antibody against a *Haemophilus* outer membrane protein. *Lancet*, **i**, 366–368.

Harboe, M., and Closs, O. (1983). Immunization with precipitates obtained by crossed immunoelectrophoresis. *Scand. J. Immunol.*, **17**, Suppl. 10, 353–359.

Hebeler, B. H., Morse, S. A., Wong, W., and Young, F. E. (1978). Evidence for peptidoglycan-associated protein(s) in *Neisseria gonorrhoeae*. *Biochem. Biophys. Res. Commun.*, **81**, 1011–1017.

Hill, J. C., (1983). Summary of a workshop on *Haemophilus influenzae* type b vaccines. *J. Infect. Dis.*, **148**, 167–175.

Hoff, G. E., and Frasch, C. E. (1979). Outer membrane antigens of *Neisseria meningitidis* Group B serotype 2 studied by crossed immunoelectrophoresis. *Infect. Immun.*, **25**, 849–853.

Hofstad, T., and Sveen, K. (1979). Endotoxins of anaerobic gram-negative rods. *Scand. J. Infect. Dis. Suppl.*, **19**, 42–45.

Hofstra, H., and Dankert, J. (1979). Antigenic cross-reactivity of major outer membrane proteins in Enterobacteriaceae species. *J. Gen. Microbiol.*, **111**, 293–302.

Hofstra, H., and Dankert, J. (1980a). Antigenic cross-reactivity of outer membrane proteins of *Escherichia coli* and *Proteus* species. *FEMS Microbiol. Lett.*, **7**, 171–174.

Hofstra, H., and Dankert, J. (1980b). Major outer membrane proteins: common antigens in Enterobacteriaceae species. *J. Gen. Microbiol.*, **119**, 123–131.

Hofstra, H., and Dankert, J. (1980c). Preparation and quantitative determination of antibodies against major outer membrane proteins of *Escherichia coli* O26K60. *J. Gen. Microbiol.*, **117**, 437–447.

Hofstra, H., and Dankert, J. (1981). Porin from the outer membrane of *Escherichia coli:* immunological characterization of native and heat-dissociated forms. *J. Gen. Microbiol.*, **125**, 285–292.

Hofstra, H., Van Tol, M. J. D., and Dankert, J. (1980). Cross-reactivity of major outer membrane proteins of Enterobacteriaceae, studied by crossed immunoelectrophoresis. *J. Bacteriol.*, **143**, 328–337.

Høiby, N. (1977). *Pseudomonas aeruginosa* infection in cystic fibrosis. *Acta Pathol. Microbiol. Scand. Sect. C Suppl.*, **262**, 1–96.

Inouye, M. (1975). Biosynthesis and assembly of the outer membrane proteins of *Escherichia coli*. In *Membrane Biogenesis, Mitochondria, Chloroplasts, and Bacteria* (Ed. A. Tzagoloff), pp.351–391. Plenum, New York.

Inouye, M. (1979). *Bacterial Outer Membranes: Biogenesis and Functions*. John Wiley, New York.

Johnson, E. M., Diena, B. B., Lior, H., Ryan, A., Krol, P., and Baron, L. S. (1982). Evaluation of two *Salmonella typhimurium* hybrids as challenge organisms in a system for the assay of typhoid vaccines. *Infect. Immun.*, **38**, 201–205.

Johnston, K. H. (1977). Surface antigens: an outer membrane protein responsible for imparting serological specificity to *Neisseria gonorrhoeae*. In *The Gonococcus* (Ed. R. B. Roberts), pp.273–283, John Wiley, New York.

Johnston, K. H. (1978). Antigenic profile of an outer membrane complex of *Neisseria gonorrhoeae* responsible for serotypic specificity. In *Immunobiology of Neisseria gonorrhoeae* (Eds. G. F. Brooks, E. C. Gotschlich, K. K. Holmes, W. D. Sawyer and F. E. Young), pp.121–129. American Society for Microbiology, Washington, DC.

Jörbeck, H. J. A., Svenson, S. B., and Lindberg, A. A. (1981). Artificial *Salmonella* vaccines: *Salmonella typhimurium* O-antigen-specific oligosaccharide–protein conjugates elicit opsonizing antibodies that enhance phagocytosis. *Infect. Immun.*, **32**, 497–502.

Kuusi, N., Nurminen, M., Saxén, H., Valtonen, M., and Mäkelä, P. H. (1979). Immunization with major outer membrane proteins in experimental salmonellosis of mice. *Infect. Immun.*, **25**, 857–862.

Kuusi, N., Nurminen, M., Saxén, H., and Mäkelä, P. H. (1981). Immunization with major outer membrane protein (porin) preparations in experimental murine salmonellosis: effect of lipopolysaccharide. *Infect. Immun.*, **34**, 328–332.

Laemmli, U. K. (1970). Cleavage of structural proteins during the assembly of the head of bacteriophage T4. *Nature*, **227**, 680–685.

Loeb, M. R., Zachary, A. L., and Smith, D. H. (1981). Isolation and partial characterization of outer and inner membranes from encapsulated *Haemophilus influenzae*. *J. Bacteriol.* **145**, 596–604.

Lugtenberg, B. (1981). Composition and function of the outer membrane of *Escherichia coli*. *Trends Biochem. Sci.*, **6**, 262–266.

Lugtenberg, B., and Van Alphen, L. (1983). Molecular architecture and functioning of the outer membrane of *Escherichia coli* and other Gram-negative bacteria. *Biochim. Biophys. Acta*, **737**, 51–115.

Lugtenberg, B., Meijers, J., Peters, R., Van der Hoek, P., and Van Alphen, L. (1975). Electrophoretic resolution of the 'major outer membrane protein' of *Escherichia coli* K12 into four bands. *FEBS Lett.*, **58**, 254–258.

Lugtenberg, B., Peters, R., Bernheimer, H., and Berendsen, W. (1976). Influence of cultural conditions and mutations on the composition of the outer membrane proteins of *Escherichia cell. Mol. Gen. Genet.*, **147**, 251–262.

Mäkelä, P. H., and Mayer, H. (1976). Enterobacterial common antigen. *Bacteriol. Rev.*, **40**, 591–632.

Mansheim, B. J., Onderdonk, A. B., and Kasper, D. L. (1979). Immunochemical characterization of surface antigens of *Bacteroides melaninogenicus. Rev. Infect. Dis.*, **1**, 263–275.

Mayer, H., and Schmidt, G. (1979). Chemistry and biology of the enterobacterial common antigen (ECA). *Curr. Top. Microbiol. Immunol.*, **85**, 99–153.

Miura, T., and Mizushima, S. (1969). Separation and properties of outer and cytoplasmic membranes in *Escherichia coli. Biochim. Biophys. Acta,* **193**, 268–276.

Mocca, L. S., and Frasch, C. E. (1982). Sodium dodecyl sulfate–polyacrylamide gel typing system for characterization of *Neisseria meningitidis* isolates. *J. Clin. Microbiol.*, **16**, 240–244.

Moxon, E. R., and Vaughn, K. A. (1981). The type b capsular polysaccharide as a virulence determinant of *Haemophilus influenzae:* studies using clinical isolates and laboratory transformants. *J. Infect. Dis.*, **143**, 517–524.

Nakamura, K., and Mizushima, S. (1976). Effects of heating in dodecyl sulfate solution on the conformation and electrophoretic mobility of isolated major outer membrane proteins of *Escherichia coli* K-12. *J. Biochem. (Tokyo)*, **80**, 1411–1422.

Nikaido, H., and Nakae, T. (1979). The outer membrane of Gram-negative bacteria. *Adv. Microbial Physiol.*, **20**, 163–250.

Nurminen, M. (1978). A mild procedure to isolate the 34K, 35K and 36K porins of the outer membrane of *Salmonella typhimurium. FEMS Microbiol. Lett.*, **3**, 331–334.

Osborn, M. J., and Munson, R. (1974). Separation of the inner (cytoplasmic) and outer membranes of Gram-negative bacteria. *Methods Enzymol.*, **31**, 642–653.

Osborn, M. J., and Wu, H. C. P. (1980). Proteins of the outer membrane of Gram-negative bacteria. *Annu. Rev. Microbiol.*, **34**, 369–422.

Overbeeke, N., and Lugtenberg, B. (1980). Major outer membrane proteins of *Escherichia coli* strains of human origin. *J. Gen. Microbiol.*, **121**, 373–380.

Overbeeke, N., Van Scharrenburg, G., and Lugtenberg, B. (1980). Antigenic relationship between pore proteins of *Escherichia coli* K12. *Eur. J. Biochem.*, **110**, 247–254.

Owen, P. (1981). Immunology of the bacterial membrane. In *Organization of Prokaryotic Cell Membranes*, Vol. 1 (Ed. B. K. Ghosh), pp.73–164. CRC Press, Boca Raton, Florida.

Owen, P. (1983a). The topological arrangement of proteins in membranes determined by electroimmunochemical methods. In *Electroimmunochemical Analysis of Membrane Proteins* (Ed. O. J. Bjerrum), pp.55–76. Elsevier, Amsterdam.

Owen, P. (1983b). Antigens of the *Escherichia coli* cell envelope. In *Electroimmunochemical Analysis of Membrane Proteins* (Ed. O. J. Bjerrum), pp.347–373. Elsevier, Amsterdam.

Owen, P., and Kaback, H. R. (1979). Immunochemical analysis of membrane vesicles from *Escherichia coli. Biochemistry*, **18**, 1413–1422.

Owen, P., and Smyth, C. J. (1977). Enzyme analysis by quantitative immunoelectrophoresis. In *Immunochemistry of Enzymes and Their Antibodies* (Ed. M. R. J. Salton), pp.147–202. John Wiley, New York.

Owen, P., Graeme-Cook, K. A., Crowe, B. A., and Condon, C. (1982). Bacterial membranes: preparative techniques and criteria of purity. In *Techniques in Lipid and Membrane Biochemistry,* Part 1 (*Biochemistry*, Vol. B4/1) (Eds. T. R. Hesketh, H. L. Kornberg, J. C. Metcalfe, D. H. Northcote, C. I. Pogson and K. F. Tipton), pp.1–69. Elsevier Biomedical, Shannon, Ireland.

Peltola, H. (1983). Meningococcal disease: still with us. *Rev. Infect. Dis.*, **5**, 71–91.

Poolman, J. T., Hopman, C. T. P., and Zanen, H. C. (1980a). Immunochemical characterization of *Neisseria meningitidis* serotype antigens by immunodiffusion and SDS–polyacrylamide gel electrophoresis immunoperoxidase techniques and the distribution of serotypes among cases and carriers. *J. Gen. Microbiol.*, **116**, 465–473.

Poolman, J. T., De Marie, S., and Zanen, H. C. (1980b). Variability of low-molecular-weight, heat-modifiable outer membrane proteins of *Neisseria meningitidis*. *Infect. Immun.*, **30**, 642–648.

Poolman, J. T., Hopman, C. T. P., and Zanen, H. C. (1982). Problems in the definition of meningococcal serotypes. *FEMS Microbiol. Lett.*, **13**, 339–348.

Robertson, S. M., Frisch, C. F., Gulig, P. A., Kettman, J. R., Johnston, K. H., and Hansen, E. J. (1982). Monoclonal antibodies directed against a cell surface-exposed outer membrane protein of *Haemophilus influenzae* type b. *Infect. Immun.*, **36**, 80–88.

Rosenbusch, J. P. (1974). Characterization of the major envelope protein from *Escherichia coli*. Regular arrangement on the peptidoglycan and unusual dodecyl sulfate binding. *J. Biol. Chem.*, **249**, 8019–8029.

Salton, M. R. J. (1971). Bacterial membranes. *CRC Crit. Rev. Microbiol.*, **1**, 161–194.

Salton, M. R. J., and Owen, P. (1976). Bacterial membrane structure. *Annu. Rev. Microbiol.*, **30**, 451–482.

Schnaitman, C. A. (1970). Examination of the protein composition of the cell envelope of *Escherichia coli* by polyacrylamide gel electrophoresis. *J. Bacteriol.*, **104**, 882–889.

Schnaitman, C. A. (1971a). Solubilization of the cytoplasmic membrane of *Escherichia coli* by Triton X-100. *J. Bacteriol.*, **108**, 545–552.

Schnaitman, C. A. (1971b). Effect of ethylenediaminetetraacetic acid, Triton X-100 and lysozyme on the morphology and chemical composition of isolated cell walls of *Escherichia coli*. *J. Bacteriol.*, **108**, 553–563.

Smyth, C. J., Friedman-Kien, A. E., and Salton, M. R. J. (1976). Antigenic analysis of *Neisseria gonorrhoeae* by crossed immunoelectrophoresis. *Infect. Immun.*, **13**, 1273–1288.

Smyth, C. J., Siegel, J. S., Salton, M. R. J., and Owen, P. (1978). Immunochemical analysis of inner and outer membranes of *Escherichia coli* by crossed immuno-electrophoresis. *J. Bacteriol.*, **133**, 306–319.

Svenson, S. B., Nurminen, M., and Lindberg, A. A. (1979). Artificial *Salmonella* vaccines. O-antigenic oligosaccharide–protein conjugates induce protection against infection with *Salmonella typhimurium*. *Infect. Immun.*, **25**, 863–872.

Towbin, H., Staehelin, T., and Gordon, J. (1979). Electrophoretic transfer of proteins from polyacrylamide gels to nitrocellulose sheets: procedure and some applications. *Proc. Natl. Acad. Sci. USA*, **76**, 4350–4354.

Tsai, C.-H., Frasch, C. E., and Mocca, L. F. (1981). Five structural classes of major outer membrane proteins in *Neisseria meningitidis*. *J. Bacteriol.*, **146**, 69–78.

Van Alphen, L., Riemens, T., Poolman, J., Hopman, C., and Zanen, H. C. (1983). Homogeneity of cell envelope protein subtypes, lipopolysaccharide serotypes and biotypes among *Haemophilus influenzae* type b from patients with meningitis in The Netherlands. *J. Infect. Dis.*, **148**, 75–81.

Van Raamsdonk, W., Pool, C. W., and Heyting, C. (1977). Detection of antigens and antibodies by an immunoperoxidase method applied on thin longitudinal sections of SDS–polyacrylamide gels. *J. Immunol. Methods*, **17**, 337–348.

Van Tol, M. J. D., Hofstra, H., and Dankert, J. (1979). Major outer membrane proteins of *Escherichia coli* analysed by crossed immunoelectrophoresis. *FEMS Microbiol. Lett.*, **5**, 349–352.

Watt, P. J., and Heckels, J. E. (1983). Prospects and strategy for immunization against gonococcal infection. In *Immunization Against Bacterial Disease* (*Medical Microbiology*, Vol. 2), (Eds. C. S. F. Easmon and J. Jeljaszewicz), pp.87–114. Academic Press, London.

Wilson, T. (1984). Engineering tomorrow's vaccines. *Biotechnology*, **2**, 29–40.

Immunology of the Bacterial Cell Envelope
Edited by D. E. S. Stewart-Tull and M. Davies
© 1985 John Wiley & Sons Ltd.

CHAPTER 8

Endotoxic Activities of Lipopolysaccharides

A. Christine McCartney* and Alastair C. Wardlaw[†]

*Department of Bacteriology,
University of Glasgow, Royal Infirmary, Glasgow G4 0SF, and
[†]Department of Microbiology, University of Glasgow, Glasgow G12 8QQ, UK

I. INTRODUCTION

This chapter attempts to distil the essence of endotoxinology from the vast literature on the subject, to highlight recent findings on the chemistry and mode of action of the bacterial lipopolysaccharides in relation to their effect on the immune system, and to discuss the continuing paradoxes associated with these substances.

Nearly 20 years ago Bennett (1964) wrote of the 'endotoxic explosion' and made the provocative remark that 'an investigator in almost any biological field is likely to obtain a "positive" result if he tries endotoxin in the experimental system he is using.' Since then, there has been an undiminishing stream of literature on endotoxins. Surprisingly, therefore, certain aspects of these substances still remain largely unexplored or unexplained. For example, despite the diversified effects of endotoxin in the whole animal and on certain types of cells, there are remarkably few observations on endotoxin causing a demonstrable change in an isolated, perfused, mammalian organ. Also, despite the high immunogenicity of endotoxins, the corresponding antibodies usually do not neutralize the toxic activities nor function protectively in infections. There seems to be no gram-negative infection for which bacteria heat-treated at 100°C make an effective vaccine yet such bacteria provide the standard antigen for raising anti-lipopolysaccharide antibodies.

In this article we shall take the terms endotoxin, lipopolysaccharide (LPS) and O-somatic antigen as essentially synonymous. They all refer to the high-molecular-weight ($\sim 0.2 \times 10^6$ to 1.0×10^6) heat-stable (100°C) substances which contain a highly characteristic lipid — lipid A — linked usually to long polysaccharide chains, and present in the outer membrane of only gram-negative bacteria. Although the original naming of these substances as *endotoxins* implied an intracellular location, it is now well established that considerable amounts of endotoxin may be liberated by intact, actively growing bacterial cells (Bishop and Work, 1965; Marsh and Crutchley, 1967; Devoe and Gilchrist, 1973; Jorgensen and Smith, 1974).

In regard to their effects in the mammalian body, endotoxins irrespective of their bacterial sources exhibit two salient features: (1) a highly diversified pattern of pathophysiological effects including fever, hypotension, changes in leucocyte count and disturbances in many other host systems (Table 1); and (2) high immunogenicity, with the resulting antibodies being specific for terminal sugars in the polysaccharide chain. In the genus *Salmonella* the number of such specificities is in the order of 2000.

Besides occurring in all mammalian pathogenic and commensal gram-negative bacteria, endotoxins are also present in other gram-negative bacteria such as thiobacilli, photosynthetic bacteria, cyanobacteria and some plant-pathogenic bacteria which have no obvious ecological links with animal hosts. Indeed, from the bacterial standpoint, the main functions of LPS probably relate to

Table 1   Biological activities of LPS

Highly specific for LPS (in order of decreasing sensitivity)
Limulus lysate gelation*
Drug-treated mouse lethality*
Pyrogenicity in rabbits*
Shwartzman reaction
Induction of tolerance to endotoxin
Characteristic but less specific (in alphabetical order)
Adjuvant activity
Bone marrow necrosis
Chick embryo lethality*
Complement activation*
Enhanced dermal reactivity to epinephrine*
Enhanced non-specific resistance to infection
Enhanced phagocytosis
Hageman factor activation
Hypoferraemia*
Hypotension
Induction of colony stimulating factor
Induction of interferon
Induction of leucopaenia
Induction of leucocytosis
Induction of plasminogen activator
Induction of prostaglandin synthesis
Lethality*
Macrophage activation
Mitogenicity for cells
Platelet aggregation
Shock
Tumour necrosis

*Used as endotoxin assays.

maintenance of structural integrity and selective permeability of the outer layer of the cell. To a considerable extent, therefore, the endotoxicity of these substances in animals should be seen as an accident of nature, and an artefact of the hypodermic syringe rather than as an influential part of the parasite–host evolutionary-adaptation strategy.

For information on other aspects and on the historical development of endotoxinology, the reader is referred to Landy and Braun (1964), Nowotny (1969), Weinbaum *et al.* (1971), Kadis *et al.* (1971), Kass and Wolff (1973).

II. BIOLOGICAL ACTIVITIES AND ASSAY

A. Biological Activities

The main interest in the biological activities of LPS has focused on their effect after parenteral administration to mammals. Endotoxins were originally recognized for their capacity to induce fever (Siebert, 1923, 1925, 1952; Siebert and Mandel, 1923; Bourn and Siebert, 1925) but pyrogenicity is only one of the manifold biological activities shown by these substances (see Table 1). It is difficult to assess differences in susceptibility among mammalian species because of the different physiological responses and endotoxin preparations which have been used. In a comprehensive study, van Miert and Frens (1968) compared parenteral administration of LPS from *E. coli* O111 B4 in 11 different mammalian species and in the chicken, measuring pyrogenicity, white cell count and gastrointestinal effects. They found the ranking susceptibility of diminishing sensitivity to be rabbit, horse, goat, dog, cow, sheep, cat, swine and chicken, with mouse, rat, and guinea pig taking a separate place by the absence of a fever reaction or a leucocyte response. Indeed it is known that LPS can induce a *hypothermic* response in mice and rats although after preconditioning the animals for 4 h at 36°C mice produce a *hyperthermic* response (Prashker and Wardlaw, 1971). Both rabbit and man exhibit a similar threshold dose for a pyrogenic response (Greisman and Hornick, 1967) which justifies the use of the rabbit pyrogen tests as mandatory for all drugs and fluids intended for parenteral administration to man. Baboons and vervets are insensitive to the acute actions of endotoxins; they can withstand intravenous injections of the order of 4–5 mg/kg without the systemic reactions seen in sensitive species such as the rabbit which responds to 0.1–1 ng/kg (Westphal, 1975).

Age is an important factor in the responsiveness of some species to endotoxin. In rabbits (Smith and Thomas, 1954), mice (Rašková and Vaněček, 1964) and man (McCabe, 1963) susceptibility increases with age. Conversely in the fowl, 8–10-day-old chick embryos are extremely sensitive and hens are very resistant to the lethal effects of endotoxin (Smith and Thomas, 1956). It was suggested that the diminishing sensitivity of chick embryos after day 11 may be due to ontogenetic changes in the synthesis of bile acids (Bertók, 1977), which appear to be important in detoxification of LPS (Bertók, 1980). There is evidence that they play a role in the prevention of absorption of endotoxin from the gastrointestinal tract (Bailey, 1976).

Pretreatment of experimental animals with agents known to depress reticulo-endothelial function may markedly increase sensitivity to endotoxin. These treatments include actinomycin-D given to mice (Pieroni *et al.*, 1970), thorotrast injected into rabbits (Rutenberg *et al.*, 1960) and lead acetate administered to rats (Selye *et al.*, 1966; Filkins, 1970).

The susceptibility to endotoxin appears to be under genetic control especially in certain mouse strains, e.g. C3H/HeJ which are markedly resistant to these substances (Sultzer, 1968) apparently because of a defect in responsiveness of both B-cells and macrophages (Rosentreich *et al.*, 1977).

In 1974 Thomas stated that 'endotoxin as such is not a toxin, it is the answer of the higher animal to it which creates toxicity.' It is now apparent that the susceptibility of any given host depends on a variety of factors such as age, environment, pharmacological conditioning, genetics, immune and hormonal status and nutritional state. Moreover, from recent work on the influence of the physicochemical state on the biological activity of both LPS and free lipid A (see p.213), it is clear that the state of dispersion of the endotoxin preparation itself markedly affects the responses produced.

B. Assay

1. Rabbit Pyrogenicity Test

The current officially recognized procedure in the European and United States' Pharmacopoeias for the detection of LPS is the rabbit pyrogenicity test. Routinely this test is used to establish absence of endotoxin but it can be adapted for assay purposes from the quantitative relationship between LPS dose and increase in rabbit body temperature (Wolff *et al.*, 1965). This test, however, has been criticized because of its high cost and poor precision (Bangham, 1971).

2. Limulus *Amoebocyte Lysate (LAL) Assay*

This assay was developed from the original observation that an aqueous extract of the amoebocytes (blood cells) of the horsehoe crab *Limulus polyphemus* formed a gel when incubated with LPS at 37°C (Levin and Bang, 1964). Compared with other *in vitro* and *in vivo* procedures for assaying endotoxin, the LAL assay has the advantages of sensitivity, convenience, reliability and cost in comparison to other *in vivo* and *in vitro* methods (Rojas-Corona *et al.*, 1969; Cooper *et al.*, 1971, 1972; Reinhold and Fine, 1971; Nowotny *et al.*, 1975; Elin *et al.*, 1976; Tomasulo *et al.*, 1977). It is now the most widely used assay for LPS and hence will be discussed in some detail.

The sensitivity of the assay, which can detect as little as 0.1 ng/ml endotoxin, together with the ubiquitous nature of these substances, necessitates stringent measures to ensure that samples to be tested are not accidentally contaminated with extraneous endotoxin. This is especially important in assessing claims of non-specificity of the LAL assay. However, there is now good evidence to show that the LAL assay is specific for LPS especially at low concentrations. No reactivity has been reported with serotonin, histamine, epinephrine, norepinephrine, bradykinin (Rojas-Corona *et al.*, 1969), 11 species of yeast (Jorgensen and Smith, 1973), streptokinase, streptodornase, streptolysin, thrombin, haemoglobin and calcium (Reinhold and Fine, 1971). Several reports do question the absolute specificity of the LAL assay (Elin and Wolff, 1973; Wildfeuer *et al.*, 1974; Brunson and Watson, 1976). Wildfeuer *et al.* (1974) reported that although cultures of viable gram-positive bacteria were LAL-negative, the isolated cell wall peptidoglycan produced gelation. However, the activity was 1000 to 400 000 times less than that of LPS. This reactivity was abolished by treatment of the peptidoglycan with lysozyme to depolymerize it. The authors interpreted this as excluding endotoxin contamination as the basis of peptidoglycan activity. However, another interpretation might be that the activity was due to LPS contamination of the peptidoglycan and that lysozyme acted as a basic protein in binding LPS, as occurs with polymyxin.

Fumarola and Jirillo (1979) demonstrated that the extreme sensitivity of the LAL assay allowed detection of LPS contamination in several commercial immunological reagents (e.g. mitogens, therapeutic antisera, cytotoxic agents) and in radiographic contrast media. This is an important finding and, as a result, investigators in biomedical research should be aware of the possibility of endotoxin contamination and the influence it may have on experimental and clinical observations.

As with all of the other biological assays for LPS, the LAL procedure measures endotoxin activity rather than endotoxin quantity and this is relative to the preparation of endotoxin used as the standard. Since LPS preparations may differ markedly in their physical, chemical and biological properties, it is important to use a defined standard preparation. Moreover, if all workers using the assay employed the same standard, it would be possible to make more meaningful comparison of results from different laboratories, even if different lysate preparations are used. Standard LPS preparations have been prepared by both the World Health Organization and the United States Pharmacopoeia. There is also a commercial preparation of *Salmonella abortus equi* LPS which has been well characterized as a protein-free preparation in the uniform Na^+ salt form with a sedimentation coefficient of 80 S (Galanos *et al.*, 1979a). It is available as NovoPyrexal in ampoules of 0.1 μg and 1 μg LPS per ml (Pyrotell Diagnostik, FRG).

From their original observations, Levin and Bang (1964) postulated an enzymatic mechanism for the gel formation produced by the LPS–LAL interaction, and further studies have confirmed this hypothesis. Young *et al.* (1972) were the first group to attempt to characterize the components of the amoebocyte lysate. Figure 1 is a schematic representation of the *Limulus* lysate gelation reaction. LPS in the presence of Ca^{2+} activates a pro-clotting enzyme (Young *et al.*, 1972; Tai and Lui, 1977) to produce an active enzyme which is a serine protease (Niwa *et al.*, 1975; Tai and Lui, 1977). The activated enzyme acts on a clottable protein (coagulogen) producing limited proteolysis of this protein followed by polymerization and gel formation. For details of the biochemical analysis of these components, see Lui *et al.* (1979), Mosesson *et al.* (1979) and Takagi *et al.* (1979).

Similarities have been demonstrated between the mammalian coagulation system and the procoagulant enzyme of the horseshoe crab and have supported the suggestion that blood coagulation in the horseshoe crab is an example of a primitive system from which human coagulation has developed (Levin and Bang, 1968; Levin, 1976). As with the other biological activities of endotoxin,

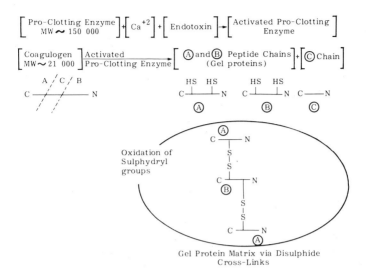

Figure 1. Schematic representation of the *Limulus* lysate gelation reaction. The pro-clotting enzyme is activated in the presence of calcium ions and endotoxin. Then the activated pro-clotting enzyme cleaves coagulogen into polypeptide subunits. The (C) chain is not incorporated into the clot. (From Mills, 1978, reproduced by permission of Mallinckrodt, Inc.)

lipid A is the active moiety in LPS activation of the lysate (Levin *et al.*, 1970a; Niwa *et al.*, 1975). The *Limulus* assay in addition to the already noted advantages also has the merit of being suitable for radiopharmaceutical preparations. (Cooper *et al.*, 1972).

In 1977 the LAL assay was accepted by the US Food and Drugs Administration for testing biological products and medical devices (Federal Register, 1977). Currently the assay has not been approved by the European Pharmacopoeia but is used by many of the pharmaceutical companies for in-process testing prior to final pyrogen testing in rabbits.

A major problem in applying the *Limulus* assay to titrating LPS in clinical blood specimens is that serum or plasma contain factors which interfere with the activation of the LAL system by LPS. Esterases (Skarnes, 1970; Skarnes and Rosen 1971), complement (Johnson and Ward, 1972), antibody (Levin *et al.*, 1970b; Young, 1975), lipoprotein (Freundenberg *et al.*, 1980) and α-globulin (Johnson *et al.*, 1977) have all been shown to inactivate the assay. Several different procedures have been developed to remove these factors but the controversy remains over the clinical value of the assay in the detection of endotoxaemia in man (Levin *et al.*, 1972; Stumacher *et al.*, 1973; Elin *et al.*, 1975; Sim and McCartney, 1980; Foulis *et al.*, 1982; McCartney *et al.*, 1983). It should be noted that this problem of inactivators does not preclude the use of the assay on other specimens such as urine or cerebrospinal fluid (CSF). Indeed the assay applied to CSF is valuable in the diagnosis of gram-negative bacterial meningitis (Nachum *et al.*, 1973; Ross *et al.*, 1975; Siegel and Nachum, 1979).

Recently the LAL assay has been modified for use with a chromogenic substrate (Iwanaga *et al.*, 1978; Scully *et al.*, 1980) which has resulted in a ten-fold increase in sensitivity and a more objective quantitation of the endpoint. The modification involves the addition of a synthetic amino acid substrate containing a *p*-nitroaniline group which is split off by the LPS-activated protease to produce a chromogen; the intensity of colour generated is proportional to the quantity of LPS.

III. STRUCTURE–FUNCTION RELATIONSHIPS

A. Preparation of LPS

Several procedures have been developed for the extraction of LPS from whole gram-negative bacteria, but only the hot, aqueous phenol method of Westphal *et al.* (1952) produces LPS free of protein and loosely bound phospholipid. The protein moiety which is retained in other extraction procedures such as the trichloracetic acid method of Boivin and Mesrobeanu (1935) has recently been shown to consist of a number of distinct proteins probably from the outer membrane of the bacterial cell (Morrison *et al.*, 1980). Their role in the immunological activities of LPS is doubtful (Izui *et al.*, 1980).

B. Chemical Structure

LPS from different genera of gram-negative bacteria share a common molecular structure (Lüderitz *et al.*, 1971). The basic molecule consists of a lipid component, the lipid A, covalently bound to a heteropolysaccharide of two

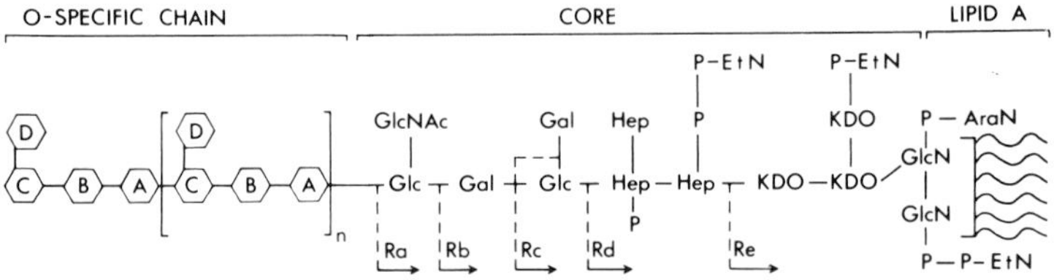

Figure 2. General structure of a *Salmonella* lipopolysaccharide. A–D sugar residues: Glc, D-glucose; Gal, D-galactose; GlcN, D-glucosamine; GlcNAc, *N*-acetyl-D-glucosamine; Hep, L-glycero-D-*manno*-heptose; KDO, 2-keto-3-deoxy-D-*manno*-octonate; Ara N, 4-amino-L-arabinose; P, phosphate; EtN, ethanolamine; ∿, hydroxy and non-hydroxy fatty acids; Ra to Re, incomplete R-form lipopolysaccharides. (From Lüderitz *et al.*, 1982, reproduced by permission of Pergamon Press.)

distinct regions: the core oligosaccharide and the O-specific chain. (Lüderitz *et al.*, 1971) (Figure 2). However, any given bacterial LPS is unlikely to be a homogeneous chemical entity and, for example, is liable to contain polysaccharide chains of variable lengths (Palva and Mäkelä, 1980; Goldman and Leive, 1980).

The O-specific chain is composed of a polymer of oligosaccharide molecules in repeating units, the nature of which is characteristic and unique for a given LPS. Several new sugar classes and unusual sugar derivatives, such as dideoxy sugars, have been discovered in these O-specific chains (Ashwell and Hickman, 1971). The O-specific chain is serotype-specific hence each serotype within a genus of gram-negative bacteria is characterized by a unique O-specific chain structure (Lüderitz *et al.*, 1971). This is exploited in the Kauffmann–White scheme for salmonellae (Lüderitz *et al.*, 1966a) in which specific antisera are used to classify the different *Salmonella* species.

In contrast, the core oligosaccharide structure is group-specific and is common among bacteria of a single genus (Galanos *et al.*, 1977a; Wilkinson, 1977; Weckesser *et al.*, 1979). The core consists of a branched oligosaccharide which contains a unique sugar, 2-keto-3-deoxy–D-mannooctonate (KDO), in addition to heptose, phosphoethanolamine and several hexoses. The O-specific chain is linked to a subterminal glucose residue in the core which in turn is covalently linked through KDO to an unusual lipid region—lipid A. Lipid A consists of a phosphorylated $\beta(1{\to}6)$-linked D-glucosamine disaccharide backbone to which long-chain fatty acids are attached (Figure 3). It is now known that the double ester is linked to position 3 of glucosamine II and the OH group at position 4 of glucosamine I is free. KDO is linked in the LPS to position 6 of glucosamine II (O. Lüderitz, personal communication, 1983).

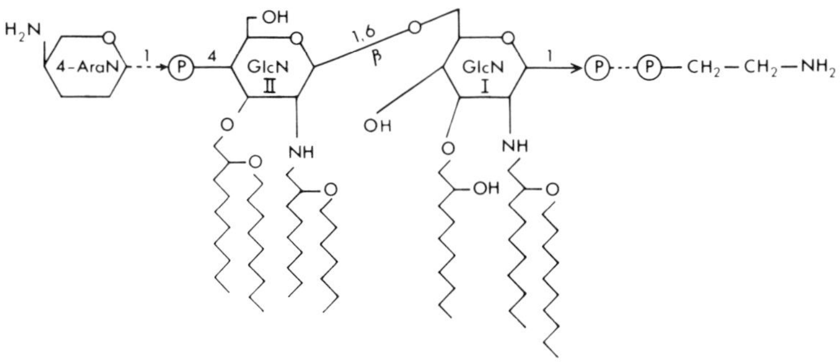

Figure 3. Proposed structure of *Salmonella lipid A*. GlcN, D-glucosamine; P, phosphate; AraN, 4-amino-L-arabinose; $\wedge\!\!\wedge\!\!\vee$, hydroxy and non-hydroxy fatty acids. (From Lüderitz *et al.*, 1982, reproduced by permission of Pergamon Press.)

Investigation of both the detailed chemical structure and biological activity of the LPS components especially the core oligosaccharide and the lipid A portions was greatly facilitated by the recognition of defective lipopolysaccharide biosynthesis in the so-called R mutants of *Salmonella* spp. (Lüderitz *et al.*, 1966b). This discovery together with the development of the phenol–chloroform–ether technique for extraction of LPS from *R* mutants by Galanos *et al.* (1969) explains why the *Salmonella* genus has provided so much information and formed the model for investigations on LPS.

There are two main groups of *R* mutants: (1) *Ra* mutants, defective in O-chain biosynthesis and producing only a complete core linked to lipid A, and (2) *Rb* and *Re* mutants, defective in core biosynthesis and which produce core fragments of varying length dependent on the blocked biosynthetic step (Figure 2). In addition, further mutants exhibiting most of the theoretically possible intermediates in core-lipid A biosynthesis have been characterized. Similar series of mutants have now also been isolated from other gram-negative genera (Jann and Westphal, 1975).

With these mutants, Lüderitz *et al.* (1966a) showed that incomplete LPS from all mutants had endotoxic activity similar to that of the complete LPS from the parent strain. This indicated that the polysaccharide part (Lüderitz *et al.*, 1971) was not essential for endotoxicity. Further work by Lüderitz and his colleagues (Rietschel *et al.*, 1971) on chemically modified *Re* glycolipids showed that the KDO portion was also not necessary. Then by mild acid hydrolysis of the ketosidic bond linking the core polysaccharide to lipid A, Galanos *et al.* (1971) were able to split off free lipid A devoid of all core sugars. Following solubilization of free lipid A in water either by coupling to bovine serum albumin (Galanos *et al.*, 1972) or by converting it to the triethylammonium salt form (Galanos and Lüderitz, 1975), the characteristic biological activities of LPS were demonstrated. Hence current attention of the chemical structure of LPS has become focused on producing further changes in the biologically active moiety—lipid A. There are only minor differences in the structures of lipid A in the LPS from different genera of bacteria. (Hase and Rietschel, 1977; Mühlradt *et al.*, 1977; Rietschel *et al.*, 1977, 1982a; Lüderitz *et al.*, 1978; Rosner *et al.*, 1979). The diphosphorylated $\beta(1\rightarrow6)$-linked D-glucosamine is a common non-variable structure in different lipid A's. Variability is mainly attributed to the number and nature of various non-acylated polar head groups bound to the phosphate residues and also the backbone (mainly fatty acids) substituents. The fatty acids of the backbone may vary in chain length, branching and degree of hydroxylation, but always the amino groups of the backbone are substituted by D-3-hydroxy fatty acids. Some photosynthetic bacteria and cyanobacteria have been shown to possess a lipid A which does not possess the otherwise common diglucosamine backbone structure. Instead it consists of a 3-amino-glucosamine structure which lacks phosphate groups and, moreover, lacks endotoxic activity either as a free entity or in the complete lipopolysaccharide (Weckesser and Drews, 1979).

C. Relationship of chemical structure to biological activity

Perhaps because of the hydrophilic and hydrophobic regions in the LPS molecule the physical state has a marked influence on the biological activities. Being amphipathic allows LPS to form micellar aggregates, while the charged groups permit formation of intermolecular ionic linkages which in turn may influence the degree of aggregation depending on the nature of ions present. Study of the effects of aggregation on the biological activities of LPS was made possible when Galanos and Lüderitz (1975) demonstrated that LPS could be converted into uniform salt forms by electrodialysis. Later it was shown that changes in the manifestations of individual biological activities of LPS were dependent on the degree of aggregation (Galanos *et al.*, 1979b).

In order to further the understanding of the relationship of structure and activity, comparative biological studies have been done with incomplete lipid A (lipid A precursor I), free lipid A derived from different bacteria, and the respective parent LPS molecules have been examined (Galanos *et al.*, 1977b; Lüderitz *et al*, 1978; Rietschel *et al.*, 1982a). The results summarized by Lüderitz *et al.* (1982) have suggested that the expression of various biological activities is related to differences in substructures and/or conformation of lipid A. The substituents of the lipid A phosphate groups — the polar head groups — are not required for lipid A endotoxicity, although they may exert an influence on the solubility of the molecule. Also it appears that lipid A precursor I (Figure 3) is the smallest lipid A substructure with endotoxic activity. The main differences between the parent *Salmonella* lipid A and the lipid A precursor I are that the latter lacks both the non-hydroxylated fatty acids and the polar head groups (Figure 3). These studies have also shown that the O-deacylated free lipid A lacks typical endotoxic activities although it is still antigenic and mitogenic. This suggested that the minimal features for endotoxic activity are the acylated diglucosamine backbone together with a suitable state of molecular dispersion.

An alternative approach for determining the molecular basis of endotoxin activity is the chemical modification of LPS by various reagents such as acid, alkali and oxidizing agents. The extensive literature on this subject is reviewed by Sultzer (1971).

IV. MECHANISM OF ENDOTOXIC ACTIVITY OF LPS

The basic mechanisms by which LPS functions involve both cellular and humoral systems and the complex inter-relationship of these systems makes it difficult to define and distinguish the primary, secondary and any incidental effects of LPS in the experimental animal. Although the mode of action of LPS at the molecular and cellular level has not yet been fully elucidated, considerable work has been done on the cellular and biochemical reactions which form the basis of the endotoxic response. The endotoxic activities of LPS in terms of levels of analysis from the whole animal through to isolated simple membranes will be discussed.

A. The Whole Animal and Isolated Organs

The numerous biological activities of injected LPS at the level of the whole experimental animal are listed in Table 1.

With regard to effects of LPS on isolated organs, a sharp distinction should be made between observations on organs taken from endotoxin-injected animals and those made on 'normal' organs exposed to LPS *in vitro*. In the former category, there is the inherent difficulty of distinguishing primary and secondary effects of the LPS. Among the major organs, the liver in particular exhibits enzymatic and metabolic changes following LPS administration to the whole animal. For example, changes in carbohydrate metabolism cause transient hyperglycaemia followed by marked hypoglycaemia. The former results from glycogenolysis due to an increased output of hepatic glucose, while hypoglycaemia arises from the increased uptake of glucose by peripheral tissues without a compensatory increase in glucose output by the liver (Wolfe *et al.*, 1977).

In the potentially more definitive category of experiments with LPS administered to normal organs *in vitro*, literature is relatively scarce. There seems to be very little direct effect of LPS on mammalian organs *in vitro*. This suggests that the major changes found in the liver and other organs of LPS-injected animals are due to secondary effects of mediators (Berry, 1971, 1975, 1977).

B. Individual Cells

In contrast to the dearth of information on perfused organs, there are numerous reports on the effects of LPS on isolated mammalian cells. Cell types that are responsive to LPS include macrophages, platelets, mast cells, polymorphonuclear leucocytes, lymphocytes, fibroblasts, and endothelial cells.

1. Polymorphonuclear Leucocytes

In marked contrast to the *in vivo* effects of LPS on polymorphonuclear leucocytes, *in vitro* effects are difficult to detect. For example, Wilson *et al.* (1981) showed that although LPS bound to polymorphonuclear leucocytes *in vitro* there was no consequential effect. However, Morrison and Ulevitch (1978) provided evidence that, in the presence of LPS, leucocytes exhibited enhanced phagocytic activity, increased glycolysis and an increased ability to reduce nitroblue tetrazolium.

LPS has a profound effect on polymorphonuclear leucocytes *in vivo*; there is an initial marked leucopaenia followed by a leucocytosis (Athens *et al.*, 1961;

Mechanic *et al.*, 1961). The initial response was shown to result from sequestration of neutrophils in capillary beds (Stetson, 1951; Athens *et al.*, 1961) while the subsequent leucocytosis was caused by release of granulocytes from the bone marrow reserves (Athens *et al.*, 1961). The role of complement in endotoxin-induced neutropaenia remains to be resolved (Morrison and Ulevitch, 1978). A role for lipid A in the observed neutropenia was suggested by Corrigan and co-workers (Corrigan and Bell, 1971; Corrigan *et al.*, 1974).

2. Platelets

The interaction of LPS and platelets *in vivo* and *in vitro* depends on the presence or absence of immune adherence sites (receptors for C3b, the split product of the complement component C3) on the platelet membrane. Des Prez and co-workers characterized the response of rabbit platelets to LPS *in vitro* and demonstrated aggregation (Des Prez *et al.*, 1961) generation of platelet factor 3 (Horowitz *et al.*, 1962a,b) and release of serotonin (Des Prez *et al.*, 1961). They also showed that LPS-induced platelet damage was dependent on a heat-labile factor in plasma (Horowitz *et al.*, 1962a; Des Prez, 1967) and on the presence of divalent cations (Des Prez and Bryant, 1966). Subsequent studies outlined a requirement for. the terminal components of complement in the endotoxin-induced lytic response in platelets (Siraganian, 1972; Brown and Lachman, 1973) and suggested that alternative rather than classical complement pathway activation was involved in this response (Morrison *et al.*, 1978; Morrison and Oades, 1979). Furthermore, Morrison and Oades (1979) provided evidence that lipid A was responsible for the binding of LPS to the platelet. However, human and primate platelets lack immune adherence receptors and their response to LPS is less well defined and, indeed, some of the literature is contradictory (Morrison and Ulevitch, 1978). It appears that LPS has little effect on human or other platelets lacking immune adherence receptors either in platelet-rich plasma or in plasma-free buffer. However, there are some reports of a secretory response in which only the granule constituents are released while the cytoplasmic membrane remains intact (Nagayama *et al.*, 1971; Hawinger *et al.*, 1975, 1977). Lipid A alone has been shown to elicit this complement-independent secretory response (Morrison *et al.*, 1981). There is evidence to suggest that *in vivo* responses of platelets to LPS also depend on the presence of receptors and on complement (Morrison and Ulevitch, 1978). Platelets have a marked affinity for endotoxin *in vivo* as demonstrated by the finding that, within minutes of injection, almost all labelled endotoxin is associated with platelets (Braude, 1964; Evans, 1971). Thereafter it accumulates in the reticuloendothelial system (Howard *et al.*, 1958; Noyes *et al.*, 1959; Das *et al.*, 1973). It would seem that by the very nature of the contents of platelets and their effects, they may play an important role in producing the endotoxic effects of LPS. Recently, Walker and Fletcher (1981) have suggested that microcirculatory events involving platelets contribute significantly to the pathophysiology of the host responses to LPS. However, induction of thrombocytopaenia *in vivo* failed to influence the development of intravascular coagulation or shock in experimental animals after the injection of LPS (Bohn and Müller-Berhaus, 1976).

3. Macrophages/Monocytes

These cells have been recognized as phagocytes since Metchinkoff's era, but only recently have they been recognized as 'secretory' cells (Unanue, 1976). On incubation with LPS, they secrete a vast array of mediators which may influence surrounding cells and tissues locally or via the circulation may reach other targets. For a review on these mediators see Schlessinger (1980). Many of these mediators can also be produced by other LPS-stimulated cells such as lymphocytes, fibroblasts or endothelial cells. Among the factors released from macrophages are endogenous pyrogen, colony stimulating factor, collagenase, leucocyte endogenous mediator, tumour necrotizing factor, lymphocyte activating factor, glucocorticoid antagonizing factor, plasminogen activator, and recently prostaglandins, which we shall now consider in more detail.

In recent years aspirin (acetylsalicyclic acid) and other non-steroid anti-inflammatory drugs have been found to inhibit some typical endotoxic activities such as fever (Feldberg, 1975), shock (Fletcher and Ramwell, 1978), abortion (Skarnes and Harper, 1972) and early hypertension (Parratt and Sturgess, 1977). Since the discovery by Vane in 1971 that these drugs are inhibitors of prostaglandin biosynthesis, the prostaglandins have been suggested as possible mediators of endotoxic activity. Chemically prostaglandins are long-chain fatty acids and as such differ from the majority of host cell derived mediators which are peptides and amines. The evidence to support an effect of LPS has been summarized by Rietschel *et al.* (1980). These workers presented results to show that LPS induces macrophages *in vitro*, on a dose- and time-dependent basis to synthesize *de novo* prostaglandins E_2 and F_2. Further evidence from two different aspects is described by Rietschel *et al.* (1982b): (1) peritoneal macrophages from C3H/HeJ mice were not stimulated by LPS to secrete enhanced levels of prostaglandins E_2 and F_2; and (2) peritoneal macrophages from mice rendered tolerant to LPS were also unable to secrete prostaglandins on incubation with LPS (Figure 4). Although further studies are needed to determine the precise role of prostaglandins in mediating toxic effects in response to LPS challenge, it seems likely that they are important.

From the pronounced sensitivity to LPS seen *in vitro* with macrophages, it seems likely that they also have a vital role in release of mediators *in vivo* in response to LPS.

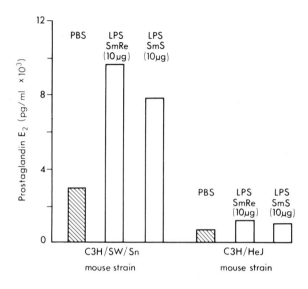

Figure 4. LPS-induced prostaglandin E₂ release by peritoneal macrophages from C3H/Sw/Sn and C3H/HeJ mice. SmS, LPS from *Salmonella minnesota* wild type (S form) bacteria; SmRe, LPS from *Salmonella minnesota Re* mutant (R595). (From Rietschel *et al.*, 1982b, reproduced by permission of the authors and Almqvist and Wiksell International.)

4. Lymphocytes

The effect of LPS on lymphocytes and the immune response has been the subject of much work over the past 20 years and a substantial amount of information on the complex interactions has resulted. Recently, Morrison and Ryan (1979) have published an extensive review of this aspect of LPS and the host immune response. The important findings may be summarized as follows.

(i) *B-lymphocytes*. LPS can have a profound effect on B-lymphocytes and can initiate both proliferative responses and antibody secretion. These events occur after injection of LPS into the experimental animal *in vivo* and also after the addition of LPS to lymphocyte cultures *in vitro*. The demonstration (Gery *et al.*, 1972) that LPS is a B-lymphocyte mitogen greatly facilitated the study of B-lymphocyte function and delineation of its role in immune responses. However, it is not a mitogen for B-lymphocytes of species other than mice. An important aspect of LPS–B-lymphocyte interaction is the phenomenon of polyclonal B-cell activation in which LPS initiates non-specifically the synthesis and secretion of antibody by immunocompetent lymphocytes in the absence of specific antigen. This was first demonstrated by Ortiz-Ortiz and Jaroslow in 1970.

(ii) *T-lymphocytes*. LPS appears not to initiate T-lymphocyte proliferative responses directly (Anderssen *et al.*, 1972; Möller *et al.*, 1972a,b; Peavy *et al.*, 1974). This contrasts with the well-characterized effects of LPS on B-lymphocyte proliferation. However, there is evidence that LPS–T-lymphocyte interactions may be involved in antigen-dependent immune responses and may influence levels of antigen-specific antibody.

5. Other Cells

After injection LPS has subsequently been found in endothelial cells but further studies are needed to determine the effect of endotoxins on these cells. The role of mast cells and basophils in producing the marked vascular changes seen in anaphylactic shock is well known (Bach, 1978). However, their contribution, if any, to the response to LPS *in vivo* or endotoxic shock is poorly defined.

The reader is referred to a comprehensive review on the significant effects of LPS on mammalian cells both *in vitro* and *in vivo* (Morrison and Ulevitch, 1978).

C. Enzyme Systems

Some of the LPS-activated cell products affect host humoral mediation systems as can LPS itself directly. Morrison and Ulevitch (1978) have reviewed the significant effects of LPS on the major humoral mediation systems, namely complement (classical and alternative pathways) and coagulation (both extrinsic and intrinsic, including kinin-forming and fibrinolytic). After injection of LPS the complement system is one of the first to be affected. It has been shown that a high degree of aggregation of LPS is essential for such activities both *in vitro* and *in vivo* (Galanos and Lüderitz, 1976). LPS activates the complement system by three distinct mechanisms and by both the classical and alternative pathway. The classical pathway is activated by LPS–antibody complexes (Möller and Michael, 1971) and also by an antibody-dependent mechanism when lipid A itself binds directly to C1 (Galanos *et al.*, 1971; Loos *et al.*, 1974; Morrison and Kline, 1977; Cooper and Morrison, 1978). The alternative pathway is activated, in the absence of antibody, by activation of C3 by the polysaccharide portion of LPS (Gewurz *et al.*, 1968; Marcus *et al.*, 1971; Morrison and Kline, 1977). As a result of complement activation, serum chemotactic factors are generated (Snyderman *et al.*, 1968, 1969), as well as activated complement components which interact with cells such as mast cells and basophils and cause further release of mediators. The well-known influences in the complement-mediated bactericidal and bacteriolytic activity of serum against smooth (S) and rough (R) strains of gram-negative bacteria can be explained readily in terms of LPS quantity and quality (Taylor, 1983). LPS can activate both the intrinsic and extrinsic coagulation pathways and the most likely sites where LPS may

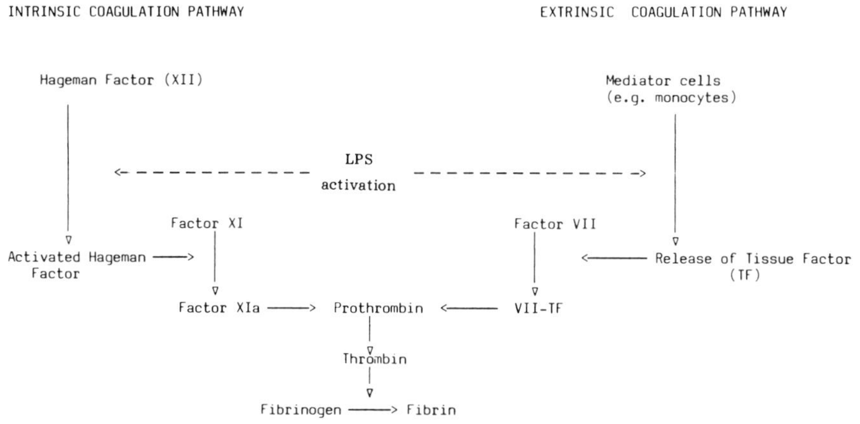

INTRINSIC COAGULATION PATHWAY   EXTRINSIC COAGULATION PATHWAY

Figure 5. Interaction of LPS with the coagulation system. (From Morrison and Ulevitch, 1978, reproduced by permission of Lippincott/Harper & Row.)

initiate coagulation are shown in Figure 5. Recent work on endotoxin-induced disseminated intravascular coagulation has been focused on the mechanism of activation of Hageman factor and the mechanism of endotoxin activity to initiate tissue factor production by leucocytes. Studies on white cell procoagulant activity have shown that the monocyte appears to be the main cellular source (Rivers *et al.*, 1975; Hiller *et al.*, 1977) and that lipid A is required to activate it (Niemetz and Morrison, 1977; Rickles and Rick, 1977). For Hagemen factor activation, it seems that LPS provides a negatively charged surface which is required to promote activation (Morrison and Cochrane, 1974). Activated Hageman factor can also activate plasma prekallikrein to form kallikrein, which is a proteolytic enzyme which converts plasminogen to plasmin and initiates fibrinolysis (Revak *et al.*, 1977). Thus LPS activation of Hageman factor can initiate both intravascular coagulation and fibrinolysis. However a major question remains to be answered: 'Does the activation of the prothrombin molecule occur predominantly by the extrinsic or intrinsic coagulation pathway?'

There are two highly characteristic types of pathological lesion produced in the whole animal by endotoxin, namely the local and generalized Shwartzman reactions (Shwartzman, 1937). Both require two injections of LPS spaced 24 h apart, and both produce vascular lesions although the mechanisms are different.

In the generalized Shwartzman reaction, two sublethal doses of LPS are given intravenously to the rabbit which then develops bilateral renal cortical necrosis. The reaction can be prevented by anticoagulant therapy which emphasizes the role of intravascular coagulation in producing the lesions (Good and Thomas, 1953). The first dose initiates coagulation with formation of the fibrin aggregates, most of which are cleared by the reticuloendothelial system. However, the second dose blocks this clearing and results in a progressive build up of fibrin which is deposited in the renal glomeruli.

In the local or dermal Shwartzman reaction, the first dose of LPS is given intradermally followed by an intravenous dose 24 h later. Both doses are small and the rabbit is again the most susceptible experimental animal. The initial dose produces an erythematous lesion at the site of injection which consists of aggregations of leucocytes and platelets. The second dose produces progressive necrosis with disintegration of leucocytes, tissue destruction and haemorrhage. Again, anticoagulants prevent this reaction, and together with polymorphonuclear leucocytes, coagulation mechanisms therefore play an important role.

D. Subcellular Particles

1. Mitochondria

Fonnesu and Severi (1956a,b) were the first to report a decrease in oxidative phosphorylation in isolated mitochondria from the livers of rats which had been given an intraperitoneal injection of endotoxin 24 h previously. The uncoupling effect was accompanied by swelling of the mitochondria. Since then it has been shown that LPS injection leads to an impairment of mitochondrial function in the whole animal, in cells in culture and also in subcellular fractions (Bradley, 1979, 1981; Mela, 1981). However, LPS does not directly inhibit the electron carriers of the respiratory chain, and the impaired coupling of oxidative phosphorylation appears to be secondary to an interaction(s) between LPS and a constituent of the mitochondria (McGivney and Bradley, 1979). In addition, the way in which endotoxin affects the respiration of isolated mitochondria varies with different substrates (McGivney and Bradley, 1980a). Changes in the ultrastructural morphology of mitochondria treated with LPS have been observed by several workers (Bradley, 1979).

McGivney and Bradley (1980b) examined mitochondrial enzyme activity in liver cells and in isolated mitochondria from both LPS-susceptible and LPS-resistant mice after exposure to LPS. They showed that both had depressed mitochondrial enzyme activities whereas only the liver cells from the LPS-susceptible mice had reduced mitochondrial enzyme activities. This suggested that resistance to LPS is an attribute of the intact cell and not of the mitochondrion itself. The same workers have also shown that changes in mitochondrial enzyme activities precede those seen for lysosomal enzymes and are associated with lower amounts of LPS (McGivney and Bradley, 1979). Although there is good correlation between *in vitro* and *in vivo* observations, work on the effects of LPS on mitochondria, the relationship between changes in mitochondrial activities and the biological activities seen after LPS administration to the intact animal remains unclear.

2. Lysosomes

In 1959 Martini observed an increase in the cathepsin activity in liver and muscle homogenates from rats injected with LPS and suggested that lysosomes may be a target of LPS. Subsequently it has been shown that LPS enhances lysosomal enzyme activities in established normal cell cultures (McGivney and Bradley, 1978, 1979). This increase in lysosomal enzyme activity is progressive with time, requires new protein synthesis, is temperature-dependent and occurs in the absence of added serum. An increase in lysosomal enzymic activity is also reported in primary culture of spleen cells from normal mice (McGivney and Bradley, 1977; Mørland, 1979) but not in primary cultures of spleen cells from genetically resistant C3H/HeJ mice or endotoxin-tolerant mice (McGivney and Bradley, 1977). Also lysosomes from mice treated with endotoxin are more fragile than those from untreated mice (Bradley and Bond, 1975). Recently McCuskey *et al.* (1982) examined the responses of the liver to endotoxin in C3H/HeJ mice, and reported that, histochemically, an apparent lysosomal enzyme deficiency existed in these mice since reduced reactions for acid phosphatase, cathepsin B and H and dipeptidylpeptidase I and II were seen. However, the role of the lysosomes and their lysosomal enzymes in the toxic effects of LPS is still unresolved. Nevertheless, Bradley suggested that mitochondria and lysosomes together play a major role in the toxic manifestations of LPS administration in the whole animal (Bradley, 1981).

E. LPS Receptor Sites

The question of whether LPS has a specific receptor in sensitive cells is still unsettled. Little is known about the mechanism by which LPS binds to cell membranes (Kabir *et al.*, 1978; Morrison and Rudbach, 1980). It is possible that any hydrophobic component of the membrane may bind lipid A to some extent. The marked affinity of endotoxin for cell mammalian membranes has prompted some workers to look for specific receptors. However, further studies are needed with purified membrane components to determine whether there are indeed specific receptors and/or non-specific binding sites involved in the interaction of LPS with cell membranes. The reader is referred to Chapter 9 for further information on the affinity of LPS and bacterial surface polysaccharides in general for mammalian cell membranes.

Bradley (1979, 1981) has proposed an ingenious model for the cellular and molecular basis of action of LPS (see Figure 6). After binding to the cell membrane, LPS is taken into the cell by endocytosis and then translocated in a vacuole to a primary lysosome which transfers the LPS to a specific receptor on the mitochondrial membrane. There the mitochondrial proton gradient is destroyed and ADP and NADH accumulate leading to enhanced glycolysis, with

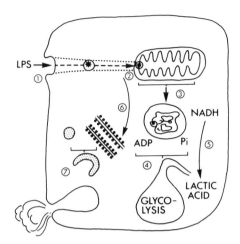

Figure 6. Cellular basis for the action of endotoxin. 1, endocytosis, and 2, translocation of endotoxin to the mitochondrion. 3, the protein gradient is destroyed, causing 4, ADP and NADH to accumulate in the cytosol, and 5, enhanced glycolysis. 6, lysosomal enzymes are induced, autophagy is stimulated and 7, lysosomal hydrolases are released. (From Bradley, 1981, reproduced by permission of Alan R. Liss, Inc.)

subsequent induction and release of lysosomal enzymes. Finally, these events produce the characteristic symptoms of endotoxicity.

F. Genetic Resistance to LPS

Recent studies of the host genetic factors that affect susceptibility to LPS have proved to be valuable in the elucidation of the biological activities of LPS. These studies were made possible by Sultzer's discovery in 1968 that the inbred mouse strain C3H/HeJ is resistant to some of the endotoxic effects of LPS. Subsequent studies showed that a single locus, named *LPS*, on chromosome 4 regulates the expression of a number of endotoxic reactions induced by lipid A (Watson and Riblet, 1974; Watson *et al.*, 1978). Thus the availability of this mouse strain has allowed genetic manipulations to separate the direct effects of LPS and LPS-sensitive cells from the indirect effects which may arise from subsequent release of mediators which activate cells which are themselves not sensitive to LPS. A second LPS-unresponsive strain of mouse, C57B1/10 Sc Cr, has been reported (Coutinho *et al.*, 1977; McAdam and Ryan, 1978; Coutinho and Meo, 1978).

It is clear that the determination of the host gene product that reacts with LPS would greatly facilitate the understanding of the biochemical basis of the initiation of cellular responses to lipid A and also contribute to our knowledge of endotoxic responses in mammals. In a review of the genetic control of endotoxic sensitivity, Watson *et al.* (1980) discuss several approaches to this problem and also outline some possible functions of the LPS responsiveness locus; namely, (A) that the LPS locus may control structural genes coding for cellular receptors for lipid A, or (B) that the LPS locus may encode for genes that influence the expression of receptors for lipid A, or (C) that the LPS 'locus' may encode for genes that are involved in expression of cellular components required to convert the binding event into a biochemical signal.

Morrison *et al.* (1981) demonstrated that LPS-initiated, calcium-dependent platelet secretory responses occurred in the C3H/HeJ mouse as well as in the endotoxin-sensitive mouse. They postulated that this is a non-specific perturbational event of the platelet membrane. However, this finding may be contrasted with the absence of a response to LPS by the macrophages, lymphocytes and fibroblasts of C3H/HeJ mice (Morrison and Ryan, 1979). Consequently they suggested that cell membranes of C3H/HeJ mice are not defective in their capacity to interact with lipid A but that for cell activation, specific recognition of binding sites is essential. Immunological evidence for such a receptor on lymphocytes has been presented by Forni and Coutinho (Forni and Coutinho, 1978a,b; Coutinho *et al.*, 1978) who showed it to be absent on lymphoid cells of the C3H/HeJ mouse.

V. ROLE IN HOST–PARASITE RELATIONSHIPS

A. Distribution of LPS in the Bacterial Kingdom

Most research on LPS has been done on the substances extracted from Enterobacteriaceae. However, LPS has been reported from a wide range of bacterial families, many of which consist of purely saprophytic organisms with no evident ecological interaction with animal hosts. Gram-negative bacteria are ubiquitous in the biosphere and, for example, constitute a significant part of the biomass in the world's oceans (Watson *et al.*, 1977). It would appear that all bacteria which stain gram-negative produce LPS although the spirochaete *Borrelia recurrentis* apparently lacks this substance (Galloway *et al.*, 1979; Butler *et al.*, 1979). Differences in LPS structure have already been discussed, but some additional examples may be cited. For example, the structure of LPS from the anaerobe *Bacteroides fragilis* seems to differ from LPS of aerobic gram-negative bacteria in lacking KDO (Kasper, 1976; Westphal, 1975). Also the lipid A region has an unusual fatty acid composition and contains no amide-linked β-hydroxymyristic acid (Wollenweber *et al.*, 1980). In addition, the biological activities of *Bacteroides fragilis* LPS also appear to differ at least in magnitude from the responses of LPS from *Salmonella* spp. (Kasper, 1976). Some of the photosynthetic bacteria have been shown to have a different type of lipid A which does not contain the glucosamine backbone but 3-aminoglucosamine instead. Neither the lipid A nor the corresponding lipopolysaccharides in either *Rhodopseudomonas viridis*, *R. palustris*, *R. sulfoviridis* or *R. sphaeroides* expressed characteristic endotoxic activities (Weckesser *et al.*, 1979; Strittmatter *et al.*, 1983). Wilkinson and Taylor (1978) reported similar findings with two saprophytic *Pseudomonas* spp. Thus it seems that not all LPS from gram-negative bacteria is endotoxic.

B. LPS in Normal Mammalian Flora

Gram-negative bacteria are present in large numbers in the environment, food and the normal commensal flora of man especially in the oropharynx, and in the genital and gastrointestinal tracts. The mammalian gut is colonized from birth onwards with gram-negative bacteria. Does the continuous presence of gram-negative bacteria influence man's reactivity to LPS? Resistance to the lethal effects of bacterial LPS has long been recognized to be higher in germ-free laboratory animals than in controls (Dubos and Schaedler, 1960; Schaedler and Dubos, 1961; Jensen *et al.*, 1963). Kiyono *et al.* (1980) showed that germ-free animals had greater mitogenic and immunologic responses to LPS *in vitro* than conventional animals and were more refractory to LPS. These observations suggest that under certain circumstances indigenous microorganisms induce immunologic tolerance to bacterial endotoxins and thus theoretically may decrease resistance to infection by pathogens producing these toxins. Melchers (1980) has postulated that LPS is necessary for the development of essential physiological systems such as the immune system.

C. Role of LPS in Gram-negative Bacterial Infections

Although there is considerable speculation, little is known of the role of LPS in gram-negative infections. Since it is a component of cell envelopes of both pathogenic and saprophytic bacteria, the possession of LPS does not in itself confer pathogenicity on a bacterium. In addition, although LPS has been shown to be an important virulence factor, it is not the sole toxic factor involved in the pathogenic activity of many gram-negative bacteria, especially those which produce a classical protein exotoxin or have a marked capacity for tissue invasion. Nevertheless, as a component of the outer surface of gram-negative bacteria, LPS must have a considerable influence on the interaction of the bacterium with its environment. Smith (1975) has suggested that most damage caused by toxic surface components like LPS depends on the extent to which they are liberated during an infection and that damage is more likely when there is extensive bacterial invasion of blood and tissues with consequently more opportunity for cell lysis and/or liberation of endotoxin.

Little is known of the factors either *in vivo* or *in vitro* which control the release from, or the retention of, LPS in the bacterial cell. Antibiotics have been shown *in vitro* to release LPS (Goto and Nakamura, 1980) but confirmatory evidence of this *in vivo* is lacking except perhaps for the observed Jarisch-Herxheimer reaction (a hypersensitivity reaction that follows the use of a rapidly acting chemotherapeutic agent which liberates toxic products of the organism) seen in syphilis (Gelfand *et al.*, 1976).

D. Antibodies to LPS

In recent years there has been a considerable increase in infections and deaths due to gram-negative bacilli especially in compromised hospital patients and despite extensive use of antibiotics. Thus interest has been aroused in immunoprophylaxis as an approach to control of gram-negative infections. An obvious common denominator in these organisms is the possession of LPS, and hence it has been explored as a possible protective antigen. Lipopolysaccharides possess a large number of antigenic determinants but not all of them are expressed in the complete molecule. In smooth (S) form LPS the immunodeterminants of the O-specific side-chain oligosaccharides are exposed. When the rough (R) mutant LPS are prepared, previously cryptic immuno-determinants of core oligosaccharides are exposed. When free lipid A is prepared by mild acid hydrolysis of lipopolysaccharides, yet further cryptic immuno-determinant structures are revealed.

Anti-R and anti-lipid A antibodies are directed against structures common to different LPS whereas anti-O antibodies are specific for individual LPS. Hence it is not surprising that antisera to smooth bacteria with the full complement of oligosaccharide side-chains are ineffective in protecting against infection by unrelated gram-negative bacteria. Antibodies against both LPS and core glycolipid protect animals against experimental infection with gram-negative bacteria (Sandford *et al.*, 1962; Kaijser and Olling, 1973). However, until recently (Ziegler *et al.*, 1982), there was practically no evidence to confirm these findings with gram-negative infections in humans (Zinner and McCabe, 1976). Titres of 'O'-specific antibody of the IgG but not IgM class against the patient's own infecting organisms correlated with a decrease in the frequency of shock and death in bacteraemia (McCabe *et al.*, 1972). Also, high titre antibody to *Re* LPS correlated with decreased frequency of shock and death. Antibody to lipid A had no protective effect in bacteraemia. Braude *et al.* (1977) demonstrated significant cross-protection against a number of gram-negative bacteria in animals immunized with the J5 mutant of *Escherichia coli* O111:B4. This mutant lacks the exogenous galactose in its LPS and, as a result, consists solely of the core determinants lipid A, *N*-acetylglucosamine, 2-keto-3-deoxyoctonate, heptose and glucose. Similar results demonstrating a cross-protection effect were also reported by McCabe *et al.* (1977) with the *Re* mutant of *Salmonella minnesota*.

Recently, Ziegler *et al.* (1982) made a randomized controlled clinical trial with antisera raised in human volunteers to the J5 mutant of *E. coli* and using preimmunization serum as control. When administered intravenously to bacteraemic patients near the onset of illness there were 39% (42 of 100) deaths in controls compared to 22% (23 of 103) in those given antiserum. Also there was a reduction in mortality in profoundly shocked patients from 77% (30 of 39) to 44% (18 of 41). It therefore appears that human J5 antiserum may have real therapeutic potential in treating gram-negative bacteraemia and septic shock. This work highlights the paradox that antisera to smooth bacteria are ineffective in protecting against infection yet antiserum to core LPS protects against infection by smooth bacteria. Ziegler *et al.* suggest that core antibody may act during early stages of cell-wall synthesis before LPS synthesis is complete.

Serum from normal subjects may contain a variety of 'natural' antibodies including antibody to core LPS (Ziegler *et al.*, 1982); hence the potential now exists to boost natural immunity in patients at risk of gram-negative septicaemia by prophylactic administration of core antiserum. This approach would be particularly attractive for immunocompromised patients.

VI. PERSPECTIVES AND GROWTH POINTS

LPS induces a vast array of effects on the host's specific and non-specific immune system. Studies on some of the individual effects of LPS on both the humoral and cellular components of the specific immune system have contributed substantially to elucidation of the immune response in general.

The unique immunological activities of LPS such as their potent intrinsic immunogenicity and their profound capacity to potentiate or suppress immune responses to unrelated antigens may explain the numerous ways that they are able to influence host immune responses. Indeed LPS may play a critical role in regulating host responsiveness to infections and neoplasia. Recently, prompted by knowledge of the immunobiology of LPS, there has been a renewed interest in the exploitation of the beneficial effects of LPS as modulators of the immune response and as immunogens in developing protective antisera for the control of gram-negative infections (Nowotny, 1983). But it remains to be seen from clinical trials whether worthwhile therapeutic measures will follow.

The question of how LPS works and what mammalian systems it affects will no doubt continue to fascinate investigators from many disciplines in the years ahead. Undoubtedly the advent of synthetic analogues of lipid A (Inage *et al.*, 1980a,b; Kiso *et al.*, 1981a,b,c) together with inbred mice of different endotoxin sensitivity should provide further refinements of insight into the molecular and cellular basis of endotoxicity.

REFERENCES

Anderssen, J., Möller, G., and Sjöberg, O. (1972). Selective induction of DNA synthesis in T and B lymphocytes. *Cell Immunol.*, **4**, 381–393.

Ashwell, G., and Hickman, J. (1971). The chemistry of the unique carbohydrates of bacterial lipopolysaccharides. In *Microbial Toxins*, Vol. IV, *Bacterial Endotoxins* (Eds. G. Weinbaum, S. Kadis, and S. J. Ajl), pp.235–266. Academic Press, London, New York.

Athens, J. W., Haab, O. P., Raab, S. O., Mauer, A. M., Ashenbrucker, H., Cartwright, G. E., and Wintrobe, M. M. (1961). Leukokinetic studies. IV. The total blood, circulating and marginal granulocyte pools and the granulocyte turnover rate in normal subjects. *J. Clin. Invest.*, **40**, 989–995.

Bach, M. K. (1978). *Immediate Hypersensitivity—Modern Concepts and Developments.* Marcel Dekker, New York.

Bailey, M. E. (1976). Endotoxin, bile salts and renal function in obstructive jaundice. *Br. J. Surg.*, **63**, 774–778.

Bangham, D. R. (1971). The dilemma of quantitation in the test for pyrogens. In *Pyrogens and Fever* (Eds G. E. W. Wolstenholme and J. Birch), pp.207–212. Churchill Livingstone, Edinburgh, London.

Bennett, I. L., Jr. (1964). Introduction: approaches to the mechanisms of endotoxin action. In *Bacterial Endotoxins* (Eds. M. Landy and W. Braun), pp.xiii–xvi. Rutgers, The State University Press, Rahway, NJ.

Berry, L. J. (1971). Metabolic effects of bacterial endotoxins. In *Microbial Toxins*, Vol. V, *Bacterial Endotoxins* (Eds. S. Kadis, G. Weinbaum, and S. J. Ajl), pp.165–208. Academic Press, New York, London.

Berry, L. J. (1975). Metabolic effects of endotoxin. In *Microbiology 1975* (Ed. D. Schlessinger), pp.315–319. American Society for Microbiology, Washington, DC.

Berry, L. J., (1977). Bacterial toxins. *CRC Crit. Rev. Toxicol.*, **5**, 239–318.

Bertók, L. (1977). Physicochemical defense of vertebrate organisms: the role of bile acids in defense against bacterial endotoxin. *Perspect. Biol. Med.*, **21**, 70–76.

Bertók, L. (1980). Role of bile in detoxification of lipopolysaccharide. In *Microbiology 1980* (Ed. D. Schlessinger), pp.91–93. American Society for Microbiology, Washington, D.C.

Bishop, D. G., and Work, E. (1965). An extracellular glycolipid produced by *Escherchia coli* grown under lysine limiting conditions. *Biochem. J.*, **96**, 567–572.

Bohn, E., and Müller-Berhaus, G. (1976). The effect of leukocyte and platelet transfusion on the activation of intravascular coagulation by endotoxin in granulocytopenic and thrombocytopenic rabbits. *Am. J. Pathol.*, **84**, 239–258.

Boivin, A., and Mesrobeanu, L. (1935). Recherches sur les antigènes somatiques et sur les endotoxins des bactéries. I. Considerations générales et exposé des techniques utilisées. *Rev. Immunol. (Paris)* **1**, 553–569.

Bourn, J. M., and Siebert, F. B. (1925). The cause of many febrile reactions following intravenous injections. II. The bacteriology of twelve distilled waters. *Am. J. Physiol.*, **71**, 652–659.

Bradley, S. G. (1979). Cellular and molecular mechanisms of action of bacterial endotoxins. *Annu. Rev. Microbiol.*, **33**, 67–94.

Bradley, S. G. (1981). Direct action of bacterial endotoxin on cells, mitochondria, and lysosomes. *Progress in Clinical and Biological Research*, Vol. 62, *Pathophysiological Effects of Endotoxin at the Cellular Level* (Eds. J. A. Majde and R. J. Person), pp.3–14. Alan R. Liss, New York.

Bradley, S. G., and Bond, J. S. (1975). Toxicity, clearance and metabolic effects of pactamycin in combination with bacterial lipopolysaccharides. *Toxicol. Appl. Pharmacol.*, **31**, 208–221.

Braude, A. I. (1964). Adsorption, distribution, and elimination of endotoxins and their derivatives. In *Bacterial Endotoxins* (Eds. M. Landy and W. Braun), pp.98–109. Rutgers, The State University, New Brunswick.

Braude, A. I. Ziegler, E. J., Douglas, H., and McCutchan, J. A. (1977). Antibody to cell wall glycolipid of gram-negative bacteria: induction of immunity to bacteraemia and endotoxaemia. *J. Infect. Dis.*, **136**, (Suppl. S), 167–173.

Brown, D. L., and Lachmann, P. J. (1973). The behaviour of complement and platelets in lethal endotoxin shock in rabbits. *Int. Arch. Allergy Appl. Immunol.*, **45**, 193–205.

Brunson, K. W., and Watson, D. W. (1976). '*Limulus* amebocyte lysate reaction with streptococcal pyrogenic exotoxin. *Infect. Immun.*, **14**, 1256–1258.

Butler, T., Hayen, P., Wallace, C. K., Awoke, S., and Habte-Michael, A. (1979). Infection with *Borrelia recurrentis:* Pathogenesis of fever and petechiae. *J. Infect. Dis.*, **140**, 665–675.

Cooper, J. F., Levin, J., and Wagner, H. N. (1971). Quantitative comparison of *in vitro* and *in vivo* methods for the detection of endotoxin. *J. Lab. Clin. Med.*, **78**, 138–148.

Cooper, J. F., Hochstein, H. D., and Seligmann, E. B., Jr. (1972). The Limulus test for endotoxin (pyrogen) in radiopharmaceuticals and biologicals. *Bull. Parenter. Drug. Assoc.*, **26**, 153–162.

Cooper, N. R., and Morrison, D. C. (1978). Binding and activation of the first component of human complement by the lipid A region of lipopolysaccharides. *J. Immunol.*, **120**, 1862–1868.

Corrigan, J. J., Jr., and Bell, B. M. (1971). Comparison between polymyxins and gentamicin in preventing endotoxin-induced intravascular coagulation and leucopenia. *Infect. Immun.*, **4**, 563–566.

Corrigan, J. J., Jr., Sieber, O. F., Jr., Ratojczak, H., and Bennett, B. B. (1974). Modification of human neutrophil response to endotoxin with polymyxin B sulfate. *J. Infect. Dis.*, **130**, 384–387.

Coutinho, A., and Meo, T. (1978). Genetic basis for unresponsiveness to lipopolysaccharide in C57BL/10 Cr mice. *Immunogenetics*, **7**, 17–24.

Coutinho, A., Forni, L., Melchers, F., and Watanabe, T. (1977). Genetic defect in responsiveness to the B cell mitogen lipopolysaccharide. *Eur. J. Immunol.*, **7**, 325–328.

Coutinho, A., Forni, L., and Watanabe, T. (1978). Genetic and functional characteristics of an antiserum to the lipid A specific triggering receptor on murine B lymphocytes. *Eur. J. Immunol.*, **8**, 63–67.

Das, J., Schwartz, A. A., and Folkman, J. (1973). Clearance of endotoxin by platelets: Role in increasing the accuracy of the *Limulus* gelation test and in combating experimental endotoxaemia. *Surgery*, **74**, 235–240.

Des Prez, R. M. (1967). The effects of bacterial endotoxin on rabbit platelets. V. Heat labile plasma factor requirements of endotoxin-induced platelet injury. *J. Immunol.*, **99**, 966–973.

Des Prez, R. M., and Bryant, R. E. (1966). Effects of bacterial endotoxin on rabbit platelets. IV. The divalent ion requirements of endotoxin-induced and immunologically induced platelet injury. *J. Exp. Med.*, **124**, 971–982.

Des Prez, R. M., Horowitz, H. J., and Hook, E. W. (1961). Effects of bacterial endotoxin on rabbit platelets. I. Platelet aggregation and release of platelet factors *in vitro*. *J. Exp. Med.*, **114**, 857–874.

Devoe, I. W., and Gilchrist, J. E. (1973). Release of endotoxin in the form of cell wall blebs during *in vitro* growth of *Neisseria meningitidis*. *J. Exp. Med.*, **138**, 1156–1167.

Dubos, R. J., and Schaedler, R. W. (1960). The effect of the intestinal flora on the growth rate of mice, and on their susceptibility to experimental infection. *J. Exp. Med.*, **111**, 407–417.

Elin, R. J., and Wolff, S. M. (1973). Nonspecificity of the *Limulus* amebocyte lysate test: positive reactions with polynucleotides and proteins. *J. Infect. Dis.*, **128**, 349–352.

Elin, R. J., Robinson, R. A., Levine, A. S., and Wolff, S. M. (1975). Lack of clinical usefulness of the *Limulus* test in the diagnosis of endotoxemia. *N. Engl. J. Med.*, **293**, 521–524.

Elin, R. J., Sandberg, A. L., and Rosentreich, D. L. (1976). Comparison of the pyrogenicity, *Limulus* activity, mitogenicity and complement reactivity of several bacterial endotoxins and related compounds. *J. Immunol.*, **117**, 1238–1242.

Evans, G. (1971). Fate of endotoxin in the circulation. *Adv. Exp. Med. Biol.*, **23**, 81–85.

Federal Register (November 4, 1977). **42**, (No. 213), 57749.

Feldberg, W. (1975). Body temperature and fever: changes in our views during the last decade. *Proc. R. Soc. London Ser. B,* **191**, 199–229.

Filkins, J. P. (1970). Bioassay of endotoxin inactivation in the lead-sensitised rat. *Proc. Soc. Exp. Biol. Med.*, **134**, 610–612.

Fletcher, J. R., and Ramwell, R. W. (1978). *E. coli* endotoxin shock in the baboon: treatment with lidocaine or indomethacin. In *Advances in Prostaglandin and Thromboxin Research*, Vol. 6 (Eds. C. Galli, G. Galli and G. Porcellati), pp.183–192. Raven Press, New York.

Fonnesu, A., and Severi, C. (1956a). Lowered P/O ratios with mitochondria isolated from livers showing cloudy swelling. *Science*, **123**, 324.

Fonnesu, A., and Severi, C. (1956b). Oxidative phosphorylation in mitochondria from livers showing cloudy swelling. *J. Biophys. Biochem. Cytol.*, **2**, 293–299.

Forni, L., and Coutinho, A. (1978a). An antiserum which recognises lipopolysaccharide reactive B cells in the mouse. *Eur. J. Immunol.*, **8**, 56–62.

Forni, L., and Coutinho, A. (1978b). Receptor interactions on the membrane of resting and activated B cells. *Nature*, **273**, 304–306.

Foulis, A. K., Murray, W. R., Galloway, D., McCartney, A. C., Lang, E., Veitch, J., and Whaley, K. (1982). Endotoxaemia and complement activation in acute pancreatitis in man. *Gut*, **23**, 656–661.

Freudenberg, M. A., Bog-Hansen, J. C., Back, U., and Galanos, C. (1980). Lipoprotein inactivation of endotoxin (lipopolysaccharides). *Infect. Immun.*, **28**, 373–380.

Fumarola, D., and Jirillo, E. (1979). Endotoxin contamination of some commercial preparations used in experimental research, In *Progress in Clinical and Biological Research*, Vol. 62, *Biomedical Applications of the Horseshoe Crab (Limulidae)* (Ed. E. Cohen), pp.379–385. Alan R. Liss, New York.

Galanos, C., and Lüderitz, O. (1975). Electrodialysis of lipopolysaccharides and their conversion to uniform salt forms. *Eur. J. Biochem.*, **54**, 603–610.

Galanos, C., and Lüderitz, O. (1976). The role of the physical state of lipopolysaccharides in the interaction with complement. *Eur. J. Biochem.*, **65**, 403–408.

Galanos, C., Lüderitz, O., and Westphal, O. (1969). A new method for the extraction of R lipopolysaccharides. *Eur. J. Biochem.*, **9**, 945–949.

Galanos, C., Rietschel, E. Th., Lüderitz, O., and Westphal, O. (1971). Interaction of lipopolysaccharides and lipid A with complement. *Eur. J. Biochem.*, **19**, 143–152.

Galanos, C., Rietschel, E. Th., Lüderitz, O., Westphal, O., Kim, B., and Watson, D. W. (1972). Biological activities of lipid A complexed with bovine serum albumin. *Eur. J. Biochem.*, **31**, 230–233.

Galanos, C. Roppel, J., Weckesser, J., Rietschel, E. Th., and Mayer, H. (1977a). Biological activities of LPS and lipid A from Rhodospirillaceae. *Infect. Immun.*, **16**, 407–412.

Galanos, C., Freudenberg, M., Hase, S., Joy, F., and Ruschmann, E. (1977b). Biological activities and immunological properties of lipid A. In *Microbiology 1977* (Ed. D. Schlessinger), pp.269–276. American Society for Microbiology, Washington DC.

Galanos, C., Lüderitz, O., and Westphal, O. (1979a). Preparation and properties of a standardized lipopolysaccharide from *Salmonella abortus equi*. *Zentralbl. Bakteriol. Hyg. Abt. I. Orig. A*, **243**, 225–244.

Galanos, C., Freudenberg, M. A., Lüderitz, O., Rietschel, E. T., and Westphal, O. (1979b). Chemical, physicochemical and biological properties of bacterial lipopolysaccharides. In *Progress in Clinical and Biological Research*, Vol. 29, *Biomedical Applications of the Horseshoe Crab (Limulidae)* (Ed. E. Cohen), pp.321–332. Alan R. Liss, New York.

Galloway, R. E., Levin, J., Butler, T., Naff, G. B., Goldsmith, G. H., Saito, H., Awoke, S., and Wallace, C. K. (1979). Activation of protein mediators of inflammation and evidence for endotoxaemia in *Borrelia recurrentis*. *Am. J. Med.*, **63**, 933–938.

Gelfand, J. A., Elin, R. J., Berry, F. W., and Frank, M. M. (1976). Endotoxaemia associated with the Jarisch-Herxheimer reaction. *N. Engl. J. Med.*, **295**, 211–213.

Gery, I., Kruger, J., and Spiesel, S. Z. (1972). Stimulation of B lymphocytes by endotoxin. Reaction of thymus deprived mice and karyotypic analysis of dividing cells in mice bearing $T_6 T_6$ thymus grafts. *J. Immunol.*, **108**, 1088–1091.

Gewurz, H., Shin, H. S., and Mergenhagen, S. E. (1968). Interactions of the complement system with endotoxic lipopolysaccharide: consumption of each of six terminal complement components. *J. Exp. Med.*, **128**, 1049–1057.

Goldman, R. C., and Leive, L. (1980). Heterogeneity of antigenic side-chain length in LPS from *E. coli* O111 and *S. typhimurium* LT2. *Eur. J. Biochem.*, **107**, 145–153.

Good, R. A., and Thomas, L. (1953). Studies on the generalised Shwartzman reactions. IV. Prevention of the local and generalised Shwartzman reaction with heparin. *J. Exp. Med.*, **97**, 871–888.

Goto, H., and Nakamura, S. (1980). Liberation of endotoxin from *Escherichia coli* by addition of antibiotics. *Jpn. Soc. Exp. Med.*, **50**, 35–43.

Griesman, S. E., and Hornick, R. B. (1967). Comparative pyrogenic reactivity of rabbit and man to bacterial endotoxin. *Proc. Soc. Exp. Biol. Med.*, **131**, 1154–1158.

Hase, S., and Rietschel, E. T. (1977). The chemical structure of the lipid A component of lipopolysaccharides from *Chromobacterium violaceum* NCTC 9694. *Eur. J. Biochem.*, **75**, 23–34.

Hawinger, J., Hawinger, A., and Timmons, S. (1975). Endotoxin-sensitive membrane component of human platelets. *Nature*, **256**, 125–127.

Hawinger, J., Hawinger, A., Steckley, S., Timmons, S., and Cheng, C. (1977). Membrane changes in human platelets induced by lipopolysaccharide endotoxin. *Br. J. Haematol.*, **35**, 285–299.

Hiller, E., Saal, J. G., Ostendorf, P., and Griffiths, G. W. (1977). The pro-coagulant activity of human granulocytes, lymphocytes and monocytes stimulation by endotoxin. *Klin. Wochenschr.*, **55**, 751–757.

Horowitz, H. I., Des Prez, R. M., and Hook, E. W. (1962a). Effects of bacterial endotoxin on rabbit platelets. II. Enhancement of platelet factor 3 activity *in vivo* and *in vitro*. *J. Exp. Med.*, **116**, 619–633.

Horowitz, H. I., Des Prez, R. M., and Hook, E.W. (1962b). Activation of platelet factor 3 by bacterial endotoxin and by immune reactions. *Blood*, **20**, 760.

Howard, J. G., Rowley, D., and Wardlaw, A. C. (1958). Investigations on the mechanisms of stimulation of non-specific immunity by bacterial lipopolysaccharides. *Immunology*, **1**, 181–203.

Inage, M., Chaki, H., Kusumoto, S., Shiba, T., Tai, A., Nakahota, M., Hanada, T., and Izumi, Y. (1980a). Chemical synthesis of bidephospholipid A of *Salmonella* endotoxin. *Chem. Lett. (Japan)*, 1373–1376.

Inage, M., Chaki, H., Kusumato, S., and Shiba, T. (1980b). Synthesis of lipopolysaccharide corresponding to fundamental structure of *Salmonella*-type lipid A. *Tetrahedron Lett.*, **21**, 3889–3892.

Iwanaga, S., Morita, T., Harada, T., Nakamura, S., Niwa, M., Takada, K., Kimura, T., and Sakakibara, S. (1978). Chromogenic substrates for horseshoe crab clotting enzyme. *Haemostasis*, **7**, 183–188.

Izui, S., Morrison, D. C., Curry, B. J., and Dixon, F. J. (1980). Effect of lipid A-associated protein on expression of lipopolysaccharide activity. I. Immunological activity. *Immunology*, **40**, 473–482.

Jann, K., and Westphal, O. (1975). Microbial polysaccharides. In *The Antigens Volume III* (Ed. M. Sela), pp.1–125. Academic Press, New York.

Jensen, S. B., Mergenhagen, S. E., Fitzgerald, R. J., and Jordan, H. V. (1963). Susceptibility of conventional and germfree mice to lethal effects of endotoxin. *Proc. Soc. Exp. Biol. Med.*, **113**, 710–714.

Johnson, K. J., and Ward, P. A. (1972). The requirement for serum complement in the detoxification of bacterial endotoxin. *J. Immunol.*, **108**, 611–616.

Johnson, K. J., Ward, P. A., Goralnick, S., and Osborn, M. J. (1977). Isolation from human serum of an inactivator of bacterial lipopolysaccharide. *Am. J. Pathol.*, **88**, 559–574.

Jorgensen, J. H., and Smith, R. F. (1973). Preparation, sensitivity and specificity of the limulus lysate for endotoxin assay. *Appl. Microbiol.*, **26**, 43–48.

Jorgensen, J., and Smith, R. (1974). Measurement of bound and free endotoxin by the *Limulus* assay. *Proc. Soc. Exp. Biol. Med.*, **146**, 1024–1031.

Kabir, S., Rosentreich, D. L., and Mergenhagen, S. E. (1978). Bacterial endotoxins and cell membranes. In *Bacterial Toxins and Cell Membranes* (Eds. J. Jeljasewicz and T. Wadstrom), pp.59–87. Academic Press, New York, London.

Kadis, S., Weinbaum, G., and Ajl, S. J. (Eds.) (1971). *Microbial Toxins*, Vol. V, *Bacterial Endotoxins*. Academic Press, New York, London.

Kaijser, B., and Olling, S. (1973). Experimental haematogenous pyelonephritis due to *Escherchia coli* in rabbits: the antibody response and its protective capacity. *J. Infect. Dis.*, **128**, 41–49.

Kasper, D. L. (1976). Chemical and biological characterization of the lipopolysaccharide of *Bacteroides fragilis* subspecies *fragilis*. *J. Infect. Dis.*, **134**, 59–66.

Kass, E. H., and Wolff, S. M. (Eds.) (1973). *Bacterial Lipopolysaccharides*. University of Chicago Press, Chicago, London.

Kiso, M., Nishiguchi, H., Murase, S., and Hasegawa, A. (1981a). A convenient synthesis of 2-deoxy-2-(D-3-hydroxytetradecanoylamino)–D-glucose; diastereoisomers of the monomeric lipid A component of the bacterial lipopolysaccharides. *Carbohydr. Res.*, **88**, C5–C9.

Kiso, M., Nishiguchi, H., Nishihari, K., and Hasegawa, A. (1981b). Synthesis of β-D-(1→6)-linked disaccharides of *N*-fatty acylated 2-amino-2-deoxy–D-glucose: an approach to the lipid A component of the bacterial lipopolysaccharide. *Carbohydr. Res.*, **88**, C10–C13.

Kiso, M. Nishiguchi, H., Hasegawa, A., Okumura, H., and Azuma, I. (1981c). Biological activities of fundamental carbohydrate skeleton of lipid A containing amide-linked 3-hydroxytetradecanoic acid. *Agric. Biol. Chem.*, **45**, 1523–1526.

Kiyono, H., McGhee, J. R., and Michalek, S. M. (1980). Lipopolysaccharide regulation of the immune response: comparison of responses to LPS in germ free *Escherichia coli* — monoassociated and conventional mice. *J. Immunol.*, **124**, 36–41.

Landy, M., and Braun, W. (Eds.) (1964). *Bacterial endotoxins*. Proceedings of a symposium held at the Institute of Microbiology of Rutgers, The State University, New Brunswick, New Jersey.

Levin, J. (1976). Blood coagulation in the horseshoe crab *(Limulus polyphemus)*: a model for mammalian coagulation and hemostasis. In *Animal Models of Thrombosis and Haemorrhagic Diseases* (Proceedings of a Symposium of the National Academy of Sciences). US Department of Health, Education and Welfare, Washington. DHEW Publication No. (NIH) 76–982, p.87.

Levin, J., and Bang, F. B. (1964). The role of endotoxin in the extracellular coagulation of *Limulus* blood. *Bull. Johns Hopkins Hosp.*, **115**, 265–274.

Levin, J., and Bang, F. B. (1968). Clottable protein in *Limulus*: Its localization and kinetics of its coagulation by endotoxin. *Thromb. Diath. Haemorrh.*, **19**, 186–197.

Levin, J., Poore, T. E., Zauber, N. P., and Oser, R. S. (1970a). Detection of endotoxin in the blood of patients with sepsis due to gram-negative bacteria. *N. Engl. J. Med.*, **283**, 1313–1316.

Levin, J., Tomasulo, P. A., and Oser, R. S. (1970b). Detection of endotoxin in human blood and demonstration of an inhibitor. *J. Lab. Clin. Med.*, **75**, 903–911.

Levin, J., Poore, T. E. Young, N. S., Margolis, S., Zauber, N. P., Townes, A. S., and Bell, W. R. (1972). Gram-negative sepsis: Detection of endotoxaemia with the *Limulus* test'. *Ann. Intern. Med.*, **76**, 1–7.

Loos, M., Bitter-Suermann, D., and Dierich, M. (1974). Interactions of the first (C1), second (C2) and fourth (C4) components of complement with different preparations of bacterial lipopolysaccharides and with lipid A. *J. Immunol.*, **112**, 935–940.

Lüderitz, O., Staub, A. M., and Westphal, O. (1966a). Immunochemistry of O and R antigens of *Salmonella* and related Enterobacteriaceae. *Bacteriol. Rev.*, **30**, 192–225.

Lüderitz, O., Galanos, C., Risse, H. J., Ruschmann, E., Schlecht, S., Schmidt, G., Schulte-Holthausen, H., Wheat, R., Westphal, O., and Schlosshardt, J. (1966b). Structural relationships of *Salmonella* O and R antigens. *Ann. N. Y. Acad. Sci.*, **133**, 349–374.

Lüderitz, O., Westphal, O., Staub, A. M., and Nikaido, H. (1971). Isolation and chemical and immunological characterisation of bacterial lipopolysaccharides. In *Microbial Toxins*, Vol. IV, *Bacterial Endotoxins* (Eds. G. Weinbaum, S. Kadis, and S. J. Ajl), pp.145–233. Academic Press, New York, London.

Lüderitz, O., Galanos, C., Lehmann, V., Mayer, H., Rietschel, E. Th., and Weckesser, J. (1978). Chemical structure and biological activities of lipid A's from various bacterial families. *Naturwissenschaften*, **65**, 578–585.

Lüderitz, O., Galanos, C., and Rietschel, E. T. (1982). Endotoxins of gram-negative bacteria. *Pharmacol. Ther.*, **15**, 383–402.

Lui, T.-Y., Seid, R. C., Jr., Tai, J. Y., Liang, S.-M., Sakmar, T. P., and Robbins, J. B. (1979). Studies on *Limulus* lysate coagulating system. In *Progress in Clinical and Biological Research*, Vol. 29, *Biomedical Applications of the Horseshoe Crab (Limulidae)* (Ed. E. Cohen), pp.147–158. Alan R. Liss, New York.

Marcus, R. L., Shin, H. S., and Mayer, M. M. (1971). An alternative complement pathway: C3-clearing activity not due to C4, 2a on endotoxic lipopolysaccharide after treatment with guinea-pig serum; relation to preparation. *Proc. Natl. Acad. Sci. USA*, **68**, 1351–1354.

Marsh, D. G., and Crutchley, M. J. (1967). Purification and physicochemical analysis of fractions from the culture supernatant of *Escherichia coli* O78K80: Free endotoxin and a non-toxic fraction. *J. Gen. Microbiol.*, **47**, 405–420.

Martini, E. (1959). Increase of the cathepsin activity of the liver and of the skeletal muscle of rats either treated with 2,4-dinitrophenol or with bacterial lipopolysaccharide. *Experientia*, **15**, 182–183.

McAdam, K. P. W. J., and Ryan, J. L. (1978). C57B1/10/Cr mice: nonresponders to activation by the lipid A moiety of bacterial lipopolysaccharide. *J. Immunol.*, **120**, 249–252.

McCabe, W. R. (1963). Endotoxin tolerance II. Its occurence in patients with pyelonephritis. *J. Clin. Invest.*, **42**, 618–625.

McCabe, W. R., Kreger, B. E., and Johns, M. (1972). Type specific and cross-reactive antibodies in Gram-negative bacteremia. *N. Engl. J. Med.*, **287**, 261–267.

McCabe, W. R., Johns, M. A., Craven, D. E., and Bruins, S. C. (1977). Clinical implications of enterobacterial antigens. In *Microbiology 1977* (Ed. D. Schlessinger), pp.293–297. American Society for Microbiology, Washington, DC.

McCartney, A. C., Banks, J. G., Clements, G. B., Sleigh, J. D., Tehrani, M., and Ledingham, I. McA. (1983). Endotoxaemia in septic shock: clinical and post mortem correlations. *Int. Care Med.*, **9**, 117–122.

McCuskey, R. S., Urbaschek, R., McCuskey, P. A., and Urbaschek, B. (1982). *In vivo* microscopic studies of the responses of the liver to endotoxin. *Klin. Wochenschr.*, **60**, 749–751

McGivney, A., and Bradley, S. G. (1977). Enhanced lysosomal enzyme activity in mouse cells treated with bacterial endotoxin *in vitro*. *Proc. Soc. Exp. Biol. Med.*, **155**, 390–394.

McGivney, A., and Bradley, S. G. (1978). Effects of bacterial endotoxin on lysosomal enzyme activities of human cells in continuous culture. *J. Reticuloendothel. Soc.*, **23**, 223–230.

McGivney, A., and Bradley, S. G. (1979). Effects of bacterial endotoxin on lysosomal and mitochondrial enzyme activities of established cell cultures. *J. Reticuloendothel. Soc.*, **26**, 307–316.

McGivney, A., and Bradley, S. G. (1980a). Action of bacterial lipopolysaccharide on the respiration of mouse liver mitochondria. *Infect. Immun.*, **27**, 102–106.

McGivney, A., and Bradley, S. G. (1980b). Susceptibility of mitochondria from endotoxin-resistant mice to lipopolysaccharide. *Proc. Soc. Exp. Biol. Med.*, **163**, 56–59.

Mechanic, R. C., Frei, E., III, Landy, M., and Smith, W. W. (1961). Quantitative studies of human leucocytic and febrile response to single and repeated doses of purified bacterial endotoxin. *J. Clin. Invest.*, **41**, 162–172.

Mela, L. (1981). Direct and indirect effects of endotoxin on mitochondrial function. In *Progress in Clinical and Biological Research,* Vol. 62, *Pathophysiological Effects of Endotoxins at the Cellular Level* (Eds. J. A. Majde and R. J. Person), pp.15–22. Alan R. Liss, New York.

Melchers, F. (1980). Interactions of bacteria with the immune system. In *Life Science Research Report: The Molecular Basis of Microbiol Pathogenicity* (Eds. H. Smith, J. J. Skehel and M. J. Turner), pp.285–306. Springer Verlag, Basel.

Mills, D. F. (1978). *Pyrogent (Limulus Amoebocyte Lysate) for Detection of Endotoxins*. Mallinckrodt Inc., St. Louis, MO.

Möller, G., and Michael, G. (1971). Frequency of antigen-sensitive cells to thymus-independent antigens. *Cell. Immunol.*, **2**, 309–316.

Möller, G., Anderssen, J., and Sjöberg, O. (1972a). Lipopolysaccharides can convert heterologous red cells into thymus-independent antigens. *Cell. Immunol.*, **4**, 416–424.

Möller, G., Sjöberg, O., and Anderssen, J. (1972b). Mitogen-induced lymphocyte-mediated cytotoxicity *in vitro*: effect of mitogens selectively activating T or B cells. *Eur. J. Immunol.*, **2**, 586–592.

Mørland, B. (1979). Studies on selective induction of lysosomal enzyme activities in mouse peritoneal macrophages. *J. Reticuloendothel. Soc.*, **26**, 749–762.

Morrison, D. C., and Cochrane, C. G. (1974). Direct evidence for Hageman factor (factor XII) activation by bacterial lipopolysaccharides (endotoxins). *J. Exp. Med.*, **140**, 797–811.

Morrison, D. C., and Kline, L. F. (1977). Activation of the classical and properdin pathways of complement by bacterial lipopolysaccharide (LPS). *J. Immunol.*, **118**, 362–368.

Morrison, D. C., and Oades, Z. G. (1979). Mechanisms of lipopolysaccharide-initiated rabbit platelet responses. II. Evidence that lipid A is responsible for binding of lipopolysaccharide to the platelet. *J. Immunol.*, **122**, 753–758.

Morrison, D. C., and Rudbach, J. A. (1980). Endotoxin–cell membrane interactions leading to transmembrane signals. *Contemp. Top. Mol. Immunol.*, **8**, 187–218.

Morrison, D. C., and Ryan, J. L. (1979). A review–bacterial endotoxins and host immune function. *Adv. Immunol.*, **28**, 293–450.

Morrison, D. C., and Ulevitch, R. J. (1978). The effects of bacterial endotoxins on host mediation systems. *Am. J. Pathol.*, **93**, 527–618.

Morrison, D. C., Kline, L. F., Oades, Z. G., and Henson, P. M. (1978). Mechanisms of lipopolysaccharide-initiated rabbit platelet responses. I. Alternative complement pathway dependence of the lytic response. *Infect. Immun.*, **20**, 744–751.

Morrison, D. C., Wilson, M. E., Raziguddin, S., Betz, S. J., Curry, B. J., Oades, Z. G., and Munkenbeck, P. (1980). The influence of lipid A-associated protein of endotoxin stimulation of non-lymphoid cells. In *Microbiology 1980* (Ed. D. Schlessinger), pp.30–35, American Society for Microbiology, Washington, DC.

Morrison, D. C., Oades, Z. G., and Di Pietro, D. (1981). Endotoxin-initiated membrane changes in rabbit platelets. In *Progress in Clinical and Biological Research*, Vol. 62, *Pathophysiological Effects of Endotoxins at the Cellular Level* (Eds. J. A. Majde and R. J. Person), pp.47–64. Alan R. Liss, New York.

Mosesson, M. W., Wolfenstein-Todel, C., Levin, J., and Bertrand, O. (1979). Structural studies of the coagulogen of amebocyte lysate from *Limulus polyphemus*. In *Progress in Clinical and Biological Research*, Vol. 29, *Biomedical Applications of the Horseshoe Crab (Limulidae)* (Ed. E. Cohen), pp.159–168. Alan R. Liss, New York.

Mühlradt, P. F., Wary, V., and Lehmann, V. (1977). A ^{31}p-nuclear magnetic resonance study of the phosphate groups in lipopolysaccharide and lipid A from *Salmonella*. *Eur. J. Biochem.*, **81**, 193–203.

Nachum, R., Lipsey, A., and Siegel, S. E. (1973). Rapid detection of gram-negative bacterial meningitis by the *Limulus* lysate test. *N. Engl. J. Med.*, **289**, 931–934.

Nagayama, M., Zucker, M. B., and Beller, F. K. (1971). Effects of a variety of endotoxins on human and rabbit platelet function. *Thromb. Diath. Haemorrh.*, **26**, 467–473.

Niemetz, T., and Morrison, D. C. (1977). Lipid A as the biologically active moiety in bacterial endotoxin (LPS)-initiated generation of procoagulant activity by peripheral blood leucocytes. *Blood*, **49**, 947–956.

Niwa, M., Hiramatsu, T., and Waguri, O. (1975). Quantitative aspects of the gelation reaction of horseshoe crab amoebocyte and bacterial endotoxin. *Jpn. J. Med. Sci. Biol.*, **28**, 98–100.

Nowotny, A. (1969). Molecular aspects of endotoxic reaction. *Bacteriol. Rev.*, **33**, 72–98.

Nowotny, A. (1983). *Beneficial Effects of Endotoxins*. Plenum Ress, New York.

Nowotny, A., Behling, U. H., and Chang, H. L. (1975). Relation of structure to function in bacterial endotoxins. VIII. Biological activities in a polysaccharide-rich fraction. *J. Immunol.*, **115**, 199–203.

Noyes, H. E., McInturf, C. R., and Blahuta, G. J. (1959). Studies on the distribution of *Escherichia coli* endotoxin in mice. *Proc. Soc. Exp. Biol. Med.*, **100**, 65–68.

Ortiz-Ortiz, L., and Jaroslow, B. N. (1970). Enhancement by the adjuvant, endotoxin, of an immune response induced *in vitro*. *Immunology*, **19**, 387–399.

Palva, E. T., and Mäkelä, P. H. (1980). Lipopolysaccharide heterogeneity in *Salmonella typhimurium* analysed by sodium dodecylsulfate–polyacrylamide gel electrophoresis. *Eur. J. Biochem.*, **107**, 137–143.

Parratt, J. R., and Sturgess, R. M. (1977). The possible roles of histamine, 5-hydroxytryptamine and prostaglandin F_2 as mediators of the acute pulmonary effects of endotoxin. *Br. J. Pharmacol.*, **60**, 209–219.

Peavy, D. L., Adler, W. H., Shands, J. W., and Smith, R. T. (1974). Selective effects of mitogens on subpopulations of mouse lymphoid cells. *Cell. Immunol.*, **11**, 86–98.

Pieroni, R. E., Broderick, E. J., Bundeally, A., and Levine, L. (1970). A simple method for the quantitation of submicrogram amounts of bacterial endotoxin. *Proc. Soc. Exp. Biol. Med.*, **133**, 790–792.

Prashker, D., and Wardlaw, A. C. (1971). Temperature responses of mice to *Escherichia coli* endotoxin. *Br. J. Exp. Pathol.*, **52**, 36–46.

Rašková, H., and Vaněček, J. (1964). Pharmacology of bacterial toxins. *Pharmacol. Rev.*, **16**, 1–45.

Reinhold, R. B., and Fine, J. (1971). A technique for quantitative measurement of endotoxin in human plasma. *Proc. Soc. Exp. Biol. Med.*, **137**, 334–340.

Revak, S. D., Cochrane, C. G., and Griffin, J. H. (1977). Initiation of coagulation by contact activation of Hageman factor. In *Kidney Disease: Hematologic and Vascular Problems* (Eds. R. M. McIntosh, S. J. Guggenheim and L. W. Schrier), pp.29–40. John Wiley, New York.

Rickles, F. R., and Rick, P. D. (1977). Structural features of *Salmonella typhimurium* lipopolysaccharides required for activation of tissue factor in human mononuclear cells. *J. Clin. Invest.*, **59**, 1188–1195.

Rietschel, E. Th., Galanos, C., Tanaka, A., Ruschmann, E., Lüderitz, O., and Westphal, O. (1971). Biological activities of chemically modified endotoxins. *Eur. J. Biochem.*, **22**, 218–224.

Rietschel, E. Th., Hase, S., King, M. T., Redmond, J., and Lehmann, V. (1977). Chemical structure of lipid A. In *Microbiology 1977* (Ed. D. Schlessinger), pp.262–268. American Society for Microbiology, Washington, DC.

Rietschel, E. Th., Schade, U., Lüderitz, O., Fischer, H., and Peskar, B. A. (1980). Prostaglandins in endotoxicosis. In *Microbiology 1980* (Ed. D. Schlessinger), pp.66–72. American Society for Microbiology, Washington, DC.

Rietschel, E. Th., Galanos, C., Lüderitz, O., and Westphal, O. (1982a). Chemical structure, physiological function and biological activity of lipid A, the lipid component of lipopolysaccharides. In *Immuno-pharmacology and the Regulation of Leukocyte Function* (Ed. D. R. Webb), pp.183–229. Marcel Dekker, New York, Basel.

Rietschel, E. Th., Schade, U., Jensen, M., Wolleweber, H.-W., Lüderitz, O., and Greisman, S. G. (1982b). Bacterial endotoxins: chemical structure, biological activity and role in septicaemia. *Scand. J. Infect. Dis. Suppl.*, **31**, 8–21.

Rivers, R. P. A., Hathaway, W. E., and Weston, W. L. (1975). The endotoxic induced coagulant activity of human monocytes. *Br. J. Haematol.*, **30**, 311–316.

Rojas-Corona, R. R., Skarnes, R., Tamakuma, S., and Fine, J. (1969). The *Limulus* coagulation test for endotoxin. A comparison with other assay methods. *Proc. Soc. Exp. Biol. Med.*, **132**, 599–601.

Rosenstreich, D. L., Glode, M., Wahl, L. M., Sandberg, A. L., and Mergenhagen, S. E. (1977). Analysis of the cellular defects of endotoxin unresponsive C3H/HeJ mice.

Microbiology 1977 (Ed. D. Schlessinger), pp.314–320. American Society for Microbiology, Washington, DC.

Rosner, M. R., Tang, J. Y., Barzilay, I., and Khorana, H. G. (1979). Structure of the lipopolysaccharide from *Escherichia coli* heptoseless mutant. I. Chemical degradations and identification of products. *J. Biol. Chem.*, **254**, 5906–5917.

Ross, S., Rodriguez, W., Contrini, G., Korengold, G., Watson, S., and Khan, W. (1975). *Limulus* lysate test for gram-negative bacterial meningitis. *J. Am. Med. Assoc.*, **233**, 1366–1369.

Rutenberg, A., Schweinburg, F. B., and Fine, J. (1960). *In vitro* detoxification of bacterial endotoxin by macrophages. *J. Exp. Med.*, **112**, 801–807.

Sandford, J. P., Hunter, B. W., and Souda, L. L. (1962). The role of immunity in the pathogenesis of experimental haemotogenous pyelonephritis. *J. Exp. Med.*, **115**, 383–410.

Schaedler, R. W., and Dubos, R. J. (1961). The susceptibility of mice to bacterial endotoxins. *J. Exp. Med.*, **113**, 559–570.

Schlessinger, D. (Ed.) (1980). Microbiology 1980, Part I: *Endogenous Mediators in Host Response*, pp.219–226. American Society for Microbiology, Washington, DC.

Scully, M. F., Newman, Y. M., Clark, S. E., and Kakkar, V. V. (1980). Evaluation of a chromogenic method for endotoxin measurement. *Thromb. Res.*, **20**, 263–270.

Selye, H., Tuchweber, B., and Bertók, L. (1966). Effect of lead acetate on the susceptibility of rats to bacterial endotoxins. *J. Bacteriol.*, **91**, 884–886.

Shwartzman, G. (1937). *The Phenomenon of Local Tissue Reactivity*. Hoeber, New York.

Siebert, F. B. (1923). Fever producing substance in some distilled waters. *Am. J. Physiol.*, **67**, 90.

Siebert, F. B. (1925). The cause of many febrile reactions following intravenous injections. *Am. J. Physiol.*, **71**, 621–651.

Siebert, F. B. (1952). Introduction to the symposium on bacterial pyrogens. *Trans. N.Y. Acad. Sci.*, **14**, 157–159.

Siebert, F. B., and Mandel, L. B. (1923). Protein fevers with special reference to casein. *Am. J. Physiol.*, **67**, 105–123.

Siegel, S. E., and Nachum, R. (1979). Indications for the use of the *Limulus* lysate assay in bacterial meningitis. In *Progress in Clinical and Biological Research*, Vol. 29, *Biomedical Application of the Horseshoe Crab (Limulidae)* (Ed. E. Cohen), pp.245–253. Alan R. Liss, New York.

Sim, A. J. W., and McCartney, A. C. (1980). The appearance of endotoxin following urethral instrumentation. *Br. J. Surg.*, **67**, 443–445.

Siraganian, R. P. (1972). Platelet requirement in the interaction of the complement and clotting systems. *Nature*, **239**, 208–210.

Skarnes, R. C. (1970). Host defense against bacterial endotoxaemia mechanism in normal animals. *J. Exp. Med.*, **132**, 300–316.

Skarnes, R. C., and Harper, M. J. K. (1972). Relationship between endotoxin-induced abortion and the synthesis of prostaglandin F. *Prostaglandins*, **1**, 191–203.

Skarnes, R. C., and Rosen, F. S. (1971). Host-dependent detoxification of bacterial endotoxin. In *Microbial Toxins*, Vol. V, *Bacterial Endotoxins* (Eds. S. Kadis, G. Weinbaum, and S. J. Ajl), pp.151–164. Academic Press, London, New York.

Smith, H. (1975). Gram-negative bacteria: the determinants of pathogenicity. In *Gram-negative Bacterial Infections and Mode of Endotoxin Actions* (Eds. B. Urbaschek, R. Urbaschek and E. Neter), pp.8–15. Springer-Verlag, Vienna, New York.

Smith, R. T., and Thomas, L. (1954). Influence of age upon response to meningococcal endotoxin in rabbits. *Proc. Soc. Exp. Biol. Med.*, **86**, 806–809.

Smith, R. T., and Thomas, L. (1956). The lethal effect of endotoxins on the chick embryo. *J. Exp. Med.*, **104**, 217–231.

Synderman, R., Gewurz, H., and Mergenhagen, S. E. (1968). Interactions of the complement system with endotoxic lipopolysaccharide. Generation of factor chemotactic for polymorphonuclear leucocytes. *J. Exp. Med.*, **128**, 259–275.

Snyderman, R., Shin, H. S., Phillips, J. K., Gewurz, H., and Mergenhagen, S. E. (1969). A neutrophil chemotactic factor from C'5 upon interaction of guinea pig serum with endotoxin. *J. Immunol.*, **103**, 413–422.

Stetson, C. A., Jr. (1951). Studies on the mechanism of the Shwartzman phenomenon. Certain factors involved in the production of the local hemorrhagic necrosis. *J. Exp. Med.*, **93**, 489–504.

Strittmatter, W., Weckesser, J., Solimath, P. V., and Galanos, C. (1983). Nontoxic lipopolysaccharides from *Rhodopseudomonas sphaeroides* ATCC 17023. *J. Bacteriol.*, **155**, 153–158.

Stumacher, R. J., Kovnat, M. J., and McCabe, W. R. (1973). Limitations of the usefulness of the *Limulus* assay for endotoxin. *N. Engl. J. Med.*, **288**, 1261–1264.

Sultzer, B. M. (1968). Genetic control of leucocyte responses to endotoxin. *Nature*, **219**, 1253–1254.

Sultzer, B. M. (1971). Chemical modification of endotoxin and inactivation of its biological properties. In *Microbiol Toxins*, Vol. V, *Bacterial Endotoxins* (Eds. S. Kadis, G. Weinbaum and S. J. Ajl), pp.91–126. Academic Press, New York, London.

Tai, J. Y., and Lui, T.-Y. (1977). Studies on *Limulus* amoebocyte lysate. Isolation of pro-clotting enzyme. *J. Biol. Chem.*, **252**, 2178–2181.

Takagi, T., Hokama, Y., Morita, T., Iwanaga, S., Nakamura, S., and Niwa, M. (1979). Amino acid sequence studies on horseshoe crab *(Tachypleus tridentatus)* coagulogen and mechanism of gel formation. In *Progress in Clinical and Biological Research*, Vol. 29, *Biomedical Applications of the Horseshoe Crab (Limulidae)* (Ed. E. Cohen), pp.169–184. Alan R. Liss, New York.

Taylor, P. W. (1983). Bactericidal and bacteriolytic activity of serum against Gram-negative bacteria. *Microbiol. Rev.*, **47**, 46–83.

Thomas, L. (1974). *The Lives of a Cell: Notes of a Biology Watcher*, p.78. Viking Press, New York.

Tomasulo, P. A., Levin, J., Murphy, P. A., and Winkelstein, J. A. (1977). Biological activities of tritiated endotoxins: correlation of the *Limulus* lysate assay with rabbit pyrogen and complement-activation assays for endotoxin. *J. Lab. Clin. Med.*, **89**, 308–315.

Unanue, E. R. (1976). Secretory function of mononuclear phagocytes: A review. *Am. J. Pathol.*, **83**, 396–417.

Vane, J. R. (1971). Inhibition of prostaglandin synthesis as a mechanism of action for aspirin-like drugs. *Nature*, **231**, 232–235.

van Miert, A. S. J. P. A. M., and Frens, J. (1968). The reaction of different animal species to bacterial pyrogens. *Zentralbl. Veterinaermed. Reihe A*, **15**, 532–543.

Walker, R. I., and Fletcher, J. R. (1981). Possible contribution of platelets to the pathophysiology of host responses to endotoxin. In *Progress in Clinical and Biological Research*, Vol. 62, *Pathophysiological Effects of Endotoxin at the Cellular Level* (Eds. J. A. Majde and R. J. Person), pp.173–185. Alan R. Liss, New York.

Watson, J., and Riblet, R. (1974). Genetic control of responses to bacterial lipopolysaccharides in mice. I. Evidence for a single gene that influences mitogenic and immunologic responses to lipopolysaccharides. *J. Exp. Med.*, **140**, 1147–1161.

Watson, J., Kelly, K., Largen, M., and Taylor, B. A. (1978). The genetic mapping of a defective LPS response gene in C3H/HeJ mice. *J. Immunol.*, **120**, 422–424.

Watson, J., Kelly, K., and Whitlock, C. (1980). Genetic control of endotoxin sensitivity. In *Microbiology 1980* (Ed. D. Schlessinger), pp.4–10. American Society for Microbiology, Washington, DC.

Watson, S. W., Novitsky, T. J., Quinby, H. L., and Valois, F. W. (1977). Determination of bacterial number and biomass in the marine environment. *Appl. Environ. Microbiol.*, **33**, 940–946.

Weckesser, J., and Drews, G. (1979). Lipopolysaccharides of photosynthetic prokaryotes. *Annu. Rev. Microbiol.*, **33**, 215–239.

Weinbaum, G., Kadis, S., and Ajl, S. J. (Eds.) (1971). *Microbial Toxins*, Vol. IV, *Bacterial Endotoxins*. Academic Press, New York, London.

Westphal, O. (1975). Bacterial endotoxins. *Int. Arch. Allergy Appl. Immunol.*, **49**, 1–43.

Westphal, O., Lüderitz, O., and Bister, F. (1952). Uber die Extraktion von Bakterien mit Phenol-Wasser. *Z. Naturforsch.*, **76**, 148–155.

Wildfeuer, A., Heymer, B., Schleifer, K. H., and Haferkamp, O. (1974). Investigations on the specificity of the *Limulus* test for the detection of endotoxin. *Appl. Microbiol.*, **28**, 867–871.

Wilkinson, S. G. (1977). Composition and structure of bacterial lipopolysaccharide. In *Surface Carbohydrates of the Prokaryotic Cell* (Ed. I. Sutherland), pp.97–175. Academic Press, London, New York, San Francisco.

Wilkinson, S. G., and Taylor, D. P. (1978). Occurrence of 2,3-diamino-2,3-dideoxy-D-glucose in lipid A from lipopolysaccharide of *Pseudomonas diminuta*. *J. Gen. Microbiol.*, **109**, 367–370.

Wilson, M. E., Munkenbeck, P., and Morrison, D. C. (1981). Influence of bacterial endotoxins on neutrophilic leukocytes: lack of a correlation between *in vivo* and *in vitro* responses. In *Progress in Clinical and Biological Research*, Vol. 62, *Pathophysiological Effects of Endotoxins at the Cellular Level* (Eds. J. A. Majde and R. J. Person), pp.157–172. Alan R. Liss, New York.

Wolfe, R. R., Elahi, D., and Spitzer, J. J. (1977). Glucose and lactate kinetics after endotoxin administration in dogs. *Am. J. Physiol.*, **232**, E180–E185.

Wolff, S. M., Rubenstein, M., Mulholland, J. H., and Alling, D. W. (1965). Comparison of hematologic and febrile response to endotoxin in man. *Blood*, **26**, 190–201.

Wollenweber, N.-W., Rietchel, E. Th., Hofstad, T., Weintraub, A., and Lindberg, A. A. (1980). Nature, type of linkage, quantity and absolute configuration of (3-hydroxy) fatty acids in lipopolysaccharides from *Bacteroides fragilis* NCTC 9343 and related strains. *J. Bacteriol.* **144**, 898–903.

Young, L. S. (1975). Opsonising antibodies, host factors and the *Limulus* assay for endotoxin. *Infect. Immun.*, **12**, 88–92.

Young, N. S., Levin, J., and Prendergast, R. A. (1972). An invertebrate coagulation system activated by endotoxin: evidence for enzymatic mediation. *J. Clin. Invest.*, **51**, 1790–1797.

Ziegler, E. J., McCutchan, J. A., Fierer, J., Glauser, M. P., Sadoff, J. C., Douglas, H., and Braude, A. I. (1982). Treatment of gram-negative bacteraemia and shock with human antiserum to a mutant *Escherichia coli*. *N. Engl. J. Med.*, **307**, 1225–1230.

Zinner, S. H., and McCabe, W. R. (1976). Effects of IgM and IgG antibody in patients with bacteraemia due to Gram-negative bacilli. *J. Infect. Dis.*, **133**, 39–45.

Immunology of the Bacterial Cell Envelope
Edited by D. E. S. Stewart-Tull and M. Davies
© 1985 John Wiley & Sons Ltd.

CHAPTER 9

The Affinity of Bacterial Polysaccharides for Mammalian Cell Membranes and its role in Immunoadjuvant Responses

Martin Davies* and Duncan E. S. Stewart-Tull[†]
*Reproductive Immunology Research Group, Department of Pathology,
The Medical School, University of Bristol, Bristol BS8 1TD, and
[†]Department of Microbiology, University of Glasgow,
Alexander Stone Building, Garscube Estate, Bearsden, Glasgow G61 1QH, UK

I. INTRODUCTION

Since 1899, there have been numerous reports of the adherence of bacteria or their products to mammalian cells (Madsen, 1899; Ginsberg *et al.*, 1948; Keogh *et al.*, 1948; Middlebrook and Dubos, 1948; Boyden, 1951; Neter, 1956). This phenomenon, termed modification, has involved primarily bacterial antigens

Table 1   Mammalian Cell Modification by Bacterial Antigens

Modifying agent	Cell type or cellular component
Tuberculin polysaccharide	Leucocytes, lymphocytes (Boyden, 1953)
Salmonella antigen	Spleen, liver and kidney cells, leucocytes (De Gregorio, 1955)
LPS from *E. coli*	Rabbit polymorphonuclear (Gimber and Rafter, 1969)
S. minnesota R-form glycolipid	Rat embryo fibroblasts (Bara *et al.*, 1973)
S. typhimurium	Rat heart and liver mitochondria (Greer *et al.*, 1973)
E. coli (whole cells)	Rabbit alveolar macrophages (Ulrich and Meier, 1973)
LPS from *E. coli, S. typhi, Shigella flexneri, Bordetella pertussis, Franciscella tularensis*	Rabbit, human, mouse erythrocytes, human white blood cells, mouse peritoneal macrophages and lymphocytes (Davies *et al.*, 1978)
Mycobacterial glycopeptides	Mouse, rabbit, sheep, horse and human erythrocytes (Stewart-Tull *et al.*, 1978)

that are polysaccharides or possess polysaccharide determinants and although the majority of studies involved erythrocyte modification by lipopolysaccharide (LPS), the phenomenon is generalized and includes a wide range of bacterial antigens and mammalian cells. Other reports were concerned with antigens from mycobacteria (Middlebrook and Dubos, 1948; Boyden and Grabar, 1954; Stewart-Tull *et al.*, 1978), rickettsiae (Chang, 1953), *Candida* (Vogel and Collins, 1955), trypanosomes (Munoz, 1950), schistosomes (Kagan, 1955), *Histoplasma* (Norden, 1949) and *Trichomonas* (McEntegart, 1952). Besides erythrocytes, modification has been reported for various other cell types including macrophages, lymphocytes, spleen cells, thymocytes, bone marrow cells and fibroblasts (De Gregorio, 1955; Gimber and Rafter, 1969; Davies *et al.*, 1978) (Table 1). Initially, this process of cell modification was thought to be a laboratory-manifested phenomenon until the demonstration by Skillman *et al.* (1955) that the *in vivo* modification of erythrocytes by streptococcal antigens occurred in patients with acute rheumatic fever. Further, in 1955 Robineaux and Nelson suggested that, in the presence of specific antibody and complement, whole bacteria attached to red cells prior to their engulfment by polymorphs. Since then, numerous studies have attempted to show that *in vitro* cellular modification has an *in vivo* basis and a biological significance.

    The bacterial components involved in the modification process were often amphipathic molecules, characterized by the possession of hydrophobic and hydrophilic moieties in their structures. Shockman and Wicken (1981) recognized the complexity of the interactions between these amphiphiles and bacterial and mammalian cells and concluded that to understand the mechanisms better, greater cooperation with biologists on the one hand and with chemists and

Table 2   Comparison of the binding and immunoadjuvant properties of gram-negative bacterial LPS and mycobacterial amphiphiles

Biological property	Amphiphiles	
	Lipopolysaccharide	Mycobacterial glycopeptide
Cell modification		
(a) new serological specificity	+	+
(b) temperature dependent	+	+
(c) dependent on incubation time	+	+
(d) dependent on composition of polysaccharide	+	+
(e) dependent on cell type	+	+
(f) effect of normal serum	Inhibits	Inhibits
(g) effect of lecithin and cholesterol	Inhibits	Inhibits
Mitogenic lymphocyte stimulation	+ + +	−
Pyrogenicity	+ + +	−
Toxicity	+ + +	−
Immunogenicity and hyper-sensitivity	+	+
Immunopotentiation	+ + +	+ + +
Macrophage stimulation	+ + +	+ + +
Effect of alkali on		
(i) modification	Increases	Increases
(ii) immunopotentiation	Decreases	Decreases
Effect of periodate on		
(i) modification	Decreases	Decreases
(ii) immunopotentiation	Decreases	Decreases

physicists on the other was needed. The chemical composition and biological properties of a variety of amphiphiles have been reviewed by Wicken and Knox (1980, 1981). The reader will recognize the importance of intermolecular interaction (ionic binding, hydrogen bonding or hydrophobic interaction) between amphiphiles and mammalian cells as the underlying theme behind various chapters in this volume. For instance, lipopolysaccharide (LPS) and lipoteichoic acid are established amphiphiles.

A membrane interaction event is a critical step in the initiation of effective immune responses, especially in the antigen handling process prior to the induction of an immune response. Macrophages were found to trap antigen in lymphoid tissue (Unanue, 1972), and Katz and Unanue (1973) showed that the binding of antigen to macrophages increased its immunogenicity when compared to the immune response against soluble antigen *in vitro*. In addition,

Vitetta and Uhr (1975a,b) provided evidence that IgM, IgG and IgD immuno-globulins acted as antigen-binding receptors on B-lymphocytes. There is also evidence for a receptor on T-lymphocytes; Cone and Marchalonis (1974) suggested that this was monomeric IgM, although other workers doubted the idea of a receptor (Vitetta *et al.*, 1972; Gery *et al.*, 1972; Hudson *et al.*, 1974.

Our own interest in this area stems from a search to discover the mode of action of some microbial immunopotentiating agents. It seemed likely that at the molecular level the initial event would involve an interaction between the amphiphilic adjuvant and the mammalian cell surface. Consequently, this chapter examines the role of two cellular amphiphiles, LPS and myco-bacterial peptidoglycolipid, and the extracellular amphiphile, mycobacterial glycopeptide, in cellular modification and in immunoadjuvant responses (Table 2).

II. CELLULAR MODIFICATION BY LIPOPOLYSACCHARIDE

A. General Considerations

The LPS of gram-negative bacteria is a complex in the outer or L-membrane of the organism (see Chapter 8, Figure 2). After extraction and purification, morphologically LPS resembles classic lipid bilayer membrane fragments of varying shape, including discs, lamellae, ribbons and vesicles (Burge and Draper, 1967; Beer *et al.*, 1966; Work *et al.*, 1966; Shands *et al.*, 1967). These LPS fragments were visualized in aqueous solutions as a bilayer, each half covalently linked with its non-polar hydrophobic lipid buried inside the structure and the polysaccharide moiety exposed to the environment (Shands, 1973). Also, dependent on the method of extraction, the LPS fragments may be associated with a mixture of cations as they occur in the bacterial cell, including alkali, alkaline earths and heavy metal ions (Lüderitz *et al.*, 1974). These LPS membranous structures possessed a natural affinity for mammalian cell membranes, especially if they were 'activated' by heat or alkali treatment (Lüderitz *et al.*, 1958; Ciznar and Shands, 1971). The majority of studies examined the association between the LPS membranous fragments and the erythrocyte membrane, although this affinity was not confined to erythrocytes (Table 1), and it was observed that the degree of modification was a function of both the mammalian cell membrane and the LPS molecule (Corvazier, 1952; Alexander *et al.*, 1950; Davies *et al.*, 1978; Stewart-Tull *et al.*, 1978). For example, LPS from *Escherichia coli* equally modified erythrocytes from human beings, dogs, rabbits, sheep, goats and rats (Corvazier, 1952) while LPS from *Franciscella tularensis* was a more effective modifier of human erythrocytes from group O individuals than those from Group A or B individuals (Alexander *et al.*, 1950).

B. Conditions for Cellular Modification

The conditions required for the optimum binding of LPS to mammalian cells are difficult to define precisely due to numerous contradictory reports in the literature. This may be due to different growth conditions of the bacteria and LPS extraction procedures. However, the degree of cell modification is also dependent on various factors including the amount of LPS available, cell concentration, electrolyte balance, pH, temperature and time.

Davies *et al.* (1978) showed that the quantity of *E. coli* LPS adsorbed by erythrocytes was dependent on the amount of LPS present, up to a saturation limit. Hence, the maximum amount of LPS that could be adsorbed by a single cell was 13.7 pg for rabbit erythrocytes and 16.12 pg for human erythrocytes. Further, the degree of LPS binding as a function of erythrocyte concentration produced a sigmoid curve which showed that only 34% of LPS molecules extracted by the phenol–water method had the potential for modifying rabbit erythrocytes. This figure agreed with the finding of Lüderitz *et al.* (1958), who demonstrated that even after alkali-activation, only 30% of LPS molecules exhibited a strong affinity for membranes with the remainder possessing slight affinity even after repeated adsorptions with fresh erythrocytes.

Table 3   Human erythrocyte modification by LPS from *E. coli* NCTC 8623: inhibition by monosaccharides

Monosaccharide (72 μg added to mixture)	Percentage inhibition of LPS uptake*
Fucose	91.0
Glucose	89.4
Arabinose	89.0
Rhamnose	86.6
Mannose	79.3
Glucosamine	64.1
Galactose	60.0

First incubation (37°C, 30 min)	Second incubation (37°C, 30 min)	Percentage inhibition of LPS uptake* Amount of glucose added (μg)		
		0	36	72
LPS + HRBC	+ glucose	0	47	66
LPS + glucose	+ HRBC	0	70	90
Glucose + HRBC	+ LPS	0	10	42
LPS + HRBC + glucose (37°C, 60 min)		0	9	17

*The uptake was measured in a reaction mixture that consisted of human erythocytes and LPS. The monosaccharide was added and the mixture incubated at 37°C for 60 min.
HRBC = human erythrocytes.

Electrolytes were also necessary for binding, since LPS from both *E. coli* and *Salmonella abortus equi* failed to modify erythrocytes in 5% glucose or sodium citrate or calcium chloride (Neter and Zalewski, 1953). However, it has been shown (Davies, 1974) that a wide range of monosaccharides are capable of inhibiting the binding of *E. coli* LPS to erythrocytes in the presence of physiological saline (Table 3). Apparently, in the case of glucose, cellular modification was partially inhibited by the glucose binding directly to the LPS, so preventing an LPS–membrane interaction. Further, LPS in phosphate buffer, pH 7.3, was far more active than LPS in normal saline, pH 6.3 (Neter and Zalewski, 1953). This effect seemed to be a reflection of the change in pH since it was also noticed that heat activation of LPS was more effective if performed in phosphate buffer at pH 7.3 than in phosphate buffer at pH 4.9 (Neter *et al.*, 1956b).

Modification of erythrocytes was also temperature dependent, occurring rapidly at 37°C and slowly at 4°C (Neter, 1956). Davies (1974) noted that maximum uptake of LPS occurred at 22°C, which is interesting in view of the observation of Ciznar and Shands (1971) that the subsequent spontaneous lysis of erythrocytes, modified at 37°C, was temperature dependent with an optimum at 22°C. However, Gimber and Rafter (1969) demonstrated that the uptake of *E. coli* LPS by polymorphonuclear leucocytes was both temperature and pH independent over the range 5.8–8.0.

Observations were made on the time course for binding and it was apparent that LPS uptake by cells was a function of time during 1–15 min, up to a maximum which was, in effect, dictated by LPS and cell concentrations. However, if LPS binding studies were extended to cover a period of several hours, cyclic variations between bound and unbound LPS were observed (Davies *et al.*, 1978) (Figure 1). The cyclic variations occurred with a wide range of cells including erythrocytes, lymphocytes and macrophages. Cyclic variations have also been reported by other workers examining the modification of mouse and pig lymphocytes by LPS (Symons and Clarkson, 1979).

Numerous substances inhibit the binding of LPS to membranes. Binding was inhibited when lecithin, cephalin, cholesterol or normal rabbit serum was added to the reaction mixture (Neter *et al.*, 1952c, 1953, 1955). In the case of lecithin, it was noted that pretreatment of the erythrocytes also caused inhibition. These inhibitors did not affect the antibody-neutralizing capacity of the LPS. With reference to the *in vitro* observation that normal rabbit serum inhibited the uptake of LPS by erythrocytes, Ulrich and Meier (1973) found that rabbit alveolar macrophages failed to phagocytose *E. coli* in the presence of 30–40% serum and that the inhibition was at the binding stage and not the ingestion stage. Binding was inhibited by EDTA (Gimber and Rafter, 1969) which tended to support the observation that electrolytes were required for optimum binding (Neter and Zalewski, 1953). No effect was noted in the presence of iodoacetate or sodium cyanide (Gimber and Rafter, 1969). Progesterone, known to associate with a red cell protein, did not affect the binding of LPS (De Venuto, 1968).

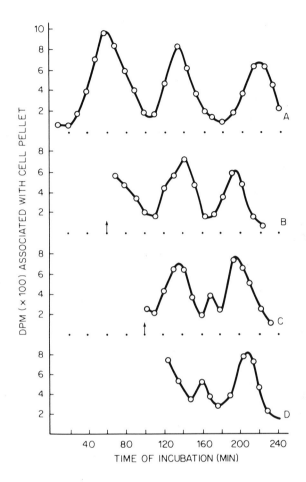

Figure 1. The variation with time of incubation on the uptake of ^{32}P-labelled LPS by rabbit erythrocytes showing the effect of interrupting the binding cycle. A, represents a complete uninterrupted test, B, C and D, were interrupted at 60, 100 and 120 min, respectively; the erythrocytes were washed and reincubated with fresh ^{32}P-labelled LPS. Note that the cyclic binding pattern was maintained even when there was interruption as in B, C and D. From Davies *et al.* (1978) reproduced by permission of Elsevier Biomedical Press B.V., Amsterdam

Pretreatment of erythrocytes altered the modifying capacity of the LPS. For example, when cells were pretreated with papain or trypsin, modification was enhanced (Skillman *et al.*, 1955). Trypsinization, which liberates sialo-glycopeptide, the major part of the membrane responsible for the surface negative charge, enhanced the uptake of *Salmonella minnesota* R-form glycolipid by rat embryo fibroblasts (Bara *et al.*, 1973). However, Ohkuma and Ikemoto

(1966) stated that pretreatment of the cells with trypsin did not alter the binding of LPS.

Finally, the binding of LPS to cell membranes was also dependent on the bacterial species used to obtain the LPS preparation and on the cell type (Alexander *et al.*, 1950; Corvazier, 1952; Davies *et al.*, 1978; Stewart-Tull *et al.*, 1978). For example, Davies and Stewart-Tull (1981) examined a range of LPS molecules and found that the degree of binding varied from molecule to molecule. In general, *Salmonella typhi* NCTC O901 LPS exhibited the greatest binding capacity for all the cell types tested and *Franciscella tularensis* LPS exhibited the least. The degree of binding was also dependent on the extraction procedure. Hence, LPS extracted from *E. coli* B with EDTA had a greater affinity for erythrocytes than the LPS extracted with ether. Similarly, a range of mouse cells was examined and the degree of binding was found to be dependent on the cell type. In general, macrophages exhibited the greatest capacity for binding, with moderate binding capacity being exhibited by thymus, bone marrow and spleen cells, and a weaker capacity by peritoneal lymphocytes and erythrocytes (Davies and Stewart-Tull, 1981).

C. Activation of LPS by Heat and Chemical Treatment

Untreated or native LPS adhered weakly to erythrocytes, and hence for most *in vitro* studies workers have used various treatments to 'activate' or increase the modifying capacity of the LPS (Neter *et al.*, 1952a, 1956b; Macpherson *et al.*, 1953). Heat or alkali treatment have proved the most popular and although the latter increased the modifying capacity of the LPS to a greater extent, both were considered to produce the same qualitative effect on the LPS (Neter *et al.*, 1956b).

1. Heat Treatment

The heat treatment consisted of either keeping the whole bacterial cells at 37°C for several days at pH 10.0, which released the somatic antigen from the cells and increased its modifying capacity (Neter *et al.*, 1954), or the LPS was extracted by conventional methods and heated at 100°C for 1–3 h (Neter *et al.*, 1956b). The degree of activation obtained by the latter procedure was dependent on the LPS used. For example, two native *Salmonella* LPS fractions had optimum modifying capacities at 1000 μg ml^{-1} and 6.0 μg ml^{-1}, whereas after heat activation, the optimum modifying capacities were 1.2 μg ml^{-1} and 1.5 μg ml^{-1}, respectively (Neter *et al.*, 1956a).

It was thought that heating affected the lipid moiety of the LPS (Neter *et al.*, 1956b) and that region of the polysaccharide not involved in the antigen–antibody reactions, since heated *Shigella dysenteriae* LPS had enhanced cellular binding capacity without altered antibody neutralization activity

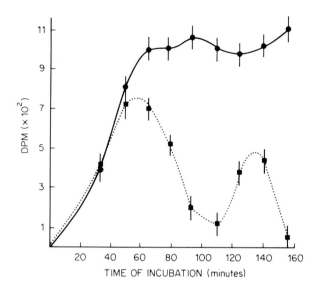

Figure 2. The effect of heat treatment on the kinetics of binding of ^{32}P-labelled LPS from *E. coli* NCTC 8623 to rabbit erythrocytes. The amount of radioactivity (dpm) associated with the erythrocytes is plotted against the incubation time (min). (. . . . . .), represents the effect with untreated LPS; (———), the effect with heat-treated LPS

(Neter and Gorzynski, 1954). This effect was reported for other lipopoly-saccharides (Neter *et al.*, 1956b).

In solution, untreated LPS was strongly opalescent and highly aggregated, having a molecular weight of 10×10^6 to 20×10^6. After heat (or alkali) treatment, the solution became clear as a result of irreversible disaggregation and change in the configuration of the molecules, which now had an average molecular weight of 200 000 (Lüderitz *et al.*, 1958; Neter *et al.*, 1956b).

We examined the kinetics of the binding of *E. coli* ^{32}P-labelled LPS to rabbit erythrocytes over a period of 160 min. The typical biphasic pattern of uptake mentioned above was obtained with untreated ^{32}P-LPS exhibiting peaks of maximum binding at 60 and 135 min. However, following heat treatment of the LPS, the pattern of binding was substantially altered so that binding gradually increased for the first 65 min of incubation in a manner similar to that of untreated ^{32}P-LPS, but attained higher levels which remained relatively constant. It appeared that heat treatment of LPS greatly enhanced its affinity for, and strengthened the bond with, the cell membrane (Figure 2) (Davies *et al.*, 1978).

2. Alkali and Periodate Treatment

Treatment of LPS with 0.25 M sodium hydroxide at 56°C for between 6 and 60 min produced the same changes in the LPS as heating, but more efficiently.

With respect to cell modifying capacity, antibody neutralization, toxicity and pyrogenicity, heating in 0.25 M sodium hydroxide for 6 min produced maximum activities compared with heating alone for 60 min when the pyrogenicity and toxicity of both LPS preparations were severely reduced (Neter *et al.*, 1956b). Contrary to this, Davies *et al.* (1958) showed that differences existed in the extent of cell modifying capacity of LPS if different incubation times were used. The reported increases in modifying capacity after alkali activation were extremely variable and ranged from 2-fold to 20-fold (Ciznar and Shands, 1971). As a quantitative example, Lüderitz *et al.* (1958) found that 1×10^9 erythrocytes were able to fix 2 μg of untreated LPS and 30–40 μg of the alkali-activated form, with the latter representing an average of 1×10^5 molecules of LPS per red cell. It should be noted, however, that although there was this apparent increase in modifying capacity after alkali treatment, Lüderitz *et al.* (1958) found that only 30% of the activated molecules actually had a strong affinity for the membranes, with the remainder of LPS molecules possessing only slight affinity even after repeated adsorptions with fresh cells. Davies *et al.* (1978) made a compatible observation and proposed a scheme to account for this which involved three subpopulations of LPS molecules (Figure 3). In addition, both heat and alkali treatment increased the ability of LPS to modify erythrocyte membranes. The extent of the membrane modification was dependent upon the LPS tested so that heat and alkali treatment had a greater effect on *S. typhi* or *S. typhimurium* LPS than on *E. coli* LPS (Table 4).

Table 4   The relative affinities of chemically treated lipopolysaccharides for human erythrocytes

Lipopolysaccharide species (unlabelled)	Treatment of LPS	Percentage inhibition at 120 μg level*	Relative affinity[†]
E. coli NCTC 8623	Untreated	24.5	1.0 (1.0)
	Heat	33.0	1.34 (1.0)
	Alkali	27.1	1.11 (1.0)
	Periodate	7.8	0.31 (1.0)
S. typhi NCTC 8393	Untreated	29.3	1.0 (1.19)
	Heat	44.9	1.53 (1.36)
	Alkali	37.8	1.29 (1.39)
	Periodate	16.0	0.54 (2.05)
S. typhimurium NCTC 5710	Untreated	18.8	1.0 (0.76)
	Heat	41.5	2.20 (1.25)
	Alkali	47.1	2.50 (1.73)
	Periodate	6.7	0.35 (0.85)

*Calculated from the formula $[(A - B)/A] \times 100$, where A = cpm associated with the erythrocytes after incubation with *E. coli* ^{32}P-LPS alone and B = cpm associated with the erythrocytes after incubation with *E. coli* ^{32}P-LPS in the presence of 120 μg of the unlabelled lipopolysaccharide preparation shown (either treated or untreated).

[†]Relative to the affinity for the untreated preparation or for untreated or heat, alkali or periodate treated *E. coli* LPS (figures in parentheses).

Erythrocytes, modified with alkali-activated LPS tended to lyse spontaneously (Ciznar and Shands, 1971). The extent of the haemolysis was dependent on the number of molecules fixed per cell. During the lytic process, the shape of the erythrocyte changed from the classical biconcave structure to a more spherical form. Untreated LPS produced little or no haemolysis (Ciznar and Shands, 1971; Davies *et al.*, 1978) but such haemolysis or 'leakage' that was observed was dependent on the concentration of the LPS (Ciznar and Shands, 1971). Davies *et al.* (1978) produced evidence that untreated LPS reacted with both positively and negatively charged liposomes in such a way that there was no increase in permeability of the liposomes to divalent anions sequestered inside the lipid bilayer sphere.

Alkali treatment of LPS cleaved ester-linked fatty acids, the amide-linked acids being resistant (Tripodi and Nowotny, 1966; Rietschel *et al.*, 1972). This cleavage caused a depolymerization, which was revealed as a change in the configuration of the LPS molecules, together with a corresponding change in molecular weight from 1 000 000 to 200 000 (Neter *et al.*, 1956b; Shands, 1971). This reduction in molecular weight was thought to remove some of the factors contributing to the steric hindrance of modification through either reduction in size or removal of inactive components. With LPS from *E. coli* or *S. abortus equi*, alkali treatment resulted in lipid degradation with the release of fatty acids and ninhydrin-positive material (Neter *et al.*, 1956b). However, lipidic groups still remained in the reaction product. Rietschel *et al.* (1972) showed that lipid A contained a complex of 3-myristomyristic acid ester-linked to glutamine and that this bond was broken by mild alkali treatment within 10 min. This observation was confirmed by Hofman and Dlabac (1974) who found 3-hydroxymyristic acid and myristic acid as the reaction products after treating LPS with 0.1 M sodium hydroxide at 30°C.

However, the actual role of the lipid is complex since *S. typhi* LPS contained approximately 30% phospholipid, most of which was removed by alkali activation, and which was required for significant membrane binding (Landy *et al.*, 1955), while *Pasteurella pestis* LPS contained 50% phospholipid (Davies, 1956), but readily adsorbed to membranes without alkali treatment (Crumpton *et al.*, 1958). Further, *Aerobacter aerogenes* LPS contained no phospholipid but required alkali treatment to activate adherence to membranes (Wilkinson *et al.*, 1955). These findings are inconclusive, but it would seem that the lipids play an important role in activation since degraded lipid-free polysaccharides, even after heat or alkali activation, failed to modify erythrocytes (Neter *et al.*, 1956b).

Finally, the involvement of *O*-acetate and *O*-acetyl groups has been suggested from data obtained from infrared spectrophotometry. The spectra revealed no differences between untreated and alkali-treated LPS with the exception of the *O*-acetyl groups; the *N*-acetyl groups were not affected (Davies *et al.*, 1958).

Alkali treatment was found to alter significantly the biological effects of LPS, especially those associated with endotoxin (Ciznar and Shands, 1970; Galanos *et al.*, 1971; Whang *et al.*, 1971; Rosenstreich *et al.*, 1973; Ciznar, 1974; Hofman and Dlabac, 1974; see also Chapter 8). Alkali treatment was observed to increase Shwartzman reactivity up to 60 min after treatment with 0.1 M sodium hydroxide while pyrogenicity increased within 5 min of treatment, but was observed to decrease if treatment was carried on for longer than 30 min (Tripodi and Nowotny, 1966). Toxicity was reported to be reduced after 60 min alkali treatment (Neter *et al.*, 1956b) and complete detoxification was achieved by 6 h (Cundy and Nowotny, 1968). Hofman and Dlabac (1974) reported that *S. typhimurium* R strain and the corresponding LPS were eliminated rapidly *in vivo*. However, if the LPS was treated with alkali or alkaline hydroxylamine, a slow elimination resulted. Mitogenicity and anti-complementary activity were completely destroyed by alkali treatment (Galanos *et al.*, 1971; Rosenstreich *et al.*, 1973), while adjuvant activity, immunogenicity and antigenicity in preparations that contained *O*-acetyl groups and monosaccharides as immunodominant groups were severely reduced (Ciznar and Shands, 1970; Whang *et al.*, 1971). In our own studies, we noticed a considerable reduction in the immunopotentiating activity of alkali-treated LPS in vaccines containing ovalbumin in saline (Table 5).

Finally, a third treatment of LPS should be briefly mentioned. LPS preparations treated with periodate lost their cell modifying capacity (Neter *et al.*, 1956b). The treatment resulted in the oxidative cleavage of each fourth sugar unit with the oxidized polysaccharide units remaining bound to the LPS so that the molecular weight remained essentially unchanged. This treatment resulted in a decrease in toxicity and antibody neutralizing capacity of the preparations. In addition, we found that 0.1 M sodium periodate also reduced adjuvant activity (Table 5).

D. Membrane Receptors for LPS

The majority of work on receptors for LPS was done by Springer and his colleagues who isolated a fraction from the erythrocyte membrane which they suggested was a lipopolysaccharide receptor (Pavlovski and Springer, 1967; Springer *et al.*, 1970, 1973; Adye *et al.*, 1973). Observations by other workers provided evidence for the nature of the receptor. LPS combined significantly with lipoproteins in the presence of alkali, and it was suggested that lipids on the erythrocyte membrane played a part in adsorption (Partridge and Morgan, 1940; Morgan, 1943), especially since lipids such as lecithin and cephalin inhibited adsorption of LPS to erythrocytes.

A receptor from human erythrocytes involved in immunoadherence haemagglutination (IAH) was released after trypsin treatment of the cells. The human erythrocyte showed a range of IAH reactions from strongly positive,

Table 5 Effect of alkali and periodate treatment on affinity for membranes and the immunopotentiating activity of bacterial lipopolysaccharides and mycobacterial glycopeptide

Bacterial component	Relative increase/decrease in affinity for sheep erythrocytes			Mean haemagglutinating antibody titre ($\log_2$ dilution)			Relative adjuvancy
	Untreated	Alkali-treated	Periodate-treated	Untreated	Alkali-treated	Periodate-treated	
Lipopolysaccharides							
E. coli NCTC 8623	1.0	1.11	0.31	8.0(1.0)	2.8(0.5)	3.6(0.8)	1.00
S. typhi NCTC 8393	1.0	1.29	0.54	10.2(0.8)	2.5(0.3)	3.8(0.5)	1.99
S. typhimurium NCTC 5710	1.0	2.50	0.35	7.2(1.0)	2.3(0.5)	1.5(0.8)	0.40
Mycobacterial glycopeptides							
ST 208	1.0	1.72	0.60	7.6(1.0)	1.5(0.8)	1.0(0.8)	0.58
ST 82	NT	NT	NT	9.8(0.44)	NT	NT	0.90
ST 210	NT	NT	NT	9.6(0.57)	NT	NT	0.95
ST 211	NT	NT	NT	8.0(1.22)	NT	NT	0.62
PPD	NT	NT	NT	9.0(0.57)	NT	NT	0.79

The haemagglutination titres were obtained after immunization of ten HAM/1CR mice per group with 20 μg of ovalbumin and 60 μg of LPS. The mean haemagglutination titre in the sera of control animals given ovalbumin in the absence of LPS was 1.0 ± 0.80 (mean $\pm$ S.D.) The adjuvancy values are for the untreated preparations relative to the untreated LPS of *E. coli* 8623. NT = not tested.

where the receptors were abundant on the cell surface, to weakly positive, where only small amounts of the receptor were present. This difference was genetically determined. Other inhibitory fractions were isolated from erythrocytes; an alcohol–ether extract from horse erythrocytes inhibited the modification of intact red cells by a filtrate from *Pfeifferella mallei* cultures (Boyden, 1950). Similarly, a glycoprotein from human erythrocytes was inhibitory to subsequent modification by *E. coli* O86 LPS (Springer *et al.*, 1966b). Neter *et al.* (1952b) reported that the A, B and Rh antigens were not blocked on erythrocytes modified by either *E. coli* or *Franciscella tulcrensis* LPS.

It is still not known whether there is more than one receptor on the membrane for LPS. The LPS from *E. coli* O8, O111 and *S. abortus equi* bound to the same receptor (Lüderitz *et al.*, 1958) and Springer *et al.* (1973) reported that the 'LPS receptor' inhibited the uptake of all LPS preparations by apparently blocking the sites on the LPS molecule that attach to the membrane. However, it was reported that more than one type of LPS may attach to the same erythrocyte (Hayes, 1951; Neter *et al.*, 1952b; Landy, 1954) and that, if one LPS was in excess, it did not block the uptake of another LPS present in minimal quantities (Neter *et al.*, 1956b).

Springer's group isolated an LPS receptor, by organic solvent treatment of erythrocyte ghosts, which inhibited the binding of LPS to erythrocytes (Springer *et al.*, 1973; Adye *et al.*, 1973). The amount of LPS required for optimal coating of erythrocytes and the amount of receptor required to give greater than 95% inhibition of uptake varied, depending on the LPS used. This particular receptor also inhibited, to a lesser extent, cellular modification by the Kunin antigen, while large amounts of the receptor were required to block Vi, Rantz and streptococcal group antigens. Results from these inhibition studies generally indicated an homologous area of the membrane to which all LPS species attach. This receptor inhibited the uptake of untreated, treated and alkali-heated S and R forms of LPS.

When the inhibitory activity of the receptor was compared with the activity of haemoglobin, gangliosides and phospholipids (Adye and Springer, 1968; Springer *et al.*, 1966a; Kimelberg and Papahadjopoulos, 1971a), it was found that the haemoglobin had 10% of the receptor activity, while the gangliosides and phospholipids possessed less than 3% of the activity. The attachment of LPS to membranes was freely reversible (Springer *et al.*, 1970; Davies *et al.*, 1978; Symons and Clarkson, 1979) and the receptor was able to remove LPS already attached to the membranes, unlike phospholipids and serum (Neter, 1956; Springer and Horton, 1964).

The receptor was heat-labile and inactivated by aldehydes, which indicated protein involvement since aldehydes form condensation products with amino acids. Furthermore, inactivation was produced by proteinase action which indicated that proteins were involved in the receptor, either as the actual determinant or as a structural component. It would seem that, for maximum activity, the receptor depends on the protein to give it size and conformation, as in the case of the human erythrocyte MN antigens (Jirgensons and Springer, 1968). The receptor was a 228-kDa lipoglycoprotein rich in *N*-acetylneuraminic acid (NANA) and galactose. It contained 61% peptide (the major amino acids were glutamic acid, aspartic acid, serine and threonine) and 10% non-covalently bound lipid. There was no indication of phospholipids in the receptor. The polysaccharide moiety contained NANA (17%), glucosamine, galactosamine, galactose, glucose, mannose and fucose. The lipid and NANA were not involved in receptor activity, since 90% of the lipid and 99% of the NANA could be removed before activity was affected.

E. LPS–membrane Interactions

The interaction between LPS and the membrane is controversial with evidence for both single bonds and double bonds. It was reported by Vogel (1957) and Hämmerling and Westphal (1967) that lipid A was necessary for the linkage between the membrane and the LPS and that this interaction was hydrophobic with an intermixing of LPS fatty acids with membrane lipids. However, Gimber and Rafter (1969) reported that the linkage was mediated by ionic bonds. For *Aerobacter aerogenes* LPS, lipids were not essential for adsorption which seemed to be a function of the size and configuration of the LPS (Davies *et al.*, 1958). It is important to remember that heat and alkali activation alters the molecular weight of the LPS as well as the configuration (Neter *et al.*, 1956b; Shands, 1971). The binding observed was also reversible, which suggested weak bonds and not a covalent hydrophobic bond (Lüderitz *et al.*, 1958).

If lipids are essential for attachment to the membrane, how is this physically achieved if they are situated within a bilayered molecule? Shands (1973) proposed two possible explanations: (a) that edge attachment occurred and the LPS fatty acids were 'solubilized' in the cell membrane; and (b) that phase transitions took place in the LPS so that hydrophobic groups became exposed in the proximity of the membrane surface. Stacking of particles (De Pamphilis, 1971; Schnaitman, 1971) and the morphological change from discs to vesicles (De Pamphilis, 1971) occurred under the appropriate conditions in the presence of lecithin. The linear association of the LPS particles after interaction with the membrane involved metallic ions and the change to the vesicle form could provide a mechanism for incorporation of LPS into membranes. Benedetto *et al.* (1973) showed that LPS bound to phospholipid monolayers and decreased their stability. They found that native LPS caused changes in the surface pressure of the phospholipid monolayer ranging from 2 to 6 dynes cm^{-1}, depending on the state of monolayer compression. This observation could account for the leakage of haemoglobin from erythrocytes (Ciznar and Shands, 1971; Davies *et al.*, 1978). This was characterized by a lipid–lipid linkage between LPS lipid A and membrane lipids. There also appeared to be a surface-adsorptive reaction, dependent on ionic bonding and inhibited by a net negative charge on the membrane. Hence Benedetto *et al.* (1973) concluded that two bonds could be observed during LPS interactions with artificial phospholipid bilayers; one of the bonds was covalent and the other involved ionic bridges. A similar observation was made with various cell types (Davies *et al.*, 1978) and it was proposed that the two bond types reflected subpopulations of LPS molecules (Figure 3). The strong lipid–lipid linkage involved the LPS$_I$ subpopulation with a proposed structure of (lipid A–heptose), while weak bonds involved the LPS$_{II}$ subpopulation with a proposed structure of either (lipid A–heptose — basal core polysaccharide) or (lipid A–heptose — basal core polysaccharide–O-specific polysaccharide). It was further proposed that heat and alkali activation, known to affect the lipid region (Tripodi and Nowotny, 1966; Rietschel *et al.*, 1972) and also to cause contraction and aggregation of polysaccharide chains (Read and Gunstone, 1958; Rees, 1967), convert LPS$_{II}$ into LPS$_I$ and hence increase the cell modifying capacity of the LPS. A further subpopulation (LPS$_{III}$), 66% of the LPS molecules, showed little or no affinity for cell membranes due to a lack of lipid in the molecule.

III. CELL MODIFICATION BY AMPHIPHILES FROM MYCOBACTERIA

A. General Considerations

Studies on the binding of bacterial polysaccharides to mammalian cell membranes have centred around the gram-negative bacteria, with similar fractions from mycobacteria being largely ignored. Although there was considerable work done on mycobacterial polysaccharides in the early 1950s, interest in such observations declined, possibly due to the fact that, although it was possible to obtain numerous active polysaccharide fractions, it was difficult to assign a structural role for them in the mycobacterial cell, as had been done for LPS in gram-negative bacteria.

In 1948, Middlebrook and Dubos observed that at least one heat-stable component present in a polysaccharide fraction of the tubercle bacillus could be adsorbed onto sheep erythrocytes, rendering them specifically agglutinable by antibodies directed against the polysaccharide fraction of the bacillus. Middlebrook (1955) found that tuberculin contained two forms of polysaccharide, one of which (40%) was capable of sensitizing sheep erythrocytes. The other polysaccharide was not involved in adsorption to erythrocytes. Sorkin *et al.* (1956) isolated a crude 'alpha haemosensitin' by alcohol fractionation of heated culture filtrates of *Mycobacterium tuberculosis* and removed the protein impurities by treatment with ammonium sulphate and trichloroacetic acid. Electrophoretic analysis of this crude preparation revealed that even the most active preparation was not homogeneous, probably because of the presence of more than one structurally related type of polysaccharide molecule. This

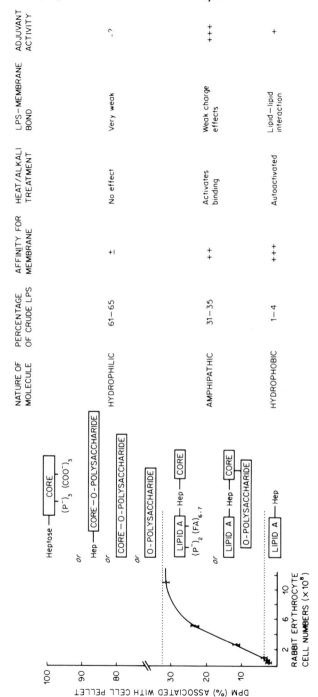

Figure 3. The relationships among binding to erythrocyte membranes, affinity for surfaces, immunopotentiating activity and charge of different molecular species of lipopolysaccharide. The curve shows the uptake of ^{32}P-labelled LPS from *E. coli* NCTC 8623 by varying numbers of rabbit erythrocytes. The graph was taken from Davies *et al.* (1978) and reproduced by permission of Elsevier Biomedical Press, B.V., Amsterdam

substance could sensitize sheep erythrocytes to antituberculous sera, resulting in a haemagglutination reaction. One of the polysaccharides in this mixture was composed of arabinose and mannose and was extremely effective in binding to erythrocyte membranes.

B. Condition for Cellular Modification

It is apparent from the literature that the binding of mycobacterial polysaccharides to mammalian cells exhibits properties similar to those observed for the binding of LPS from gram-negative bacteria (Table 2). Boyden and Andersen (1955) examined the binding of mycobacterial components to erythrocyte membranes by means of the Middlebrook–Dubos test in which the cells were rendered specifically agglutinable by sensitization with the mycobacterial fraction. They observed that with purified protein derivative (PPD) the antigenic determinants of the PPD were still available after cell modification and that, in the form of an antigen–antibody complex, the PPD still retained an affinity for the cell surface. The sensitization step was ten times more rapid at 37°C than at 20°C, while at 4°C the reaction was negligible; the haemagglutination step was independent of temperature over the range 4–37°C. Heat treatment of the PPD at 100°C for 60 min failed to destroy its cell modifying capacity, but completely abrogated the haemagglutination reaction. However, trypsin treatment of the PPD destroyed its affinity for the erythrocyte membranes. The affinity reaction was also inhibited in the presence of normal serum (Boyden and Andersen, 1955), lecithin, cephalin or cholesterol (Boyden and Grabar, 1954). The inhibition by lecithin and cephalin could be greatly increased if the mycobacterial polysaccharide was incubated with these membrane components prior to the incubation with erythrocytes. Stewart-Tull *et al.* (1978) showed that the degree of binding of mycobacterial polysaccharides was dependent on the polysaccharide itself, the mammalian cell, and on time of incubation. As a general rule, polysaccharide preparations that contained a high carbohydrate content also possessed a high degree of affinity for erythrocyte membranes (Fleming *et al.*, 1984). Further, the mycobacterial preparations were shown to bind to a wide range of cells, including erythrocytes, lymphocytes and macrophages and that the degree of binding was dependent on the cell type. While examining the binding of a glycopeptide to sheep erythrocytes, it was found that the normal carbohydrate content of the erythrocytes varied over a period of time and that erythrocytes with a relatively high carbohydrate content adsorbed relatively less of the glycopeptide. In addition, the quantitative binding of a glycopeptide to erythrocytes at 37°C exhibited a cyclic fluctuation with time similar to that shown in Figure 1. Throughout the incubation period a portion of the glycopeptide remained firmly bound while another fraction bound reversibly. Since some of the glycopeptide remained bound throughout the experimental period, it was apparent that different molecular forms were present in the mycobacterial preparation and that different chemical bonds were involved in the adsorption of these to the cell. The binding of mycobacterial glycopeptide to cell membranes increased after alkali treatment and decreased after periodate treatment (Table 5). This situation is identical to that encountered for LPS.

C. Mycobacterial Amphiphile–membrane Interactions

The mycobacterial polysaccharides appear to bind to the mammalian cell membranes in a manner similar to that observed for the LPS preparations. As with LPS, the binding of mycobacterial polysaccharides to membranes can be inhibited with normal serum, lecithin and cholesterol (Boyden and Grabar, 1954; Boyden and Andersen, 1955). Davies and Stewart-Tull (1973) reported that glycopeptide bound reversibly to sheep erythrocyte membranes and that, after a period of 48 h at 4°C, a major portion of the glycopeptide was lost from the cell surface. Stewart-Tull *et al.* (1978) suggested that two types of bonds were involved, one being strong and the other relatively weak. The strong bonds might be due to a covalent or hydrophobic interaction, while the weak bonds, which readily dissociate, might be due to weak electrostatic interactions in a situation analogous to LPS binding. In studies with whole erythrocytes and with artificial lipid bilayers (liposomes), evidence was found for a small amount of membrane disruption, as shown by the leakage of a small amount of haemoglobin from the erythrocytes and of potassium chromate sequestered inside the liposomes (Stewart-Tull *et al.*, 1978). With negatively charged liposomes of lecithin–dicetyl phosphate–cholesterol, some of the mycobacterial preparations caused membrane disruption, resulting in leakage of the sequestered chromate ions; some had no effect on the liposomes and a few protected the liposomes from 'spontaneous' leakage. A similar effect was observed with positively charged liposomes. Peptidoglycolipid fractions caused an increase in permeability and leakage in both types of liposomes while proteinaceous fractions did not react adversely with the positively charged liposomes, but did cause leakage from the negatively charged liposomes. Proteins will bind to artificial lipid bilayers containing anionic lipids until the net charge of bound protein neutralizes that of the lipid aggregate (Das *et al.*, 1965; Steinemann and Läeuger, 1971). Sweet and Zull (1970) showed that serum albumin bound to vesicles composed of phosphatidylcholine, cholesterol and dicetyl phosphate below the isoelectric pH where the protein had a positive charge. This binding increased in proportion to the negative charge on the vesicle. Kimelberg and Papahadjopoulos (1971a,b) showed that basic proteins increased the permeability of liposomes at neutral pH and low ionic strength. An initial electrostatic attraction between protein and phospholipid was required as a prerequisite of the increased permeability due to subsequent hydrophobic interaction, penetration and distortion of the hydrocarbon region of the lipid bilayer. These observations could explain the results with negatively charged liposomes and proteïnaceous preparations. Peptidoglycolipid preparations might react with the bilayer via lipid–lipid hydrophobic bonds in addition to the protein interactions. The mycobacterial glycopeptides contain the charged hydrophilic amino acids, aspartic, glutamic and diaminopimelic acid, and the hydrophobic amino acid, alanine, together with the hydrophilic carbohydrate moiety, and would bind to the surface predominantly through coulombic attraction between oppositely charged ionic groupings and through hydrophobic interactions to a much lesser extent. Glycopeptides containing high levels of carbohydrate significantly reduced the leakage of chromate by coating the surface of both types of liposome.

   With regard to studies concerning a receptor molecule, very little work has been done although Boyden and Grabar (1954) reported that an alcohol–ether extract from red cells was able to inhibit the binding of mycobacterial preparations to erythrocytes.

IV. AMPHIPHILES AS IMMUNOADJUVANTS

As mentioned earlier, the cell modifying activity of bacterial amphiphiles was examined in attempts to define their immunopotentiating activity (see also Chapters 3 and 10).

   It has to be generally supposed that the interaction between immunoadjuvants and cell membranes is of prime importance and a prerequisite for influencing the immunoadjuvant response. The cells involved in this interaction, such as macrophages and lymphocytes, could play a central role in the immune responses, thus providing the adjuvant with a direct mode of action. Alternatively, the cells involved could be secondary to the immune system so that after interaction with the adjuvant, factors are released (e.g. interferon, polynucleotides) which influence the immune response. This latter involvement would indicate an indirect role for immunoadjuvants. Both direct and indirect modes of adjuvant action could be attributed to both LPS and mycobacterial polysaccharide adjuvants (Stewart-Tull, 1983a,b). Direct evidence for the interaction of adjuvants with cell membranes as the first step in the adjuvant response is not readily available in the literature. However, there are several sources of indirect evidence which can be explored and possibly interpreted in terms of cell membrane–adjuvant interactions. It has already been suggested that the binding of LPS to receptors on the membranes of host tissue cells is a prerequisite for most, if not all, of its physiological effects. Hill and Weiss (1964) stated that there was a direct relationship between the lethal effects of endotoxin in various strains of mice and LPS affinity for erythrocytes from these strains. Also, *in vivo* modification of erythrocytes was reported after the injection into guinea pigs of large amounts of the Vi antigen (De Gregorio, 1955) and a polysaccharide fraction from tuberculin (Boyden, 1953). Hence, it was possible that, since the binding of these bacterial components to membranes was more than just a surface phenomenon as evidenced by membrane instabilities (Ciznar and Shands, 1971; Davies *et al.*, 1978; Stewart-Tull *et al.*, 1978), the membrane disorganization acted as a stimulatory mechanism analogous to the effect of phytohaemagglutinin in binding to carbohydrate structures on the cell membrane and causing a mitogenic effect while still external to the cell (Greaves and Bauminger, 1972).

Gimber and Rafter (1969) reported that after endotoxin bound to leucocytes, the LPS was partially degraded, and Cooper *et al.* (1960) showed that new pyrogenic material was released from the cells. Such treated leucocytes showed increased glucose metabolism via the hexose monophosphate pathway (Hohnadel and Stjernholm, 1966; Graham *et al.*, 1967) and ATP hydrolysis was inhibited in intact cells (Tenney and Rafter, 1968).

Betz and Morrison (1977) found that the butanol-extracted LPS from *E. coli* lost its ability to mitogenically stimulate C_3H/HeJ mouse lymphocytes after the removal, by phenol, of a protein-rich fraction known as the lipid A-associated protein (LAP). The LAP was a potent mitogen, although this effect was dose dependent since LAP proved to be toxic at high doses. Although in its mitogenic action LAP was similar to intact LPS, it was observed that LAP activity was destroyed after mild alkali treatment in direct contrast to LPS. In other structure and function studies (Behling *et al.*, 1976) synthetic glycolipids similar to those of the lipid moiety of LPS (*N*-acetylated D-glucosamine derivatives) were shown to be potent B-cell mitogens. These glycolipids, especially the lauroyl derivative, showed comparable or even superior enhancement to LPS in an adjuvant assay which measured the numbers of plaque-forming cells (PFC) and rosette-forming cells (RFC) produced in response to human gamma globulin (HGG) or sheep erythrocytes. However, in the radioprotection assay, LPS exhibited an 80% protection, unlike the best protection (40%) afforded by the synthetic glycolipid.

Rook and Stewart-Tull (1976), using an *in vitro* culture, found that mycobacterial peptidoglycolipids and PPD were B-cell mitogens and that this mitogenicity was almost completely destroyed by splitting off the glycopeptide fraction of these preparations. However, in this system the adjuvant-active glycopeptides were non-mitogenic, in direct contrast to the adjuvant-active LPS preparations which were found to be potent B-cell mitogens (Gery *et al.*, 1972; Shinohara and Kern, 1976).

Mayer *et al.* (1978) examined over 50 LPS preparations but found that significant binding to mammalian cells occurred with only eight of these. They found that some preparations bound only to Ig-negative cells or only to Ig-positive cells, whilst others bound to both types of cell. On the basis of this binding they were able to describe three subpopulations of B-cells (B_1–B_3) and three subpopulations of T-cells (T_1–T_3). However, Zimmerman *et al.* (1977) showed that lipid A bound preferentially to spleen cells rather than to thymocytes and that T-cell-enriched spleen cells after passage through nylon wool columns showed a loss of specific binding of the lipid A. Thus, it appeared from this that whilst the adjuvant activity of LPS preparations is a widely accepted phenomenon, the binding to mammalian membranes is not. A relationship existed between the adjuvant activity of a preparation and the ability to cause the fusion of avian erythrocytes (Ahkong *et al.*, 1974). They suggested that the membrane instabilities caused by the binding of LPS fractions were the basis for both adjuvant activity and fusogenic action. However, the direct relationship of adjuvant activity to fusogenic activity is somewhat tenuous since some fusogenic agents do not possess the ability to stimulate antibody production.

However, the interaction between cells, especially lymphocytes, is the basis of all immune reactions, and Roseman (1970) showed that these interactions were conditioned by the sugar residues of the plasma membrane glycoproteins and glycolipids. Mammalian cells modified with LPS or mycobacterial polysaccharide acquire new serological specificities (Springer and Horton, 1964) and the current evidence suggested that the polysaccharide fraction will be exposed to the environment. These cells will not only alter their interactions with other cells, but will also acquire altered migration pathways throughout the body. Gesner and Ginsberg (1964) have shown that the cell surface glycoproteins are important for lymphocyte migration and alteration of these components results in different distribution throughout the body. It is interesting to note that R-strain gram-negative bacteria and the extracted LPS tended to localize mainly in the spleen, while S-strain bacteria and the LPS were found predominantly in the lungs (Hofmann and Dlobac, 1974). As mentioned before, differences between S and R strains of bacteria depended upon the carbohydrate composition of their LPS fractions. Although this indicates an important role for the carbohydrate moiety, evidence from other sources (Betz and Morrison, 1977) has demonstrated an activity associated with the protein fraction of these bacteria.

Studies with *Bacteroides melaninogenicus* (Mansheim *et al.*, 1978) revealed that extracted LPS was deficient in the basal sugars, heptose and 2-keto-3-deoxy–D-mannooctonate (KDO) together with a fatty acid, β-hydroxymyristic acid. This resulted in a low biological activity as judged by skin reactions and the chick embryo lethality test. The activity of this LPS was dependent on the method of extraction.

From the above evidence, it is apparent that the biological activities of polysaccharide preparations are dependent on several factors, including method of extraction (Mansheim *et al.*, 1978), chemical composition (Betz and Morrison, 1977) and state of activation by either heat or alkali treatment (Neter and Gorzynski, 1954; Neter *et al.*, 1956a; Johnson *et al.*, 1956; Tripodi and Nowotny, 1966; Cundy and Nowotny, 1968). These parameters also cause a marked effect on the degree of binding or affinity that these preparations have for cell membranes. Initial observations were made by comparing the adjuvant activity of the bacterial preparations before and after treatments shown to alter the natural affinity for cell membranes. In 1956, Johnson *et al.* investigated the effect of alkali treatment on the adjuvancy of *Salmonella typhi* LPS in rabbits and noted a decrease in the adjuvant activity. However, the alkali-treated LPS was used at $20\,\mu g$ and $200\,\mu g$ levels, while the untreated native LPS was used at a $5\,\mu g$ level. Hence, the relatively decreased antibody levels with the alkali-treated LPS could be due to the suppressive effect of excess LPS. However, these observations were confirmed by the findings of Davies and Stewart-Tull (1981), who examined several species of gram-negative LPS and mycobacterial glycopeptides and found that at equivalent concentrations the adjuvant effect of the polysaccharides on haemagglutination titres produced in response to ovalbumin in mice decreased after alkali treatment (Table 5). The same treatment, however, corresponded with an increase in the erythrocyte-binding capacity of the LPS and mycobacterial preparations. Similar experiments were performed with periodate-treated preparations. As expected, a decrease in the affinity of the preparations for erythrocyte membranes was observed, together with a marked decrease in the adjuvant activity. Stewart-Tull *et al.* (1965), while attempting to find an explanation of mycobacterial adjuvancy, demonstrated a molecular interaction between a mycobacterial glycopeptide and guinea pig IgG_2. It was suggested that the mycobacterial peptidoglycolipid (wax D) might combine with newly synthesized IgG and act as a specific derepressor for the ribonucleic acid template in the plasma cell. The preparation with high concentrations of arabinose and muramic acid were shown to possess the affinity for the IgG_2 (Stewart-Tull and Wilkinson, 1973). It was proposed that, since the mycobacterial glycopeptide possessed an affinity for cell membranes, the glycopeptide–IgG_2 complex could be held at the surface of cells providing a cell-bound combining site for antigen. The IgG_2 bound by this method could be accounted for by the small early peak of antibody production that sometimes precedes the main adjuvant-stimulated responses (French *et al.*, 1970; White, 1973). This theory would require that the mycobacterial glycopeptide possessed a dual affinity, one for cell membranes and the other for IgG_2. Further, either property must be able to be expressed without interfering with the other. In 1973, Davies and Stewart-Tull demonstrated that, by means of a glycopeptide bridge, guinea pig IgG_2 could be held at the surface of erythrocytes and still function as an antibody. Other explanations of the observed affinities were expressed, and White (1973) proposed that the mycobacterial constituent, by combining with the antibody produced in the early peak, interfered with the negative feedback suppression of the homeostatic response.

Hence, stimulated by these latter observations, Davies and Stewart-Tull (1981) attempted to provide a direct correlation between the natural affinity of bacterial polysaccharides and the adjuvant activity of these preparations. In a series of experiments, we examined the affinities that different polysaccharide preparations had for different cell types and compared them to the affinity possessed by a standard bacterial polysaccharide preparation (*E. coli* NCTC

8623, phenol-extracted LPS). By both radioactive and chemical methods, we were able to obtain a set of relative affinity values for the preparations. By this comparison method the standard LPS preparation was assigned a relative affinity value of 1.0. Similarly, by examining the adjuvant effect of the preparations on the production of passive haemagglutinating antibodies in response to ovalbumin in mice and comparing them with the standard LPS, a series of relative adjuvant activities was obtained. For each cell type examined, the relative affinity value of a preparation was plotted against the appropriate relative adjuvant activity value. A direct relationship existed between the affinity that a bacterial polysaccharide possessed for peritoneal lymphocytes and the adjuvant activity of the polysaccharides. This relationship was true for both bacterial LPS and the mycobacterial glycopeptides and exhibited a correlation coefficient (r) of 0.92. Some LPS preparations, notably those from *Bordetella pertussis* and *Franciscella tularensis* did not fit into this scheme. On the other hand, with peritoneal macrophages, an inverse relationship existed ($r = 0.86$) between affinity and adjuvancy with most preparations. For the other cell types examined, no significant relationship appeared to exist. Hence, both gram-negative LPS and the mycobacterial polysaccharide fractions seemed to act through very similar mechanisms, and the best adjuvant active compounds possessed a low affinity for macrophages and a high affinity for peritoneal lymphocytes. However, it should be remembered that, on average, quantitatively ten times more of the bacterial fraction was adsorbed by the macrophages, although phagocytosis and subsequent digestion may have reduced the effective amount of the bacterial component available. It is possible that the polysaccharides with low affinity for macrophages act initially, at least, by escaping phagocytic destruction. This would explain the earlier observations (Johnson *et al.*, 1956) that polysaccharides whose affinity was greatly increased by alkali treatment possessed markedly decreased adjuvant activity. The most efficient adjuvants also possessed a high affinity for the lymphocyte preparation and could be explained by a direct mode of action, either by supplying a 'second signal' in the case of B-cells or by the induction of non-specific help in the case of T-cells. It is interesting to note that all the polysaccharide fractions tested (with the exceptions mentioned earlier) possessed a high lymphocyte, low macrophage affinity property; i.e. a high level of affinity for lymphocytes was always accompanied by a low level of affinity for macrophages. The results obtained with periodate can be explained in terms of reduced binding to the lymphocytes. The various cell modifying and immunoadjuvant properties associated with LPS and the mycobacterial glycopeptides are summarized in Table 2.

Evidence in the literature is sparse concerning direct data on relationship between affinity for cell membranes and bioactivity, but such evidence that does exist suggests that this is an area of molecular immunological research worthy of greater attention.

REFERENCES

Adye, J. C., and Springer, G. F. (1968). Mode of inhibition of endotoxin coating of human red cells by compounds of known structure. *Fed. Proc.*, **27**, 267.

Adye, J. C., Springer, G. F., and Murthy, J. R. (1973). On the nature and function of the lipopolysaccharide receptor from human erythrocytes. *Z. Immun.-Forsch.*, **144**, 491–496.

Ahkong, Q. F., Howell, J. I. Tampion, W., and Lucy, J. A. (1974). The fusion of hen erythrocytes by lipid-soluble and surface-active immunological adjuvants. *FEBS Lett.*, **41**, 206.

Alexander, M. M., Wright, G. C., and Baldwin, A. C. (1950). Observations on the agglutination of polysaccharide-treated erythrocytes by tularemia antisera. *J. Exp. Med.*, **91**, 561–566.

Bara, J., Lallier, R., Brailovsky, C., and Nigam, V. N. (1973). Fixation of *Salmonella minnesota* R-form glycolipid on the membrane of normal and transformed rat embryo fibroblasts. *Eur. J. Biochem.*, **35**, 489–494.

Beer, H., Braude, A. I., and Brinton, C. C. (1966). A study of particle sizes, shapes and toxicities present in a Boivin-type endotoxin preparation. *Ann. N.Y. Acad. Sci.*, **133**, 450–475.

Behling, U. H., Campbell, B., Chang, C.-M., Rumpf, C., and Nowotny, A. (1976). Synthetic glycolipid adjuvants. *J. Immunol.*, **117**, 847–851.

Benedetto, D. A., Shands, J. W., and Shah, D. O. (1973). The interaction of bacterial lipopolysaccharide with phosopholipid bilayers and monolayers. *Biochim. Biophys. Acta*, **298**, 145–157.

Betz, S. J., and Morrison, D. C. (1977). Chemical and biologic properties of a protein-rich fraction of bacterial lipopolysaccharides. I. The *in vitro* murine lymphocyte response. *J. Immunol.*, **119**, 1475–1481.

Boyden, S. V. (1950). Adsorption by erythrocytes of antigens of *Pfeifferella mallei* and *Pfeifferella whitmori*. *Proc. Soc. Exp. Biol. Med.*, **73**, 289–291.

Boyden, S. V. (1951). The adsorption of proteins on erythrocytes treated with tannic acid and subsequent haemagglutination by anti-protein sera. *J. Exp. Med.*, **93**, 107–120.

Boyden, S. V. (1953). Fixation of bacterial products by erythrocytes *in vivo* and by leucocytes. *Nature*, **171**, 402–403.

Boyden, S. V., and Andersen, M. E. (1955). Agglutination of normal erythrocytes in mixtures of antibody and antigen, and haemolysis in the presence of complement. *Br. J. Exp. Pathol.*, **36**, 162–170.

Boyden, S. V., and Grabar, P. (1954). Rôle des lipides dans la sensibilisation des érythrocytes par les constituants de la tuberculine. *Ann. Inst. Pasteur*, **87**, 257–267.

Burge, R. E., and Draper, J. C. (1967). The structure of the cell wall of the gram-negative bacterium *Proteus vulgaris*. III. A lipopolysaccharide 'unit membrane'. *J. Mol. Biol.*, **28**, 205–210.

Chang, R. S. (1953). A serologically-active erythrocyte-sensitizing substance from typhus rickettsiae. *J. Immunol.*, **70**, 212–214.

Ciznar, I. (1974). Reactivity of modified lipopolysaccharide with erythrocyte membranes. *J. Hyg. Epidemiol. Microbiol. Immunol.*, **18**, 415–419.

Ciznar, I., and Shands, J. W. (1970). Effect of alkali on the immunological reactivity of lipopolysaccharide from *Salmonella typhimurium*. *Infect. Immun.*, **2**, 549–555.

Ciznar, I., and Shands, J. W. (1971). Effect of alkali-treated lipopolysaccharide on erythrocyte membrane stability. *Infect. Immun.*, **4**, 362–367.

Cone, R. E., and Marchalonis, J. J. (1974). Surface proteins of thymus-derived lymphocytes and bone-marrow-derived lymphocytes. *Biochem. J.*, **140**, 345–354.

Cooper, K. E., Cranston, W. I., and Fessler, J. H. (1960). Interactions of a bacterial pyrogen with rabbit leucocytes and plasma. *J. Physiol.*, **154**, 22P–23P.

Corvazier, P. (1952). Etude de l'antigene Vi a l'aide d'une technique d'hémagglutination passive. *Ann. Inst. Pasteur.*, **83**, 173–179.

Crumpton, M. J., Davies, D. A. L., and Hutchison, A. M. (1958). The serological specificities of *Pasteurella pseudotuberculosis* somatic antigens. *J. Gen. Microbiol.*, **18**, 129–139.

Cundy, K. R., and Nowotny, A. (1968). Comparisons of five toxicity parameters of *Serratia marcescens* endotoxins. *Proc. Soc. Exp. Biol. Med.*, **127**, 999–1003.

Das, M. L., Haak, E. D., and Crane, F. L. (1965). Proteolipids. IV. Formation of complexes between cytochrome *c* and purified phospholipids. *Biochemistry*, **4**, 859–865.

Davies, D. A. L. (1956). A specific polysaccharide of *Pasteurella pestis*. *Biochem. J.*, **63**, 105–116.

Davies, D. A. L., Crumpton, M. J., MacPherson, I. A., and Hutchison, A. M. (1958). The adsorption of bacterial polysaccharides by erythrocytes. *Immunology*, **2**, 157–171.

Davies, M. (1974). The affinity of bacterial polysaccharides for mammalian cell surfaces and its relationship to adjuvant activity. *Ph.D. Thesis*, Glasgow University.

Davies, M., and Stewart-Tull, D. E. S. (1973). The dual affinity of a mycobacterial glycopeptide for sheep erythrocyte membranes and guinea-pig gamma-globulin. *Immunology*, **25**, 1–9.

Davies, M., and Stewart-Tull, D. E. S. (1981). The affinity of bacterial polysaccharide-containing fractions for mammalian cell membranes and its relationship to immunopotentiating activity. *Biochim. Biophys. Acta*, **643**, 17–29.

Davies, M., Stewart-Tull, D. E. S., and Jackson, D. M. (1978). The binding of lipopolysaccharide from *Escherichia coli* to mammalian cell membranes and its effect on liposomes. *Biochim. Biophys. Acta*, **508**, 260–276.

De Gregorio, M. (1955). Fissazione di antigeni sulla superficie cellulare. *Boll. Ist. Sieroter. Milan.*, **34**, 118–122.

De Pamphilis, M. L. (1971). Dissociation and reassembly of *Escherichia coli* outer membrane and of lipopolysaccharide and their reassembly onto flagellar basal bodies. *J. Bacteriol.*, **105**, 1184–1199.

De Venuto, F. (1968). Osmotic fragility and spontaneous lysis of human red cells preserved with addition of progesterone. *Proc. Soc. Exp. Biol. Med.*, **128**, 997–1000.

Fleming, W. A., Stewart-Tull, D. E. S., McClure, S., and McKee, A. (1984). Cellular responsiveness *in vitro*: the effect of mycobacterial glycopeptides, glycolipids and peptidoglycolipids on the *in vitro* growth of haemopoietic colony-forming cells. *Immunology*, **51**, 1–7.

French, V. I., Stark, J. M., and White, R. G. (1970). The influence of adjuvants on the immunological response of the chicken. II. Effects of Freund's complete adjuvant on later antibody production after a single injection of immunogen. *Immunology*, **18**, 645–655.

Galanos, C., Rietschel, E. T., Lüderitz, O., and Westphal, O. (1971). Interaction of lipopolysaccharides and lipid A with complement. *Eur. J. Biochem.*, **19**, 143–152.

Gery, I., Krüger, J., and Spiesel, S. Z. (1972). Stimulation of B lymphocytes by endotoxin. Reactions of thymus-deprived mice and karotypic analysis of dividing cells in mice bearing T6T6 thymus grafts. *J. Immunol.*, **108**, 1088–1091.

Gesner, G. M., and Ginsberg, V. (1964). Effect of glycosidases in the fate of transfused lymphocytes. *Proc. Natl. Acad. Sci. USA*, **52**, 750–755.

Gimber, P. E., and Rafter, G. W. (1969). The interaction of *Escherichia coli* endotoxin with leukocytes. *Arch. Biochem. Biophys.*, **135**, 14–20.

Ginsberg, H. S., Goebel, W. F., and Horsfall, F. L. (1948). The effect of polysaccharides on the reaction between erythrocytes and viruses, with particular reference to mumps virus. *J. Exp. Med.*, **87**, 411–424.

Graham, R. C., Karnovsky, M. J., Shafer, S. W., Glass, E. A., and Karnovsky, M. L. (1967). Metabolic and morphological observations on the effect of surface-active agents of leukocytes. *J. Cell Biol.*, **32**, 629–647.

Greaves, M. F., and Bauminger, S. (1972). Activation of T and B lymphocytes by insoluble phytomitogens. *Nature*, **235**, 67–70.

Greer, C. G., Epps, N. A., and Vail, W. J. (1973). Interaction of lipopolysaccharides with mitochondria. I. Quantitative assay of *Salmonella typhimurium* lipopolysaccharides with isolated mitochondria. *J. Infect. Dis.*, **127**, 551–556.

Grey, H. M., Kubo, R. T., and Cerottini, J. C. (1972). Thymus-derived (T) cell immunoglobulins. Presence of a receptor site for IgG and absence of large amounts of 'buried' Ig determinants on T cells. *J. Exp. Med.*, **136**, 1323–1328.

Hämmerling, U., and Westphal, O. (1967). Synthesis and use of *O*-stearoyl polysaccharides in passive haemagglutination and haemolysis. *Eur. J. Biochem.*, **1**, 46–50.

Hayes, L. (1951). Specific serum agglutination of sheep erythrocytes sensitized with bacterial polysaccharides. *Aust. J. Exp. Biol. Med. Sci.*, **29**, 51–62.

Hill, G. J., and Weiss, D. W. (1964). Relationships between susceptibility of mice to heat-killed *Salmonellae* and endotoxin and the affinity of their red blood cells for killed organisms. In *Bacterial Endotoxins* (Eds. M. Landy and W. Braun), pp.422–427. Institute of Microbiology of Rutgers University.

Hofman, J., and Dlabac, V. (1974). The role of lipid A in phagocytosis of Gram-negative bacteria and their lipopolysaccharides. *J. Hyg. Epidemiol. Microbiol. Immunol.*, **18**, 447–453.

Hohnadel, V., and Stjernholm, R. (1966). The influence of endotoxin on the glucose metabolism of normal human polymorphonuclear leukocytes. *Fed. Proc.*, **25**, 760.

Hudson, L., Sprent, J., Miller, J. F. A. P., and Playfair, J. H. L. (1974). B cell-derived immunoglobulin on activated mouse T lymphocytes. *Nature*, **251**, 60–62.

Jirgensons, B., and Springer, G. F. (1968). Conformation of blood-group and virus receptor glycoproteins from red cells and secretions. *Science*, **162**, 365–367.

Johnson, A. G., Gaines, S., and Landy, M. (1956). Studies on the O antigen of *Salmonella typhosa*. V. Enhancement of antibody response to protein antigens by the purified lipopolysaccharide. *J. Exp. Med.*, **103**, 225–246.

Kagan, I. G. (1955). Haemagglutination after immunization with schistosome antigens. *Science*, **122**, 376–377.

Katz, D. H., and Unanue, E. R. (1973). Critical role of determinant presentation in the induction of specific responses in immunocompetent lymphocytes. *J. Exp. Med.*, **137**, 967–990.

Keogh, E. V., North, E. A., and Warburton, M. F. (1948). Adsorption of bacterial polysaccharides to erythrocytes. *Nature*, **161**, 687–688.

Kimelberg, H. K., and Papahadjopoulos, D. (1971a). Interactions of basic proteins with phospholipid membranes. Binding and changes in the sodium permeability of phosphatidylserine vesicles. *J. Biol. Chem.*, **246**, 1142–1148.

Kimelberg, H. K., and Papahadjopoulos, D. (1971b). Phospholipid–protein interactions: Membrane permeability correlated with monolayer 'penetration'. *Biochim. Biophys. Acta*, **233**, 805–809.

Landy, M. (1954). On haemagglutination procedures utilizing isolated polysaccharide and protein antigens. *Am. J. Public Health*, **44**, 1059–1064.

Landy, M., Trapani, R. J., and Clark, W. R. (1955). Studies on the O antigen of *Salmonella typhosa*. *Am. J. Hyg.*, **62**, 54–65.

Lüderitz, O., Westphal, O., Sievers, K., Kröger, E., Neter, E., and Braun, O. H. (1958). Über die Fixation von P^{32} markiertem Lipopolysaccharide (Endotoxin) aus *Escherichia coli* an menschlichen Erythrocyten. *Biochem. Z.*, **330**, 34–46.

Lüderitz, O., Galanos, C., Lehmann, V., and Rietschel, E. T. (1974). Recent findings on the chemical structure and biological activity of bacterial lipopolysaccharides. *J. Hyg. Epidemiol. Microbiol. Immunol.*, **18**, 381–390.

MacPherson, I. A., Wilkinson, J. F., and Swain, R. H. A. (1953). The effect of *Klebsiella aerogenes* and *Klebsiella cloacae* polysaccharides on haemagglutination by and multiplication of the influenza group of viruses. *Br. J. Exp. Pathol.*, **34**, 603–615.

Madsen, T. (1899). Über Tetanolysin. *Z. Hyg.*, **32**, 214–238.

Mansheim, B. J., Onderdonk, A. B., and Kasper, D. L. (1978). Immunochemical and biologic studies of the lipopolysaccharide of *Bacteroides melaninogenicus* subspecies *asaccharolyticus*. *J. Immunol.*, **120**, 72–78.

Mayer, E. P., Chen, W.-Y., Dray, S., and Teodorescu, M. (1978). The identification of six mouse lymphocyte subpopulations by their natural binding of bacteria. *J. Immunol.*, **120**, 167–173.

McEntegart, M. G. (1952). The application of a haemagglutination technique to the study of *Trichomonas vaginalis* infections. *J. Clin. Pathol.*, **5**, 275–280.

Middlebrook, G. (1955). In *Experimental Tuberculosis. Bacillus and host with an addendum on leprosy* (*Ciba Found. Symp.*, Eds. G. E. W. Wolstenholme, M. P. Cameron assisted by C. M. O'Connor), p.171. London.

Middlebrook, G., and Dubos, R. J. (1948). Specific serum agglutination of erythrocytes sensitized with extracts of tubercle bacilli. *J. Exp. Med.*, **88**, 521–528.

Morgan, W. T. J. (1943). An artificial antigen with blood group A specificity. *Br. J. Exp. Pathol.*, **24**, 41–49.

Munoz, J. (1950). On the value of 'conditioned haemolysis' for the diagnosis of American trypanosomiasis. *O Hospital*, **38**, 685–691.

Neter, E. (1956). Bacterial haemagglutination and haemolysis. *Bacteriol. Rev.*, **20**, 166–188.

Neter, E., and Gorzynski, E. A. (1954). Erythrocyte-modifying capacity of *Shigella dysenteriae* (Shiga) antigen and its polysaccharide component. *Proc. Soc. Exp. Biol. Med.*, **85**, 503–506.

Neter, E., and Zalewski, N. J. (1953). The requirements of electrolytes for the adsorption of *Escherichia coli* antigen by red blood cells. *J. Bacteriol.*, **66**, 424–428.

Neter, E., Bertram, L. F., and Arbesman, C. E. (1952a). Demonstration of *Escherichia coli* O55 and O111 antigens by means of haemagglutination test. *Proc. Soc. Exp. Biol. Med.*, **79**, 255–257.

Neter, E., Zak, D. A., Zalewski, N. J., and Bertram, L. F. (1952c). Inhibition of bacterial (*Escherichia coli*) modification of erythrocytes. *Proc. Soc. Exp. Biol. Med.*, **80**, 607–610.

Neter, E., Bertram, L. F., Zak, D. A., Murdock, M. R., and Arbesman, C. E. (1952b). Studies on haemagglutination and haemolysis by *Escherichia coli* antisera. *J. Exp. Med.*, **96**, 1–15.

Neter, E., Zalewski, N. J., and Zak, D. A. (1953). Inhibition by lecithin and cholesterol of bacterial (*Escherichia coli*) haemagglutination and haemolysis. *J. Immunol.*, **71**, 145–151.

Neter, E., Westphal, O., and Lüderitz, O. (1955). Effects of lecithin, cholesterol and serum on erythrocyte modification and antibody neutralisation by enterobacterial lipopolysaccharides. *Proc. Soc. Exp. Biol. Med.*, **88**, 339–341.

Neter, E., Westphal, O., Lüderitz, O., and Gorzynski, E. A. (1956a). The bacterial haemagglutination test for the demonstration of antibodies to Enterobacteriaceae. *Ann. N.Y. Acad. Sci.*, **66**, 141–156.

Neter, E., Westphal, O., Lüderitz, O., Gorzynski, E. A., and Eichenberger, E. (1956b). Studies of enterobacterial lipopolysaccharides. Effects of heat and chemicals on erythrocyte-modifying, antigenic, toxic and pyrogenic properties. *J. Immunol.*, **76**, 377–385.

Neter, E., Gorzynski, E. A., Zalewski, N. J., Rachman, R., and Gino, R. M. (1954). Studies on bacterial haemagglutination. *Am. J. Pub. Health*, **44**, 49–54.

Norden, A. (1949). Agglutination of sheep's erythrocytes sensitized with histoplasmin. *Proc. Soc. Exp. Biol. Med.*, **70**, 218–220.

Ohkuma, S., and Ikemoto, S. (1966). A sialoglycopeptide liberated from human red cells by treatment with trypsin. *Nature*, **212**, 198–199.

Partridge, S. M., and Morgan, W. T. J. (1940). Immunization experiments with artificial complexes formed from substances isolated from the antigen of *Bact. shigae*. *Br. J. Exp. Pathol.*, **21**, 180–195.

Pavlovski, O., and Springer, G. F. (1967). Lipopolysaccharide receptor from human erythrocytes. *Fed. Proc.*, **26**, 801.

Read, J., and Gunstone, F. D. (1958). *A Textbook of Organic Chemistry*, p.318. Bell, London.

Rees, D. A. (1967). *The Shapes of Molecules*. Oliver and Boyd, Edinburgh, London.

Rietschel, E. T., Gottert, H., Lüderitz, O., and Westphal, O. (1972). Nature and linkages of the fatty acids present in the lipid A component of *Salmonella* lipopolysaccharides. *Eur. J. Biochem.*, **28**, 166–173.

Robineaux, R., and Nelson, R. S. (1955). Etude par la microcinematographie en contraste de phase et a l'accelere du phenomene d'immune adherence et de la phagocytose secondaire. *Ann. Inst. Pasteur*, **89**, 254–256.

Rook, G. A. W., and Stewart-Tull, D. E. S. (1976). The dissociation of adjuvant properties of mycobacterial components from mitogenicity and from the ability to induce the release of mediators from macrophages. *Immunology*, **31**, 389–396.

Roseman, S. (1970). The synthesis of complex carbohydrates by multiglycosyl transferases and their potential function in intercellular adhesion. *Chem. Phys. Lipids*, **5**, 270–276.

Rosenstreich, D. L., Nowotny, A. Chused, T., and Mergenhagen, S. E. (1973). *In vitro* transformation of mouse bone-marrow-derived (B) lymphocytes induced by the lipid component of endotoxin. *Infect. Immun.*, **8**, 406–411.

Schnaitman, C. A. (1971). Effect of ethylenediaminetetra acetic acid, Triton-X100 and lysozyme on the morphology and chemical composition of isolated cell walls of *Escherichia coli*. *J. Bacteriol.*, **108**, 553–563.

Shands, J. W. (1971). Evidence for a bilayer structure in Gram-negative lipopoly-saccharide; Relationship to toxicity. *Infect. Immun.*, **4**, 167–172.

Shands, J. W. (1973). Affinity of endotoxin for membranes. *J. Infect. Dis.*, **128**, S197–S201.

Shands, J. W., Graham, J. A., and Nath, K. (1967). The morphologic structure of isolated bacterial lipopolysaccharide. *J. Mol. Biol.*, **25**, 15–21.

Shinohara, N., and Kern, M. (1976). Differentiation of lymphoid cells: B cell as a direct target and T cell as a regulator in lipopolysaccharide-enhanced induction of immunoglobulin production. *J. Immunol.*, **116**, 1607–1612.

Shockman, G. D., and Wicken, A. J. (Eds.) (1981). *Chemistry and Biological Activities of Bacterial Surface Amphiphiles*. Academic Press, London.

Skillman, R. K., Spurrier, W., Friedman, I. A., and Schwartz, S. O. (1955). Rheumatic fever activity determination by two correlative methods. *Arch. Intern. Med.*, **96**, 51–60.

Sorkin, E., Boyden, S. V., and Rhodes, J. M. (1956). Chemische und biologische Untersuchungen über ein hämosensitin aus *Mycobacterium tuberculosis*. *Helv. Chim. Acta*, **39**, 1684–1697.

Springer, G. F., and Horton, R. E. (1964). Erythrocyte sensitization by blood group specific bacterial antigens. *J. Gen. Physiol.*, **47**, 1229–1250.

Springer, G. F., Nagai, Y., and Teg-Meyer, H. (1966a). Isolation and properties of human blood group NN and meconium-V_G antigens. *Biochemistry*, **5**, 3254–3272.

Springer, G. F., Wang, E. T., Nichols, J. M., and Shear, J. M. (1966b). Relations between bacterial lipopolysaccharide structures and those of human cells. *Ann. N.Y. Acad. Sci.*, **133**, 566–579.

Springer, G. F., Huprikar, S. V., and Neter, E. (1970). Specific inhibition of endotoxin coating of red cells by a human erythrocyte membrane component. *Infect. Immun.*, **1**, 98–108.

Springer, G. F., Adye, J. C., Bezkorovainy, A., and Murthy, J. R. (1973). Functional aspects and nature of the lipopolysaccharide-receptor of human erythrocytes. *J. Infect. Dis.*, **128**, S202–S212.

Steinemann, A., and Läeuger, P. (1971). Interaction of cytochrome c with phospholipid monolayers and bilayer membranes. *J. Membr. Biol.*, **4**, 74–86.

Stewart-Tull, D. E. S., and Wilkinson, P. C. (1973). The affinity of mycobacterial glycopeptides for guinea-pig gamma-2 immunoglobulin and its fragments. *Immunology*, **24**, 205–216.

Stewart-Tull, D. E. S. (1983a). Immunologically important constituents of mycobacteria: Adjuvants. In *Biology of Mycobacteria*, Vol. 2 (Eds. C. Ratledge and J. L. Stanford), pp.3–84. Academic Press, London.

Stewart-Tull, D. E. S. (1983b). Immunopotentiating products of bacteria. In *Medical Microbiology*, Vol. 2, *Immunization Against Bacterial Disease* (Eds. C. S. F. Easmon and J. Jeljaszewicz), pp.1–42. Academic Press, London.

Stewart-Tull, D. E. S., Wilkinson, P. C., and White, R. G. (1965). The affinity of a mycobacterial glycopeptide for guinea-pig gamma-globulin. *Immunology*, **9**, 151–160.

Stewart-Tull, D. E. S., Davies, M., and Jackson, D. M. (1978). The binding of adjuvant active mycobacterial peptidoglycolipids and glycopeptides to mammalian cell membranes and their effect on artificial lipid bilayers. *Immunology*, **34**, 57–67.

Sweet, C., and Zull, J. E. (1970). The binding of serum albumin to phospholipid liposomes. *Biochim. Biophys. Acta*, **219**, 253–262.

Symons, D. B. A., and Clarkson, C. A. (1979). The binding of LPS to the lymphocyte surface. *Immunology*, **38**, 503–508.

Tenney, S. R., and Rafter, G. W. (1968). Leukocyte adenosine triphosphatases and the effect of endotoxin on their activity. *Arch. Biochem. Biophys.*, **126**, 53–58.

Tripodi, D., and Nowotny, A. (1966). Relation of structure to function in bacterial O-antigens. V. Nature of active sites in endotoxic lipopolysaccharides of *Serratia marcescens*. *Ann. N.Y. Acad. Sci.*, **133**, 604–621.

Ulrich, F., and Meier, F. M. (1973). Inhibition of phagocytosis; effects of normal rabbit serum on *E. coli* uptake by rabbit alveolar macrophages. *J. Reticuloendothel. Soc.*, **14**, 8–17.

Unanue, E. R. (1972). The regulatory role of macrophages in antigenic stimulation. *Adv. Immunol.*, **15**, 95–165.

Vitetta, E. S., and Uhr, J. W. (1975a). Immunoglobulin receptors revisited. A model for the differentiation of bone-marrow-derived lymphocytes is described. *Science*, **189**, 964–969.

Vitetta, E. S., and Uhr, J. W. (1975b). Immunoglobulins and alloantigens on the surface of lymphoid cells. *Biochim. Biophys. Acta*, **415**, 253–264.

Vitetta, E. S., Bianco, C., Nussenzweig, V., and Uhr, J. W. (1972). Cell surface immunoglobulin. IV. Distribution among thymocytes, bone-marrow cells and their derived populations. *J. Exp. Med.*, **136**, 81–93.

Vogel, R. A. (1957). Role of lipid in haemagglutination by *Candida albicans* and *Saccharomyces cerevisiae*. *Proc. Soc. Exp. Biol. Med.*, **94**, 279–283.

Vogel, R. A., and Collins, M. E. (1955). Haemagglutination test for detection of *Candida albicans* antibodies in rabbit antiserum. *Proc. Soc. Exp. Biol. Med.*, **89**, 138–140.

Whang, H. Y., Mayer, H., and Neter, E. (1971). Differential effects on immunogenicity and antigenicity of heat, freezing and alkali treatment of bacterial antigens. *J. Immunol.*, **106**, 1552–1558.

White, R. G. (1973). Immunopotentiation by mycobacteria in complete Freund-type adjuvant as the failure of normal immunological homeostasis. In *Immunopotentiation (Ciba Found. Symp.*, No. 18), pp.47–68. Elsevier, Amsterdam.

Wicken, A. J., and Knox, K. W. (1980). Bacterial cell surface amphiphiles. *Biochim. Biophys. Acta*, **604**, 1–26.

Wicken, A. J., and Knox, K. W. (1981). Chemical composition and properties of amphiphiles. In *Chemistry and Biological Activities of Bacterial Surface Amphiphiles* (Eds. G. D. Shockman and A. J. Wicken), pp.1–9. Academic Press, London.

Wilkinson, J. F., Dudman, W. F., and Aspinall, G. O. (1955). The extracellular polysaccharide of *Aerobacter aerogenes*. A3(51) (*Klebsiella* type 54). *Biochem. J.*, **59**, 446–457.

Work, E., Knox, K. W., and Vesk, M. (1966). The chemistry and electron microscopy of an extracellular lipopolysaccharide from *Escherichia coli*. *Ann. N.Y. Acad. Sci.*, **133**, 438–449.

Zimmerman, D. H., Gregory, S., and Kern, M. (1977). Differentiation of lymphoid cells: The preferential binding of the lipid A moiety of lipopolysaccharides to B lymphocyte populations. *J. Immunol.*, **119**, 1018–1023.

Immunology of the Bacterial Cell Envelope
Edited by D. E. S. Stewart-Tull and M. Davies
© 1985 John Wiley & Sons Ltd.

CHAPTER 10

Immunopotentiating Activity of Lipopolysaccharides

Martin Davies

Reproduction Immunology Research Group, Department of Pathology
The Medical School, University of Bristol, Bristol, BS8 1TD, UK

I. INTRODUCTION

The immunopotentiating or adjuvant properties of gram-negative bacteria have been recognized since the discovery that the therapeutic value of vaccines could be enhanced if they were administered in conjunction with certain, suitably killed, gram-negative bacteria. For example, up to five times more tetanus antitoxin could be produced in man if the tetanus toxoid was administered as a mixture with heat-killed *Salmonella typhi* and *S. paratyphi* (MacLean and Holt, 1940). The ability of these bacteria to potentiate immune responses has invariably been found to be associated with the bacterial cell envelope complex termed the lipopolysaccharide (LPS).

Although the majority of studies concerned with the immunopotentiating properties of LPS have centred on their ability to modulate humoral responses, it is now apparent that LPS can also affect the range of responses that are normally associated with the cellular arm of the immune system including antibody-dependent cellular cytotoxicity (ADCC) (Ralph and Nakoinz, 1977a), anti-tumour immunity (Parr *et al.*, 1973; Ribi *et al.*, 1975. Bober *et al.*, 1976)

271

and natural cytotoxicity, possibly related to natural killer (NK) cell activity (Schacter *et al.*, 1981).

Although the well-documented immunopotentiating activity is an intrinsic property of LPS, it was recognized early on that the property was very much dependent on the conditions of administration after it was observed that large amounts of LPS resulted in suppression, rather than stimulation, of the immune system (Condie *et al.*, 1955). Since then it has become apparent that even subtle changes in the conditions of administration of the LPS can have profound consequences on the effectiveness of the component as an immunopotentiator: the dose of LPS, the number, timing and route of injections are all critical (Johnson *et al.*, 1956; Chester *et al.*, 1971; Davies, 1974; Behling and Nowotny, 1977). Using the dose component as an example, Johnson *et al.* (1956) showed that by using a constant dose of ovalbumin and varying the amount of LPS, a straightforward dose–response curve was not produced in NZW rabbits when the serum anti-ovalbumin levels were examined. The serum antibody levels (μg antibody nitrogen per ml) increased from 11 μg ml^{-1} to 215 μg ml^{-1} as the quantity of LPS was increased from 0 μg to 5 μg. However, further increases in the amount of LPS resulted in a decrease in the antibody level, so that 10 μg of LPS produced 167 μg ml^{-1} antibody nitrogen. This dose-dependent variation is not confined to LPS but can be observed with most biological agents that modulate immune responses (Davies, 1983). Hence, in the following account it is particularly important to consider the 'external' conditions used for LPS administration since they will have a significant effect, either favourable or adverse, on the outcome of the intervention with LPS.

The role of LPS as an immunopotentiator, especially of the humoral response, has been thoroughly reviewed elsewhere (Neter, 1971; Morrison and Ryan, 1979). The following represents a brief account of selected examples of LPS-stimulated responses together with an examination of the underlying mechanisms involved, particularly the cell targets and the influence of LPS–membrane interactions on intracellular events.

II. LPS AS A POTENTIATOR OF HUMORAL RESPONSES

The immunopotentiating effect of LPS was studied as far back as 1926 (Ramon and Zoeller, 1926) and after observations with heat-killed microorganisms (MacLean and Holt, 1940), Johnson *et al.* (1956) identified the LPS as the active fraction in *S. typhi-, Escherichia coli-, Pseudomonas aeruginosa-,* and *Proteus vulgaris*-stimulated antibody responses to ovalbumin in NZW rabbits. Under their conditions of administration the antibody response was up to 20 times greater when the antigen was administered in conjunction with LPS compared with the levels obtained with the antigen alone. This basic observation that the addition of LPS to an injection mixture resulted in an enhanced antibody response directed against a defined antigen has now been reported on countless occasions.

Although the LPS does not have to be administered at the same time or at the same site as the antigen, it has emerged that certain conditions of administration have to be satisfied in order for LPS to act as an effective immunopotentiator. The adjuvant effect was observed if the LPS was administered within several days of the antigen challenge. Enhanced antibody responses to human serum albumin (HSA) in NZW rabbits were obtained if the LPS from *S. typhi* was injected at $+6$, $+12$, $+24$ or $+48$ h after the antigen administration, but no potentiating effect could be detected when the LPS was injected at -24, -12, -6, $+72$ or $+96$ h (Kind and Johnson, 1959). Leucke and Sibal (1962) reported a similar phenomenon with *S. abortus equi* LPS in White Rock chickens using bovine serum albumin (BSA) as the antigen. They further demonstrated that the LPS enhanced all phases of the anti-BSA response, so that the period of antibody induction (lag phase) was shortened and the response, which was several times greater than that observed with the antigen alone, persisted for a longer period. These properties, which represent a functional definition of the humoral immunopotentiating activity of LPS, are associated with immunopotentiation studies in general with a wide variety of agents. In NZW rabbits responding to bovine gamma-globulin (BGG), the addition of LPS from *E. coli* O111:B4 shortened the lag phase (the first day antibodies could be detected in the serum by a haemagglutination assay) from 8 days to 4 days. At the same time the titre at the peak response was increased from 2560 to 10 240 (Ward *et al.*, 1959).

In BALB/c mice challenged with trinitrophenol (TNP)-modified homologous erythrocytes (BALB/c RBC), the recipients failed to recognize the non-immunogenic carrier and produced only a poor anti-TNP plaque-forming cell (PFC) response (75 PFC/spleen) (Schmidtke and Dixon, 1972). However, if the TNP–RBC conjugates were injected with *Serratia marcescens* LPS, the combination proved to be extremely immunogenic producing a greater than 100-fold increase in the anti-TNP PFC response (10 981 PFC/spleen). This response was produced following the injection of $10\,\mu g$ LPS per mouse, but if the dose was decreased to $1\,\mu g$ or increased to $100\,\mu g$ then the effect was diminished from the peak response (7871 and 8531 PFC/spleen, respectively).

These *in vivo* effects could also be readily mirrored with the use of *in vitro* cultures. Normal DBA/1 spleen cells cultured in the presence of sheep erythrocytes (SRBC) produced an anti-SRBC response, which peaked at day 6, and which could be increased significantly if *S. typhi* LPS was present during the first 12–24 h of culture. If the LPS was added at other times then no potentiating effect was observed. However, if the spleen cells were incubated with the LPS prior to the addition of the SRBC, then a depressed anti-SRBC response was obtained (Ortiz-Ortiz and Jaroslow, 1970). The LPS effect seemed to coincide with an initial phase of RNA synthesis, seemingly independent of DNA synthesis which was not detected during the first 24 h of culture.

LPS is able to serve as an immunopotentiator of responses involving all the major classes of antibody (IgM, IgG and IgE). For example, in an outbred guinea pig system challenged with ovalbumin (OVA) the day 10 homocytotrophic antibody response was examined (Perni and Mota, 1973). It was observed that the response was mediated by both IgE and IgG_1 antibodies and that the early response (less than 10 days) was LPS dose dependent, with low doses favouring the preferential production of IgE; larger doses or even the antigen alone favoured IgG_1 production. As the response progressed (more than 10 days) the IgG_1 became the predominant antibody class. Although LPS from *S. typhi* was more effective at inducing an IgE response than LPS from either *E. coli* or *Bordetella pertussis*, the low dose preferential production was only obtained if the LPS was injected at the same time as the antigen. If the injection was delayed for 24 h, there was a loss of the preferential IgE production, which was compensated for by increased production of IgG_1, so that the overall response was mediated equally by both classes.

Hence, depending on the conditions of administration, LPS therapy was able to shorten the lag phase of antibody induction, preferentially induce different immunoglobulin classes, increase the total amount of antibody produced and prolong the appearance of the antibodies in the serum. These properties are all concerned with the effect of LPS on the immune response to a specific antigen challenge; however, it has also been observed that LPS can induce antibodies in the absence of any known antigenic stimulus as well as acting as an immunogen itself.

Polyclonal activation of B-cells by LPS was reported by Andersson *et al.* (1972b), who indicated that only IgM-producing cells were induced in mouse spleen in numbers corresponding to the LPS-induced DNA synthesis. The IgM antibody was directed against a wide range of antigens selected randomly and coupled to indicator erythrocytes.

Further work extended this observation and demonstrated that LPS-induced polyclonal activation could be observed in mouse cell cultures independently of T-cells, using cells from a variety of lymphoid tissues including Peyer's patches, lymph nodes, thoracic duct and spleen (Kearney and Lawton, 1975) and, provided that the cell density was low, IgM, IgG_1 and IgG_2 antibody production could be detected (Kearney and Lawton, 1975; Andersson *et al.*, 1978). Further LPS was found to induce the 'characteristic switch' in an antibody response from IgM to IgG production (Van Der Loo *et al.*, 1979). To emphasize the observation that polyclonal B-cell activation by LPS was independent of T-cell influence, Izui *et al.* (1981) demonstrated that LPS from *S. minnesota* R595 induced a prolonged IgM and IgG polyclonal response in athymic nude C57B1/6 (*nu/nu*) mice. In man the polyclonal activation of spleen lymphocytes, but not peripheral blood lymphocytes (PBL), in response to *S. typhi* LPS was also reported with the synthesis of IgG, IgA and IgM. Immunoglobulin production by PBL could be achieved if the cells were preincubated for 24 h

Table 1 The effect of LPS on the humoral response

Lipopolysaccharide species	Animal/antigen	System	Assay	Effect of LPS	Reference
S. typhi	NZW rabbit/ ovalbumin	in vivo	Kjeldahl	Increased serum antibody levels up to 20-fold. LPS dose dependent	Johnson et al., 1956
E. coli O111:B4	NZW rabbit/BGG	in vivo	Haemag- glutination	Increased serum antibody up to 16-fold	Ward et al., 1959
S. typhi	NZW rabbit/HSA	in vivo		Increased serum antibody levels dependent on timing of LPS injection	Kind and Johnson, 1959
S. abortus equi	White Rock chickens/ BSA	in vivo		Several-fold increase in serum antibody levels dependent on timing of LPS injection	Leucke and Sibal, 1962
S. typhi O901	DBA/1 spleens/SRBC	in vitro	PFC	Enhanced peak PFC response dependent on timing of addition of LPS	Ortiz-Ortiz and Jaroslow, 1970
Serratia marcescens	BALB/c mice/TNP– MRBC	in vivo	PFC	Converts non-immuno- genic carrier into effective immunogen, LPS dose dependent	Schmidtke and Dixon, 1972
S. typhi, E. coli B. pertussis	Outbred guinea pigs/ ovalbumin	in vivo	PCA	Increases antibody levels, preferential antibody class production, LPS dose dependent	Perni and Mota, 1973
E. coli O111:B4	A/J mice/HGG or BSA	in vivo	PFC	Increased serum antibody level	Chiller et al., 1973

prior to the exposure to the LPS. The authors interpreted this as either suppressor cell inactivation or the maturation of LPS responding cell populations (Ilfield *et al.*, 1981).

Several reports have been concerned with LPS as an immunogen. In mice it is possible to stimulate both primary and secondary humoral responses, provided that the first injection of LPS was a low dose and that a minimum interval of 10–14 days was observed between the primary and secondary challenge. The heightened secondary response was quantitatively related to the LPS dose in the booster injection (Rudbach, 1971). In Swiss mice which exhibited 'naturally' high titres of bactericidal antibody directed against LPS from *E. coli* O127:B8, it was possible to alter these levels non-specifically with an injection of *Pseudomonas aeruginosa* LPS or specifically with *E. coli* LPS. If the latter was used a linear increase followed by a decline in the anti-*E. coli* LPS PFC response was observed. However, the *Pseudomonas* spp. LPS produced a cyclic pattern to the PFC response, characterized by an initial decline in the levels followed by an enhanced response and subsequent decline (Michael, 1966). Finally, patients suffering from typhoid exhibit an increase in their serum levels of IgG$_1$ IgM and IgA as measured by single radial immunodiffusion with anti-immunoglobulin antisera, as well as increased levels of antibody reactive against *S. typhi* LPS (Tsang *et al.*, 1981).

Under these circumstances the ability of an animal to respond to LPS was dependent on the 'history' of that animal. Kiyono *et al.* (1980) reported that conventional BALB/c mice responded to an injection of *E. coli* K235 LPS with an anti-LPS response that peaked at day 14 and then declined over the next 2 weeks. The animals were found to respond in this manner over the fairly limited dose range of 10–100 µg. However, germ-free animals (caesarian-derived) responded over a broader dose range, including much lower doses, 0.1–500 µg, and the response peaked at 4 weeks and was in general greater than that observed in the conventional animals. *E. coli* K235-monoassociated BALB/c mice (i.e. germ-free mice in which *E. coli* K235 was introduced into the drinking water) gave an intermediate response.

The effect of LPS on the humoral response is summarized in Table 1 by means of a few selected examples.

III. LPS AS A POTENTIATOR OF CELL-MEDIATED RESPONSES

There is now considerable evidence available to indicate that LPS is able to potentiate a variety of phenomena that are manifestations of the cellular arm of the immune system, e.g. anti-tumour immunity (Parr *et al.*, 1973; Bober *et al.*, 1976; Schacter *et al.*, 1981).

One of the earliest recognized forms of interaction between LPS and cellular activity associated with the immune system was the ability of the polysaccharide to act as a stimulant of the reticuloendothelial system, which resulted in increased

Table 2 The effect of LPS on anti-tumour immunity

Lipopolysaccharide species	Animal/tumour system	Effect of LPS	Reference
S. marcescens O8	A/HeHa mouse/TA3-HA spontaneous mammary adenocarcinoma *in vivo*	Tumour rejected if LPS injected prior to tumour challenge	Groshman and Nowotny,
Shigella spp., S. minnesota S lipid A	DBA/2 mouse/lymphoma L5178Y *in vivo* and peritoneal macrophages *in vitro*	Non-specific cytotoxicity generated	Alexander and Evans, 1971
Salmonella spp. (Re mutants)	Sewall-Wright strain 2 guinea-pigs/line 10 hepatocarcinoma	Enhanced tumour rejection when injected IL in combination with cord factor from BCG	Ribi *et al.*, 1975
E. coli	W/Fu rat spleen cells/gross virus-induced lymphoma (C58NT)D	Enhances non-specific cytotoxicity and ADCC activity	Glaser *et al.*, 1976
E. coli	BALB/c mouse/mineral oil-induced 315 PCT	Tumour rejected if LPS injected prior to tumour challenge and continuous therapy	Bober *et al.*, 1976
S. typhi WO901	Macrophage cell line RAW264/ lymphoma EL4	Enhanced ADCC activity in the presence of specific antibody	Ralph and Nakoinz, 1977a
S. typhi O901	BALB/c mouse/syngeneic B-cell tumour BCL1	No effect on tumour, but mice showed increased susceptibility to lethal effects of LPS	Muirhead *et al.*, 1981

non-specific phagocytosis (Nowotny, 1969; Neter, 1971). It was suggested that this property of LPS was the basis of its immunopotentiating activity (Biozzi *et al.*, 1955; Rubenstein *et al.*, 1962). Since these observations LPS has been found to potentiate several cellular immune functions of which the most studied is its ability to promote tumour rejection. The main body of evidence is summarized in Table 2.

The effectiveness of LPS against tumour challenges is dependent on the same basic rules of administration as observed for the LPS-induced potentiation of antibody responses. For example, the timing of the LPS injection affected its efficacy against tumours implanted at different sites. Using BALB/c mice challenged with a mineral oil-induced 315 plasma cell tumour (PCT), Bober *et al.* (1976) found that their immunotherapeutic regimen (*E. coli* O55:B5 LPS) was effective against tumours implanted subcutaneously only if an LPS injection prior to the tumour challenge was incorporated into the regimen. This condition of LPS pretreatment did not apply if the PCT was implanted intraperitoneally. Similarly, the protection of A/HeHa mice with *Serratia marcescens* O8 LPS against a challenge with a spontaneous mammary adenocarcinoma, TA3-Ha, required that the LPS was injected prior to the tumour challenge. The TA3 tumour, which was found to be weakly immunogenic but lethal to mice, was rendered an effective immunogen by the prior injection of the LPS (Grohsman and Nowotny, 1972).

The efficacy of the LPS treatment could be significantly increased if the LPS was incorporated into a combined therapy programme. In Sewall-Wright strain 2 guinea pigs challenged intradermally with a lethal dose of line 10 hepatocarcinoma, a 90% cure rate could be achieved if the LPS was administered in combination with trehalose mycolate (cord factor) from *Bacillus Calmette-Guérin* and injected intradermally; the cure rate was greater than the rate achieved with either of the components alone, and the combined therapy allowed for the treatment of well-established tumours (Ribi *et al.* 1975). In these experiments the most successful LPS preparations were obtained from the rough strains of *Salmonella* (*Re* mutants).

The ability to affect well-established tumours is regarded as the exception in trials with immunotherapeutic agents, although Parr *et al.* (1973) previously reported this effect with LPS. Parr *et al.* (1973) demonstrated that DBA/2 mice could successfully resist the growth of a syngeneic lymphoma (L5178Y) if the LPS was injected intralesionally some time after the tumour was established. In their system the LPS was ineffective if administered at the time of the tumour challenge. Although the authors postulated that the LPS effect could be due to the direct damage of the blood vasculature of the tumour, they also observed that the beneficial effect was abrogated in anti-lymphocyte serum (ALS) immunosuppressed mice, indicating that the immune system was somehow involved.

The anti-tumour effect of LPS could also be demonstrated quite successfully *in vitro* using cultures of isolated lymphoid cells. In general the cultures generated a form of non-specific immunity that was active against a wide range of tumour cell lines. Non-immune spleen cells from C57B1 mice became cytotoxic against a DBA/2 lymphoma, L5178Y, following incubation with LPS. After 48 h in culture with LPS the spleen cells produced up to 70% inhibition of tumour growth that was dependent on a subpopulation of spleen cells that were adherent to glass surfaces, sensitive to anti-macrophage serum (AMS) and resistant to anti-Thy.1 serum and complement (Grant and Alexander, 1974). Cytotoxicity against the L5178Y lymphoma (and the SL2 lymphoma) could also be generated in syngeneic DBA/2 peritoneal macrophage cell cultures by incubation with either *Shigella* spp. LPS or lipid A, prepared by acid hydrolysis of LPS from *S. minnesota* S (Alexander and Evans, 1971). This effect was also achieved *in vivo*. Similar effects were observed in rat cell cultures. Normal W/Fu rat spleens were rendered cytotoxic against Gross virus induced lymphoma, (C58NT)D, by prior incubation with LPS. This non-specific activity was independent of T-cells but required the presence of macrophages. At the same time LPS was found to augment antibody-dependent cellular cytotoxicity (ADCC) of the normal spleen cells against (C58NT)D (Glaser *et al.*, 1976). Throughout the culture experiments the LPS effect seemed to be dependent on the presence of macrophages and this was reflected in the observation that LPS could exert a direct cytostatic effect on monocytic and histiocytic tumour cell lines while having no effect on myelomas, T-lymphomas and mastocytomas (Ralph and Nakoinz, 1977b).

The increased ADCC activity has also been a consistent finding although Ralph and Nakoinz (1977a) found that the activity mediated by macrophages and directed against erythrocyte targets could be increased by *S. typhi* WO901, LPS, but no similar increase was observed against tumour targets. In man the weak spontaneous cell-mediated cytotoxicity of PBL observed against a non-B-cell lymphoblastoid cell line (CCRF-CEM) was elevated in the presence of *E. coli* O26:B6 LPS. This activity was mediated by both adherent and non-adherent cells and an increased binding of the non-adherent cells to the target cells was observed. Concomitant with this increased activity was an elevation in the natural cytotoxicity directed against K562 target cells, and possibly mediated by natural killer (NK) cells (Schacter *et al.*, 1981).

Although beneficial effects of LPS on tumour growth have been consistently observed, there are a few reports dealing with deleterious effects following LPS administration. For example, Muirhead *et al.*, (1981) found that the susceptibility of BALB/c mice to the lethal action of LPS (endotoxin) was increased ten-fold if the animals were challenged with a syngeneic B-cell tumour (BCL1). The increased susceptibility paralleled tumour growth in the liver and spleen and manifested itself 2–3 weeks after the tumour implant. The authors suggested several possible explanations for this phenomenon including the tumour-induced elevation in release of prostaglandins by macrophages which may be involved in endotoxic shock.

Finally, LPS has been observed to affect one of the definitive forms of the manifestations of the cellular arm of the immune system, i.e. delayed-type hypersensitivity (DTH). Studies have demonstrated that LPS is able to affect both the afferent and efferent arms of the response depending on the time of the LPS injection relative to that of the antigen challenge. Lagrange *et al.* (1975) found that 1×10^8 SRBC sensitized specific pathogen free CD-1 mice to respond to a subsequent footpad challenge with the specific antigen. The response peaked 4 days after sensitization. If the LPS (*S. enteritidis*) was injected prior to the sensitizing dose of SRBC, an increase in the anti-SRBC antibody response was obtained, which corresponded to a depression in the T-cell-mediated activity, i.e. the footpad swelling. Although LPS caused hyperplasia in the reticuloendothelial system, with a subsequent reduction in the effective immunogenic dose of SRBC, the authors considered that the reduction in the DTH activity was due to the premature inhibition of the T-cell response by the accelerated production of antibodies causing an earlier onset in the inhibitory mechanisms which regulate the T-cell response. To a certain extent this postulate was confirmed by the fact that cyclophosphamide, a B-cell inhibitor, was able to abolish the LPS-induced suppression of DTH, although cyclophosphamide has also been implicated with suppressor cell activity. Lagrange and Mackaness (1975) studied the effect of LPS on the efferent arm of the response following the injection of the SRBC into the specific pathogen free CD-1 mice. If LPS was injected into the draining lymph node 24–72 h after sensitization, the swelling response was considerably enhanced. The authors examined other injection schedules and found that the relationship between the induction and expression of DTH and LPS was complex. LPS caused DTH to appear transiently if the SRBC were administered in a T-cell blocking dose (1×10^9 SRBC), while injection of LPS at the height of the response produced a short-lived and reversible suppression of the DTH reaction.

Hence, LPS has been shown to affect a wide variety of cellular activities. However, since current evidence has revealed that antibody plays a central role in the induction and expression of cellular activity, it is unclear whether the LPS affects the cells directly or controls them through its influence on antibody expression. For instance, under the conditions where LPS acted as an *in vivo* anti-tumour agent, it is uncertain whether LPS acts by directly enhancing the anti-tumour cytotoxic cell activity or whether it acts by suppressing the production of blocking factor antibody, which could result in a seemingly enhanced cellular response and the destruction of the tumour.

IV. CELLULAR TARGETS OF LPS

The preceding sections have indicated that under the appropriate conditions LPS can stimulate the whole range of responses associated with the immune system. However, it is unclear whether the diversity of action is a result of LPS interacting with all the different cell types of the immune system (T-cells, B-cells, macrophages, K-cells and NK-cells), or if it is because of the direct interaction between LPS and a 'common denominator' type of cell, involved as a basic component of all the different types of immune responses.

It has long been understood that LPS is able to interact physically with the plasma membranes of a wide variety of mammalian cells including erythrocytes, thymocytes, spleen cells, bone marrow cells and macrophages (see Chapter 9). It has been postulated that the LPS is able to insert itself into the lipid bilayer of these membranes. However, despite this seemingly wide choice of cellular targets, the interactions with the lymphocytes and the macrophages are of prime importance (Davies and Stewart-Tull, 1981).

However, the majority of reports have indicated that LPS affects a wide spectrum of immunocompetent cells rather than a single type, although this statement probably reflects the nature of the scientific inquiries rather than a biological mechanism. In reality, LPS quantitatively affects the results of assays for specific cells including B-cells (Schmidtke and Dixon, 1972; Sultzer and Nilsson, 1972; Skidmore *et al.*, 1975), T-cells (Allison and Davies, 1971; Hamaoka and Katz, 1973; Shinohara and Kern, 1976; Norcross and Smith, 1977), K-cells (Forman and Möller, 1973), NK-cells (Schacter *et al.*, 1981) and macrophages (Nowotny, 1969; Grant and Alexander, 1974).

A large body of evidence, especially from the earlier studies, showed that the B-cell was the prime target for LPS. This statement was supported by evidence which demonstrated that LPS was a potent B-cell mitogen, a polyclonal B-cell activator and that it could function as a T-independent antigen (Skidmore *et al.*, 1975; Chiller *et al.*, 1973). Further, it was observed that LPS was able to reverse tolerance to human gamma-globulin (HGG) in responder mouse strains, even in the presence of suppressor T-cells (Louis *et al.*, 1973; Skidmore *et al.*, 1976), but was unable to effect tolerance reversal to HGG in C3H/HeJ mice, which are known to have an autosomal gene defect. This results in the lack of expression of a B-cell membrane component whose function has been postulated to be related to their interaction with LPS (Sultzer and Nilsson, 1972; Watson and Riblet, 1974, 1975; Coutinho *et al.*, 1975; Skidmore *et al.*, 1975). Finally, LPS was shown to be able to bypass the requirement for helper T-cells, by enhancing anti-hapten responses in mice when the hapten was presented on a non-immunogenic carrier (Schmidtke and Dixon, 1972; Hoffmann *et al.*, 1977).

The involvement of LPS with B-cells has now been demonstrated on several occasions by techniques of *in vivo* depletion and reconstitution or by the use of the genetic matrix of the inbred mouse strains. Jones and Kind reported in 1972 that BD_1 mice, lethally irradiated (1000 Rad), could produce an antibody response to a subsequent challenge with SRBC if the animals were reconstituted with thymocytes and bone marrow cells. The reconstituted response required both T- and B-cells. However, the authors reported that anti-SRBC responses could also be obtained if the animals were reconstituted with B-cells mixed with LPS from *S. typhi*. The LPS was able to replace T-cell function in the antibody reponse, even after the bone marrow cells were treated with anti-theta serum and complement, although this procedure could not be guaranteed to have removed all the T-cell precursors. A similar finding that LPS was able to bypass the helper T-cell effect and exert its influence directly on B-cells was also reported by Schmidtke and Dixon (1972), who used a different experimental approach. They observed that BALB/c mice were unable to generate an effective anti-TNP PFC response (75 PFC/spleen) if the hapten was injected coupled to a non-immunogenic carrier, i.e. BALB/c erythrocytes, which failed to be recognized by the T-cell system. However, a concurrent injection of *S. marcescens* LPS with the hapten-carrier conjugate stimulated the generation of an effective anti-hapten response (10 981 PFC/spleen).

Further if the hapten (TNP) was directly coupled to *E. coli* O111:B4 LPS and injected into C57B1/6 mice, an anti-TNP response was generated which upon rechallenge exhibited the characteristics of a secondary anamnestic antibody response, i.e. the response was produced faster and was mediated by antibodies of the IgG class. The generation of B-cell memory, as expressed by the IgG production, did not require functional T-cells since the same response could be obtained in lethally irradiated mice reconstituted with T-depleted spleen cells (Motta *et al.*, 1981). The secondary response, 15 times greater than the predominantly IgM primary response, could also be generated *in vitro* in T-depleted spleen cell cultures. Hence the interaction of bone marrow derived cells with LPS, independently of T-cell influence, leads not only to the differentiation of B-cells into antibody forming cells (AFC) but also into memory cells.

Similarly, Campbell *et al.* (1966) directly examined the influence of the thymus upon the antibody response to BGG in CBA mice. In intact animals, by the use of *S. typhi* LPS, an enhanced anti-BGG response was obtained which was mediated by 7 S immunoglobulin. The rate of antigen elimination and the antibody titre was the same in adult sham-thymectomized or in thymectomized mice. Neonatal thymectomy, however, did reduce the antibody production and perhaps indicated a role for the thymus, other than the supply of mature T-cells in the development of lymphoid cells of bone marrow origin. Contrary to this, however, Scibienski and Gershwin (1977) found that poor responses to lysozyme–LPS (from *S. enteritidis*) conjugates were obtained in thymectomized CBA mice, unless they were reconstituted with splenic T-cells. In a further experiment, however, they found that N:NIH(S) (*nu/nu*) mice responded as well as normal +/*nu* animals. Although this seemingly contradicted their earlier result, the response in both *nu/nu* and +/*nu* animals was severely depressed by treatment with anti-lymphocyte serum (ALS). The effect of ALS on the *nu/nu* animals appears anomalous, but Scheid *et al.* (1973) have reported the appearance of theta-positive cells in nude mice following an injection of LPS. The involvement of T-cells in LPS-influenced antibody responses was also reported by Uchiyama and Jacobs (1978). They found that the anti-TNP response in C57Bl/6 spleens following a challenge with TNP–SRBC and *E. coli* O55:B5 LPS was controlled by two T-cell subpopulations, one of which exerted a helper effect and the other a suppressive effect. The helper cells were characterized as Thy.1$^+$, radioresistant and non-adherent to nylon wool, while the suppressor cells were Thy.1$^+$, radiosensitive and nylon wool adherent.

In cultures of lymphoid cells, the LPS-induced proliferation, characterized by the incorporation into the cells of radiolabelled thymidine, was attributed solely to the stimulation of the B-cell population, with no direct action on T-cells (Gery *et al.*, 1972b). Further, Andersson *et al.* (1972a) found that *E. coli* O55:B5 LPS was unable to exert a mitogenic effect on normal thymocytes, cortisone-treated thymocytes or educated peripheral T-cells, but was able to stimulate DNA synthesis, to equal degrees, in normal spleen cells, anti-Thy.1-treated spleen cells, spleen cells from athymic nude mice and normal bone marrow cells. The mitogenic activity of *E. coli* O111:B4 LPS was attributable to the lipid A fraction, which acted as a mitogen for splenic B-cells from athymic nude mice but not for thymocytes from normal animals (Chiller *et al.*, 1973). Similarly, Bruynzeel *et al.* (1978) found that the *E. coli* LPS mitogenic activity could be detected in spleen cell populations from BALB/c mice and from athymic nude B10.LP (*nu/nu*) animals; the levels of stimulation were similar in each population. However, recent evident has demonstrated by the analysis of spleen cell growth, at different cell densities in response to *E. coli* O55:B5 LPS, that there is a requirement for cell–cell interaction, with the cell–LPS interaction not exhibiting single-hit kinetics (Wetzel and Kettman, 1981).

The polyclonal activation of B-cells by LPS to induce antibody formation also exhibited characteristics which suggested an independence from T-cell influence. In C57Bl/6 (*nu/nu*) athymic nude mice low levels of IgG$_1$ and IgG$_{2a}$ are found in the serum which by treatment with *S. minnesota* LPS can be elevated as a result of polyclonal activation, so that the levels are similar to control values found in normal mice (Izui *et al.*, 1981). However, Goodman and Weigle (1981) found that B-cell polyclonal activation by *E. coli* O55:B5 LPS was regulated by T-cells which exerted both helper and suppressor influences. The activation of C3H/HeN B-cells by LPS could be enhanced if low numbers of T-cells were added to the cultures. In normal spleens the T:B ratio was at an optimum level to observe this helper effect, with any suppressive activity being non-existent or at such low levels as to be undetectable. This helper effect was mediated by Lyt 1$^+$23$^-$ T-cells. However, if the T:B ratio was increased significantly then a suppression of the polyclonal response to LPS was observed. This suppression could also be detected in splenic T-cells activated by concanavalin A. If unstimulated spleens cell suspensions were subjected to ultrasonication, then the sonicate contained two factors: one, 15–23 kDa, was derived from Lyt 1^+23^- T-cells and exerted the helper effect; the second factor, 68–84 kDa, came from Lyt 1^-23^+ T-cells, and produced the suppressive effect.

In A/J mice challenged with HGG, the antibody response was abrogated if the animals were previously thymectomized and reconstituted with anti-theta serum and complement-treated bone marrow cells. The response was restored either by adding syngeneic thymocytes to the reconstitution mixture or by adding LPS from *E. coli* O111:B4 Chiller and Weigle, 1973). They found that in normal intact A/J mice it was possible to induce tolerance in the animals by an injection of the monomeric, deaggregated, form of HGG. For the first 25 days after the tolerizing injection, the tolerant state was maintained solely by B-cells, while after 50–60 days the condition was maintained by T-cells. If HGG, in an immunogenic form, was injected alone or in combination with *E. coli* LPS during the first 25 days of the tolerant state, no antibody response was observed, i.e. LPS was unable to break B-cell-maintained tolerance. However, if the injection was delayed for 50 days, the T-cell-maintained tolerant state was broken in the presence of LPS, and an anti-HGG response was induced.

Despite the evidence that the B-cell is the primary target for LPS action, there are reports in the literature which implicate other cells, especially T-cells and macrophages.

The mitogenic effect seen with LPS on thymus-derived cells has either been extremely low or has been attributable to an indirect action. Gery and Waksman (1972) found that the stimulation of T-cells was dependent on the presence of adherent cells in the culture, which were stimulated by the LPS to produce a lymphocyte activating factor (LAF). Further, using CBA/J mice that were thymectomized, irradiated and reconstituted, Gery *et al.* (1972b) found that reconstitution with bone marrow cells resulted in the recipient's splenic response being normal to *E. coli* O55:B5 LPS but depressed when the mitogens used were phytohaemagglutinin (PHA) and concanavalin A. However, if the animals were reconstituted with a mixture of bone marrow cells and thymocytes, that carried the T6T6 chromosome marker, then 1.2% of the splenic cells responding to LPS, by increased DNA synthesis, were of thymic origin. Further, Mizuguchi *et al.* (1980) found that thymocytes responded well to PHA if the cells were precultured for up to 24 h in the presence of LPS. The response was poor if fresh cells or cells precultured in the absence of LPS were substituted. In all cases the kinetics and the PHA dose–response profiles were unaltered. The LPS effect was, however, strain dependent, being present in BALB/c.Cr, AKR/Jms and DDD/1 mice and absent from C3H/HeJms and C57B1/6J animals.

With the hapten–carrier model, Newburger *et al.* (1974) demonstrated that LPS from *E. coli* O26:B6 appeared to exert an influence on the carrier-primed helper T-cells, rather than on the hapten-primed B-cells. In their basic model, BALB/c recipient mice were lethally irradiated and reconstituted with syngeneic spleen cells from donors primed with a 2,4-dinitrophenyl conjugate of *Ascaris* protein (DNP–ASC). The reconstituted recipients were then challenged with a DNP–ASC and LPS mixture. The secondary anti-DNP response was under adjuvant control, being mediated by IgE and IgG antibodies, of which the former seemed to be more sensitive to the enhancing effects of LPS. The authors took this procedure a step further to determine which primed population the LPS acted on. In all cases the irradiated recipients were first reconstituted with DNP–ASC-primed syngeneic spleen cells. If they were challenged with DNP–ovalbumin (DNP–OVA) conjugates alone or in combination with LPS, no anti-DNP response of either class could be detected. In the absence of carrier-primed T-cells, LPS failed to elicit a response. However, if the reconstituted recipients were also injected with spleen cells from donors primed with OVA, then upon subsequent challenge with DNP–OVA and LPS, an enhanced secondary response mediated by both IgE and IgG was observed, and was LPS dose dependent. Hence LPS was able to exert its effect only in the presence of carrier-primed cells, indicating an involvement of the LPS with T-cells. Finally, an increased response upon challenge with DNP–OVA was also observed in those recipients which were reconstituted with DNP–ASC-primed spleen cells and with spleen cells from donors primed with OVA and LPS.

LPS is also a well-known stimulant of macrophage activity (Nowotny, 1969; Neter, 1971). The identification of the macrophage as a target for LPS has been derived from studies which have demonstrated increased levels of phagocytosis and lysosomal enzymes (Jenkin and Palmer, 1960; Weiner and Levanon, 1968) and the inhibition of tumour growth (Grant and Alexander, 1974; Glaser *et al.* 1976) following the exposure of macrophages to LPS.

The cytotoxicity directed against tumour targets was found to be mediated by cells that were sensitive to anti-macrophage serum and complement but were resistant to treatment with anti-Thy.1 serum and complement (Grant and Alexander, 1974). W/Fu rat spleen cells, that exerted non-specific cytotoxicity against a lymphoma, (C58NT)D, following incubation with LPS, also depended on macrophages for the expression of this activity; the activity was independent of T-cells (Glaser *et al.*, 1976). Besides this direct cytotoxic activity, Ralph and Nakoinz (1977a) reported that the macrophage cell line RAW 264 exhibited a 70–80% increase in ADCC activity against erythrocyte targets following exposure to *S. typhi* WO901 LPS. These cells, however, showed no evidence of increased phagocytosis or increased ADCC activity directed against tumour targets. This increased form of ADCC activity induced by LPS was also attributed to cells other than macrophages, probably K-cells, which were non-adherent, non-phagocytic and bore receptors for the Fc region of immunoglobulin (FcR^+) and had immunoglobulin on their surface (SIg^+) (Forman and Möller, 1973).

A final cell type that has been reported as a target for LPS action is the natural killer (NK)-cell. Shacter *et al.* (1981) found that the spontaneous cell-mediated cytotoxicity of human PBL against the 'standard' K562 target cell could be elevated from 30% to 50% at an attacking cell-to-target cell ratio of 12.5:1 if *E. coli* O26:B6 LPS was added to the assay medium. If the target was changed to CCRF-CEM, a non-B lymphoblastoid cell line, the activity, mediated by both adherent and non-adherent cells, was markedly elevated by the addition of LPS, from 1% to 16% at a 25:1 ratio.

Hence the primary cellular target for LPS would appear to be B-cells and macrophages, depending on the conditions of the experiment. However, there is also enough experimental evidence to indicate that under the appropriate circumstances LPS can interact with T-cells and possibly K- and NK-cells.

V. MECHANISM OF ACTION OF LPS AS AN IMMUNOPOTENTIATOR

As with other types of biological immunopotentiators, such as Freund's adjuvant or BCG, the exact mechanism by which LPS enhances immune responses still remains to be determined. From an examination of the evidence concerned with the cellular targets, it could be argued that LPS exerts its influence by directly activating B-cells and/or possibly macrophages. However, although this 'simple' direct interaction could be postulated, LPS, or endotoxin, has been observed to affect many physiological processes so that the mechanism of the LPS adjuvant action is certainly more complex.

From the early work, several mechanisms of action were postulated. Unlike Freund's adjuvant, LPS does not act either by local proliferation of the cells at the injection site or by a depot effect, since the injection of LPS does not have to be concurrent with that of the antigen (Leucke and Sibal, 1962; Freedman *et al.*, 1967). However, the distribution and retention of the antigen could still be influenced by haemodynamic changes caused by the LPS, since *B. pertussis* LPS or *S. enteritidis* LPS increased vascular permeability in CFW mice as measured by the disappearance of Evans Blue dye from the circulation (Munoz, 1961). A related feature is also the ability of LPS to cause a redistribution of lymphoid cells, with decreased lymph node and increased splenic localization (Freitas and De Sousa, 1976). Cohen *et al.* (1964) postulated a further mechanism based on the non-specific ability of LPS to break tolerance. They suggested that this ability exerted an influence in immunopotentiation by making available more cells responsive to the antigen. Watson *et al.* (1973) proposed that LPS acted by supplying the 'second signal' to B-cells, bypassing the need for helper T-cells, while Nakano *et al.* (1973) thought that LPS might facilitate the cooperation between the thymus-derived antigen reactive cells (ARC) and the bone marrow-derived antigen sensitive cells (ASC). In 1963, Talmage and Pearlman postulated that complement, might act as an inhibitor of cell division, which led Pearlman *et al.* (1963) to put forward the hypothesis that the fixation (inactivation) of complement by LPS could be a vital step in the adjuvant action of the polysaccharide. Further, several authors advanced the postulate that LPS caused cellular damage, similar to Freund's adjuvant, with the subsequent release of oligonucleotides, which were known to enhance immune responses (Jaroslow, 1960; Plescia and Braun, 1968), while others proposed that the cellular damage, especially to the adrenal gland and the liver, released enzymes (e.g. beta-glucuronidase, cathepsin) or possibly hormones that exerted an effect on the immune system (Havens, 1959; Weissman and Thomas, 1962). Finally, Solliday *et al.* (1967) proposed that LPS overcame the immunosuppressive effects of antibody by modulating the feedback inhibition mechanisms. Hence, while some of these mechanisms suggested that LPS acted directly on the cells of the immune system, others proposed that the LPS affected the immune system indirectly following interaction with other types of cells.

Since these early observations and postulates, several complex studies involving either the interaction between LPS and cells, or the genetic control of LPS responsiveness and factor production, have been attempted and a series of hypotheses have emerged from them. In the following section some of these studies will be examined in more detail.

Since 1971 it has been considered that LPS acted by replacing the need for the helper T-cell effect in the generation of humoral responses, by interacting directly with the precursors of the antibody producing cells, supplying a 'signal' which was recognized by the B-cells and which induced and directed antibody formation.

Specific antibody production by B-cells in response to many antigens (T-dependent) is under the control of two signals, one derived from the antigen itself and the other from the specialist helper T-cells. Involvement of the T-cells and their 'helper signal' is vital to ensure that an adequate antibody response is generated and that the 'switch' is made to the appropriate antibody class. It was proposed that LPS was able to replace or 'mimic' this T-cell function without affecting either the quality or the quantity of the resulting antibody response (Jones and Kind, 1972; Schmidtke and Dixon, 1972; Motta *et al.*, 1981).

The interaction of LPS with the B-cells, in its T-cell replacing role, led to the proposal of two hypotheses of the mechanism to account for the observed events; these are termed the 'one-signal' and the 'two signal' hypotheses.

The supporters of the one-signal hypothesis proposed that the LPS supplied a mitogenic signal to the cells, which resulted in the differentiation of the precursor cells into antibody-forming cells (AFC). In this model the surface immunoglobulin (SIg) receptors acted passively as focusing devices to localize antigen on the specific cells. In support of this, Coutinho *et al.* (1974) examined anti-hapten (4-hydroxy-3,5-dinitrophenol, NNP) responses in spleen cell cultures of A strain mice in the presence of *E. coli* O55:B5 LPS. When NNP–LPS was used as the immunogenic stimulus, polyclonal activation, as well as the induction of anti-NNP responses, resulted. However, the induction of a specific anti-NNP response required a concentration of NNP–LPS that was several orders of magnitude lower than the concentration required for polyclonal activation. At higher concentrations, optimal for polyclonal activation, the NNP-specific cells were paralysed. This paralysis could be abolished, and specific activation take place, if free hapten was added to the cultures. Further, they found that if free hapten was added initially to the cultures, no specific or non-specific activation of the B-cells could be detected, even though the NNP could be found bound to the spleen cells. If an optimum concentration of NNP–LPS was added, activation resulted. This suggested that the activation was due to one non-specific signal, produced by the mitogenic properties of the LPS, which meant that the surface receptors responsible for triggering the cells were not the surface immunoglobulin molecules which were presumably occupied by the free hapten determinants.

If this model is relevant in the context of LPS as an immunopotentiator then several assumptions and conclusions must be made. If at low concentrations of the hapten–LPS complex specific activation takes place, then presumably the complex is bound preferentially by specific cells so that the surface 'triggering concentration' reaches an optimum on these cells compared with the non-specific cells. At high concentrations the polyclonal activation observed would imply that direct LPS–cell membrane interactions take place involving non-specific cells. In terms of an *in vivo* model for immunopotentiation, since the LPS does not have to be injected at the same time or at the same site as the antigen, in order to be effective as an adjuvant there has to be an *in vivo* mechanism by which either LPS–antigen or LPS–antigenic determinant complexes are formed directly or via an intermediary carrier such as an accessory cell or macrophage. This would ensure that LPS contact with the hapten specific cells results, which in turn would lead to specific B-cell activation. In this model the potentiation of a specific response by LPS is dependent on the ability of the hapten units to 'guide' the LPS to the hapten-sensitive B-cells.

The two-signal hypothesis, which is equally complex, proposed that there are two independent signals involved in the activation of specific B-cells. One is supplied by the interaction between the SIg and the antigenic determinants and the other is supplied by the LPS through an interaction of the multiple repeating determinants of the polysaccharide with surface receptors; this latter signal would normally be supplied by T-cells. Watson *et al.* (1973) examined the antibody response to SRBC in spleen cell cultures from C57B1/6 (*nu/nu*) mice. In control cultures they found that no anti-SRBC response could be detected with SRBC alone and only a poor response with *S. typhi* WO901 LPS in the absence of SRBC (less than 200 PFC/culture). However, if the LPS and the SRBC were combined, the response increased to 3000–4000 PFC/culture. Hence it was established that LPS stimulated an antibody response which was independent of T-cell influence. They extended this basic model and replaced the SRBC with a TNP-derivative (2,3,4-trinitrophenylleucyltyrosine; TNP–Leu–Tyr). This molecule was considered too small to interact with more than one receptor combining site at a time, which meant that it could not participate in the normal cooperative interactions required for the induction of antibody synthesis. They found that anti-TNP responses could be stimulated in *nu/nu* spleen cell cultures in the presence of LPS. Lipid A, prepared from the LPS, produced the same result. The authors proposed two explanations for this finding and favoured the second one. First, they suggested that the TNP–Leu–Tyr bound non-specifically to the LPS and the TNP–Leu–Tyr–LPS complex presented an immunogenic array of TNP units to the antigen receptors on the APC precursors. This arrangement and density of the 'cross-linked' TNP units was such that a specific activation of the B-cells resulted. This was an explanation of the results based on a variant of the one-signal hypothesis. However, their second, favoured, explanation proposed that since the LPS and the TNP–Leu–Tyr were uncoupled, i.e. physically separate, then the TNP–Leu–Tyr concentrated at the cell surface by interaction with specific SIg receptors and transmitted a transmembrane signal as did the LPS which was independently held on the surface membrane of the precursor APC by an LPS receptor. Both signals were needed for induction. This represents the two-signal hypothesis. Trenkner (1974) extended these ideas with BALB/c spleen cell cultures and DNP or TNP conjugates and compared their activation in the presence of LPS or alloreactive T-cells. The results were similar to the earlier work with the activated cells in the splenic cultures being of B-cell origin; these data were interpreted in terms of the two-signal hypothesis. However, it was found that whereas the alloreactive T-cells (C57B1/6 cells educated in an irradiated BALB/c host) activated at best 8% of the total spleen cell population, the LPS stimulated 23% of the cells. As a further piece of evidence in favour of the two signal hypothesis, Jacobs and Morrison (1975) found that the mitogenic activity of TNP–LPS could be inhibited in the presence of a low concentration of the antibiotic polymyxin B. However, under the same conditions the TNP–LPS conjugate was still immunogenic. Since the one-signal hypothesis relied on the supply of a LPS-directed mitogenic signal to the precursor cells, the apparent dissociation of the mitogenicity and immunogenicity appeared to favour the two-signal mechanism interpretation of the data. In terms of its biological significance *in vivo*, the two-signal hypothesis does not require that the LPS and the antigen are injected together, at the same site or at the same time. This would fit with the experimental evidence for the immunopotentiation of immune responses by LPS.

From the current results concerning B-cell activation by LPS, it is difficult to be categorical about which mechanism is likely to represent the true biological events. In each case the hapten is held at the surface by an interaction with specific SIg receptors, but the LPS–membrane contact is dependent on the hapten in the one-signal hypothesis and is independent of such influence in the two-signal hypothesis. Even though both models require the two conditions of membrane contact to be satisfied, they diverge over the question of 'what happens next?'. Do the intracellular processes 'see' two distinct signals or only one from the hapten–LPS complex?

From the above, and from evidence previously cited, it is apparent that LPS can act by supplying a stimulus to the AFC precursors and thus replacing the need for helper T-cells. However, there is a body of data which seems to indicate that LPS acts through the helper T-cells, either directly or indirectly, and does not bypass them. Notably Newburger *et al.* (1974) showed, using lethally irradiated animals reconstituted with syngeneic cells, that LPS exerted its effect through the helper T-cells (see section IV). Similarly, Parks *et al.* (1981) found evidence of an interaction between LPS and helper T-cells. They induced in A/J mice a tolerant state to HGG by an injection of deaggregated (ultracentrifuged) HGG. However, if the animals were exposed to *E. coli* O111:B4 LPS 3 h after the tolerogenic stimulus, the tolerant state failed to develop for both B- and T-cells, as demonstrated by the presence of both primary and secondary responses. By the use of transfer experiments, they demonstrated that the secondary B-cell response was T-cell dependent and that helper T-cells could be primed with an injection of deaggregated (tolerogenic) HGG and LPS. LPS also injected together with immunogenic or tolerogenic HGG facilitated the priming of helper T-cells for exposure to the hapten–carrier, DNP–HGG. They interpreted their data to indicate that exposure to the antigen alone resulted in tolerance, but an immunogenic signal could be achieved by the use of LPS; therefore the T- and B-cells received two stimuli—one from the antigen, the other from the LPS. Although LPS could interfere with the induction of tolerance in this manner, it is interesting to note, as reported earlier, that once tolerance is induced, LPS can only break that state which is maintained by T-cells, i.e. it is able to bypass T-cell influence (Chiller and Weigle, 1973).

From the evidence in the literature, the macrophage would appear to be another major target for LPS. This was especially noticeable in the studies involving the immune destruction of tumour cell targets (Alexander and Evans, 1971; Grant and Alexander, 1974; Glaser *et al.*, 1976; Ralph and Nakoinz, 1977b). However, it has also been reported that LPS is able to induce the production of monokines, especially lymphocyte activating factor (LAF) or interleukin-1 (IL-1) (Gery *et al.*, 1972a; Gery and Waksman, 1972; Oppenheim and Gery, 1982). Gery *et al.* (1972a) observed that human or mouse (CBA/J) lymphoid cells cultured in the presence of *E. coli* O55:B5 LPS produced a factor that was demonstrable, in the supernatant fluid, by its ability to induce mitogenic activity in thymocytes and peripheral T-cells. They proposed that the factor with this ability should be termed LAF. They subsequently showed that this factor was a monokine (i.e. produced by macrophages) (Gery and Waksman, 1972). LAF is now termed interleukin-1 and a minireview of its properties and effects has recently appeared (Oppenheim and Gery, 1982). IL-1 is genetically unrestricted and has a molecular weight of 12 000–16 000. Its production can be induced by a variety of stimuli including LPS and the components of the mycobacterial adjuvants, e.g. muramyl-dipeptide. In its effects, besides inducing the formation of biologically active factors by lymphocytes (i.e. lymphokines),

IL-1 is also able to influence the generation of helper T-cells. The production of this factor can be modulated by other stimuli — LAF can be induced by another factor termed colony stimulating factor (CSF) or its production can be inhibited by prostaglandins, PGE_2. However, LPS has been reported to stimulate both the production of CSF and PGE_2 (Kurland and Bockman, 1978; Moore *et al.*, 1980). Further, with respect to the anti-tumouricidal activity of macrophages, it has been observed that in C3H/HeN spleen cell cultures, the induction of this activity in macrophages by lymphokines took place only in the presence of LPS (Pace and Russell, 1981). Finally, it is interesting to note that C3H/eB mouse spleen cell cultures will generate high levels of interferon (IF) in response to *S. abortus equi* LPS, which are dependent on the presence of macrophages. Hence LPS is able to influence the production of both IF and PGE_2, which are two of the factors known to control the activity of NK-cells against tumour cell targets (Gidlund *et al.*, 1978; Oehler *et al.*, 1978; Tracey and Adkinson, 1980).

Finally, in considering the mechanisms of action of LPS it is worth examining the genetic control of the responses induced by LPS. In terms of mitogenicity and immunopotentiating activity, some inbred strains of mice have been found to be low or non-responders to these LPS-induced effects, e.g. C3H/HeJ, C57B1/10ScR, CBA/N (Watson and Riblet, 1974, 1975; Ness *et al.*, 1976; Gregory *et al.* 1980). In the C3H/HeJ mice there is a defect in a single autosomal locus, *Lps*, which maps to chromosome 4 and whose product is normally expressed on B-cells. An intact locus was thought to be required for the synthesis of a membrane component which serves as a functional receptor for LPS (Watson *et al.* 1978). The CBA/N mouse has an X-linked defect affecting responsiveness to LPS.

Skidmore *et al.* (1975) observed the antibody response to BSA in the presence of *E. coli* O111:B4 LPS and found that in responder strains, e.g. A/J, a positive correlation was obtained between mitogenicity for B-cells and immunopotentiating activity. However, in non-responder animals, e.g. C3H/HeJ, LPS failed to function as an adjuvant, and the B-cells were unresponsive to LPS-induced mitogenesis. Also, the induction of tolerance to HGG, which was B-cell-dependent early in the response, could be interfered with in responder strains but not in non-responder strains by LPS. Further, in adult thymectomy and reconstitution experiments, Watson and Riblet (1975) were able to demonstrate that the non-responsive state in C3H/HeJ mice was not due either to non-specific LPS-induced suppressive events or to a lack of the appropriate accessory cell types. Similar data were obtained with *in vitro* cultures (Slowe and Waldmann, 1975). The unresponsiveness was due to a defect in a membrane component in the B-cell population, not related to the H-2 or heavy chain allotypic loci. It was proposed that interaction between the LPS and this membrane component normally initiated intracellular events that lead to cell proliferation. Mating experiments (Watson and Riblet, 1974) showed that responsiveness was dominant, i.e. in responder × non-responder crosses the F1 hybrid progeny were all of the responder phenotype. Further by back-crossing they were able to establish that mitogenicity and immune responsiveness to LPS were genetically linked and were due to a single autosomal gene not linked to the H-2 locus.

These experiments with responder/non-responder strains have clearly shown that LPS exerts an influence through the B-cell, since defective B-cells (i.e. B-cells unresponsive to LPS) render the animal resistant to the immunopotentiating effects of LPS. However, other reports have demonstrated that a T-cell and/or macrophage influence is also present, together with possibly a T-cell defect in non-responder strains.

With primary cultures of responder and non-responder cells challenged with TNP–SRBC or SRBC in the presence of *E. coli* K235 LPS, McGhee *et al.* (1979) found that the LPS adjuvant effect required both T-cells and macrophages. If responder spleen cells (C3H/HeN) were mixed with responder macrophages, the LPS enhanced the antibody response to SRBC, while no response was obtained if non-responder spleen cells (C3H/HeJ) were substituted for the responder spleen cells. This represented the basic experiment and indicated that the spleen cells (either T- or B-cells) from non-responder animals were defective. They expanded this system, using TNP–SRBC as the immunogen. LPS was able to enhance the anti-TNP response in cultures containing spleen cells from athymic nude mice C3H (*nu/nu*) and responder T-cells (C3H/HeN) but not in cultures containing responder *nu/nu* spleen cells and non-responder T-cells. This pair of cultures indicated that LPS exerted its effect through T-cells, which were defective in non-responder strains. Finally, they compared the effect of LPS in a pair of cultures. The first culture contained responder T-cells, responder macrophages and non-responder B-cells, while the second culture contained responder T-cells, responder macrophages and responder B-cells. In both types of cultures LPS acted as an effective immunogen. These cultures revealed that non-responder B-cells became responsive in the presence of responder T-cells and macrophages, but that non-responder spleen cells remained unresponsive after the addition of responder macrophages. Hence there appeared to be a defect in the T-cell system which prevented the LPS from exerting a potentiating effect.

These slightly contrasting effects of LPS in responder/non-responder strains could arise from different activities in different parts of the LPS molecule. *E. coli* LPS was reported as non-mitogenic for B-cells from the non-responsive strain, C3H/HeJ. However, if the lipid A-associated protein (LAP) was removed from the LPS by extraction with phenol, then the protein-free LPS preparation was mitogenic for B-cells from both responder and non-responder mice (Betz and Morrison, 1977).

Ness *et al.* (1976) have reported data that support the notion of the involvement of T-cells, with strains that were low (B10.BR, C3H) and high

(C57B1/10, C57B1/6) responders for the synthetic polypeptide of tyrosine, glutamine, alanine and leucine, (TG)–A–L$_{420}$. It was observed that LPS enhanced the primary IgM response to (TG)–A–L in both low and high responders. Hence LPS enhanced the IgM response regardless of the *Ir* gene status of the mouse. In general LPS enhanced secondary responses in both low and high responders, but only in the latter was there some evidence that the antibody produced was resistant to 2-mercaptoethanol, i.e. was IgG. However, in a few low responder strains, notably BALB/c and NIH Swiss Albino mice, a LPS-induced secondary response was obtained which exhibited a switch to IgG. If, in the Swiss mice, athymic nude animals (*nu/nu*) were compared with normal animals (+ /*nu*), then only in the latter was it possible to obtain a LPS-influenced switch to IgG production. Hence low responder mice which have the tendency to make IgM antibody to (TG)–A–L can be influenced by LPS to switch to IgG production if appropriate T-cells are available.

Table 3   Mechanisms of action of LPS as an immunopotentiator

1. Direct action on B-cells (antibody-forming cell precursors) — bypass of helper T-cell function
2. Direct action on helper T-cells — facilitates priming
3. Converts signals tolerogenic to T- and B-cells into immunogenic signals
4. Induces the production of factors (e.g. interleukin-1, colony stimulating factor) which influence T-cell function
5. Direct action on macrophages to exhibit direct cytotoxicity, increased antibody-dependent cellular cytotoxicity, increased intracellular enzyme activity, etc.

From the above data it is evident that LPS in all probability acts through more than one mechanism, exerting its influence on B-cells, macrophages and T-cells. These mechanisms are summarized in Table 3. Hence, when an antibody response is enhanced in the presence of LPS, the observed response is probably a summation of the effects of all these mechanisms. Further, each mechanism is probably independent of any other mechanism, which would explain why LPS is able to function perfectly well regardless of the presence or absence of T-cells. What is probably critical, however, in immunopotentiation are the conditions used for administration of the LPS so that all the available mechanisms become fully functional. Further, from the literature it can be seen that LPS, in its role as an immunopotentiator, has many properties in common with other biological agents which are known to modulate immune responses (Davies, 1982).

VI. CONCLUSIONS

Lipopolysaccharides derived from the cell envelope of gram-negative bacteria have been shown to possess the intrinsic ability to enhance both the cellular and humoral arms of the immune system. In the humoral response, the primary cellular target for the LPS is the B-cell and although there is evidence to suggest that this can be a direct interaction, there are also substantial data to indicate that the interaction could be indirect, being mediated through T-cells and/or macrophages. The direct influence exerted on B-cells has been postulated to be mediated through one of two mechanisms. A single mitogenic signal from the LPS molecule was proposed as the activation signal, with the antigenic determinants from the specific antigenic stimulus being 'passive', acting merely as a 'guide' for the LPS to identify the specific APC precursor cells. The second postulate is based on a two-signal approach, one signal derived from the LPS molecule and the other from the antigenic determinant; both signals are necessary for B-cell activation. Although there is evidence for both of these mechanisms it is difficult to determine which is correct since both require the antigenic determinant and the LPS molecule to be held at the cell surface.

There are also considerable data to indicate that LPS is able to influence events associated with the cellular arm of the immune system. Although *in vitro* cultures have shown that the macrophage is a 'target cell' for LPS in its effects on anti-tumour immunity, it is uncertain, whether *in vivo* the LPS directly enhances the cellular activity or whether it influences it indirectly by controlling the production of antibodies which are known to modulate cellular responsiveness.

REFERENCES

Alexander, P., and Evans, R. (1971). Endotoxin and double-stranded RNA render macrophages cytotoxic. *Nature*, **232**, 76–78.

Allison, A. C., and Davies, A. J. S. (1971). Requirement of thymus-dependent lymphocytes for potentiation by adjuvants of antibody synthesis. *Nature*, **233**, 330–332.

Andersson, J., Möller, G., and Sjöberg, O. (1972a). Selective induction of DNA synthesis in T and B lymphocytes. *Cell. Immunol.*, **4**, 381–393.

Andersson, J., Sjöberg, O., and Möller, G. (1972b). Induction of immunoglobulin and antibody synthesis *in vitro* by lipopolysaccharides. *Eur. J. Immunol.*, **2**, 349–353.

Andersson, J., Coutinho, A., and Melchers, F. (1978). Stimulation of murine B lymphocytes to IgG synthesis and secretion by mitogens lipopolysaccharide and lipoprotein and its inhibition of anti-immunoglobulin antibodies. *Eur. J. Immunol.*, **8**, 336–346.

Behling, U. H., and Nowotny, A. (1977). Immune adjuvancy of lipopolysaccharide and a nontoxic hydrolytic product demonstrating oscillating effects with time. *J. Immunol.*, **118**, 1905–1907.

Betz, S. J., and Morrison, D. C. (1977). Chemical and biologic properties of a protein-rich fraction of bacterial lipopolysaccharide. I. The *in vitro* murine lymphocyte response. *J. Immunol.*, **119**, 1475–1481.

Biozzi, G., Benacerraf, B., and Halpern, B. N. (1955). The effect of *Sal. typhi* and its endotoxin on the phagocytic activity of the reticuloendothelial system in mice, *Br. J. Exp. Pathol.*, **36**, 226–235.

Bober, L. A., Kranepool, M. J., and Hollander, V. P. (1976). Inhibitory effect of endotoxin on the growth of plasma cell tumour. *Cancer Res.*, **36**, 927–929.

Bruynzeel, D. P., Ettekoven, H., and Kreeftenberg, J. G. (1978). The synergistic activity of BCG on the stimulation of lymphocytes with concanavalin A and lipopolysaccharide. *Cancer Immunol. Immunother.*, **3**, 253–258.

Campbell, P. A., Rowlands, D. T., Harrington, M. J., and Kind, P. D. (1966). The adjuvant action of endotoxin in thymectomised mice. *J. Immunol.*, **96**, 849–853.

Chester, T. J., De Clercq, E., and Merigan, T. C. (1971). Effect of separate and combined injections of poly rI:poly rC and endotoxin on reticuloendothelial activity, interferon and antibody production in the mouse. *Infect. Immun.*, **3**, 516–520.

Chiller, J. M., and Weigle, W. O. (1973). Termination of tolerance to human gamma globulin in mice by antigen and bacterial lipopolysaccharide (endotoxin). *J. Exp. Med.*, **137**, 740–750.

Chiller, J. M., Skidmore, B. J., Morrison, D. C., and Weigle, W. O. (1973). Relationship of the structure of bacterial lipopolysaccharides to its function in mitogenesis and adjuvanticity. *Proc. Natl. Acad. Sci. USA*, **70**, 2129–2133.

Cohen, E. P., Crosby, L. K., and Talmage, D. W. (1964). The effect of endotoxin on the antibody response of transferred spleen cells. *J. Immunol.*, **92**, 223–226.

Condie, R. M., Zak, S. J., and Good, R. A. (1955). The effect of meningococcal endotoxin on resistance to bacterial infection and the immune response of rabbits. *Fed. Proc.*, **14**, 459.

Coutinho, A., Gronowicz, E., Bullock, W. W., and Möller, G. (1974). Mechanisms of thymus-independent immunocyte triggering mitogenic activation of B-cells results in specific immune responses. *J. Exp. Med.*, **139**, 74–92.

Coutinho, A., Gronowicz, E., and Sultzer, B. M. (1975). Genetic control of B-cell responses I. Selective unresponsiveness to lipopolysaccharide. *Scand. J. Immunol.*, **4**, 139–143.

Davies, M. (1974). The affinity of bacterial polysaccharides for mammalian cell surfaces and its relationship to adjuvant activity. *Ph.D. Thesis*, University of Glasgow.

Davies, M. (1982). BCG as an anti-tumour agent: Interaction with cells of the mammalian immune system. *Biochim. Biophys. Acta*, **651**, 143–174.

Davies, M. (1983). Phase variations in the modulation of the immune response. *Immunol. Today*, **4**, 103–106.

Davies, M., and Stewart-Tull, D. E. S. (1981). The affinity of bacterial polysaccharide-containing fractions for mammalian cell membranes and its relationship to immunopotentiating activity. *Biochim. Biophys. Acta*, **643**, 17–29.

Forman, J., and Möller, G. (1973). The effector cell in antibody-induced cell-mediated immunity. *Transplant. Rev.*, **17**, 108–149.

Freedman, H. H., Fox, A. E., and Schwartz, B. S. (1967). Antibody formation at various times after previous treatment of mice with endotoxin. *Proc. Soc. Exp. Biol. Med.*, **125**, 583–587.

Freitas, A. A., and De Sousa, M. (1976). Control mechanisms of lymphocyte traffic. Altered distribution of ^{51}Cr-labelled mouse lymph node cells pretreated *in vitro* with lipopolysaccharide. *Eur. J. Immunol.*, **6**, 269–273.

Gery, I., and Waksman, B. H. (1972). Potentiation of the T-lymphocyte response to mitogens. II. The cellular source of potentiating mediator(s). *J. Exp. Med.*, **136**, 143–155.

Gery, I., Gershon, R. K., and Waksman, B. H. (1972a). Potentiation of the T lymphocyte response to mitogens. I. The responding cell. *J. Exp. Med.*, **136**, 128–142.

Gery, I., Krüger, J., and Spiessel, S. Z. (1972b). Stimulation of B lymphocytes by endotoxin. Reactions of thymus-deprived mice and karyotypic analysis of dividing cells in mice bearing T6T6 thymus grafts. *J. Immunol.*, **108**, 1088–1091.

Gidlund, M., Orn, A., Wigzell, H., Senik, A., and Gresser, I. (1978). Enhanced NK cell activity in mice injected with interferon and interferon inducers. *Nature*, **273**, 759–761.

Glaser, M., Djeu, J. Y., Kirchner, H., and Herberman, R. B. (1976). Augmentation of cell-mediated cytotoxicity against syngeneic Gross virus-induced lymphoma in rats by phytohaemagglutinin and endotoxin. *J. Immunol.*, **116**, 1512–1519.

Goodman, M. G., and Weigle, W. O. (1981). T-cell regulation of polyclonal B-cell responsiveness. III. Overt T helper and latent T suppressor activities from distinct subpopulations of unstimulated splenic T-cells. *J. Exp. Med.*, **153**, 844–856.

Grant, C. K., and Alexander, P. (1974). Nonspecific cytotoxicity of spleen cells and the specific cytotoxic action of thymus-derived lymphocytes *in vitro*. *Cell. Immunol.*, **14**, 46–51.

Gregory, S. H., Zimmerman, D. H., and Kern, M. (1980). The lipid A moiety of lipopolysaccharide is specifically bound to B-cell subpopulations of responder and nonresponder animals. *J. Immunol.*, **125**, 102–107.

Grohsman, J., and Nowotny, A. (1972). The immune recognition of TA3 tumour, its facilitation by endotoxin and abrogation by ascites fluid. *J. Immunol.*, **109**, 1090–1095.

Hamaoka, T., and Katz, D. H. (1973). Cellular site of action of various adjuvants in antibody responses to hapten–carrier conjugates. *J. Immunol.*, **111**, 1554–1563.

Havens, W. P. (1959). Haemagglutination in viral hepatitis. *Trans. Assoc. Am. Physicians*, **72**, 218–224.

Hoffmann, M. K., Galanos, C., Koenigs, S., and Oettgen, H. F. (1977). B-cell activation by lipopolysaccharides. Distinct pathways for induction of mitosis and antibody production. *J. Exp. Med.*, **146**, 1640–1647.

Ilfield, D. N., Cathcart, M. K., Krakauer, R. S., and Blaese, M. (1981). Human splenic and peripheral blood lymphocytes response to lipopolysaccharide. *Cell. Immunol.*, **57**, 400–407.

Izui, S., Eisenberg, R. A., and Dixon, F. J. (1981). Subclass restricted IgG polyclonal antibody production in mice injected with lipid A rich lipopolysaccharide. *J. Exp. Med.*, **153**, 324–338.

Jacobs, D. M., and Morrison, D. C. (1975). Dissociation between mitogenicity and immunogenicity of TNP–lipopolysaccharide, a T-independent antigen. *J. Exp. Med.*, **141**, 1453–1458.

Jaroslow, B. N. (1960). Factors associated with initiation of the immune response. *J. Infect. Dis.*, **107**, 56–64.

Jenkin, C., and Palmer, D. L. (1960). Changes in the titre of serum opsonins and phagocytic properties of mouse peritoneal macrophages following injection of endotoxin. *J. Exp. Med.*, **112**, 419–429.

Johnson, A. G., Gaines, S., and Landy, M. (1956). Studies on the O antigen of *Salmonella typhosa*. V. Enhancement of antibody response to protein antigens by the purified lipopolysaccharide. *J. Exp. Med.*, **103**, 225–246.

Jones, J. M., and Kind, P. D. (1972). Enhancing effect of bacterial endotoxin on bone marrow cells in the immune response to SRBC. *J. Immunol.*, **108**, 1453–1455.

Kearney, J. F., and Lawton, A. R. (1975). B lymphocyte differentiation by lipopolysaccharide. I. Generation of cells synthesizing four major immunoglobulin classes. *J. Immunol.*, **115**, 671–676.

Kind, P., and Johnson, A. G. (1959). Studies of the adjuvant action of bacterial endotoxin on antibody formation. I. Time limitation of enhancing effect and restoration of antibody formation in X-irradiated rabbits. *J. Immunol.*, **82**, 415–427.

Kiyono, H., McGhee, J. R., and Michalek, S. M. (1980). Lipopolysaccharide regulation of the immune response: Comparison of responses to LPS in germ-free, *Escherichia coli*-monoassociated and conventional mice. *J. Immunol.*, **124**, 36–41.

Kurland, J. I., and Bockman, R. (1978). Prostaglandin E production by human blood monocytes and mouse peritoneal macrophages. *J. Exp. Med.*, **147**, 952–957.

Lagrange, P. H., and Mackaness, G. B. (1975). Effects of bacterial lipopolysaccharides on the induction and expression of cell-mediated immunity. II. Stimulation of the efferent arc. *J. Immunol.*, **114**, 447–451.

Lagrange, P. H., Mackaness, G. B., Miller, T. E., and Pardon, P. (1975). Effects of bacterial lipopolysaccharides on the induction and expression of cell-mediated immunity. I. Depression of the afferent arc. *J. Immunol.*, **114**, 442–446.

Leucke, D. H., and Sibal, L. R. (1962). Enhancement by endotoxin of the primary antibody response to bovine serum albumin in chickens. *J. Immunol.*, **89**, 539–544.

Louis, J. A., Chiller, J. M., and Weigle, W. O. (1973). The ability of bacterial lipopolysaccharide to modulate the induction of unresponsiveness to a state of immunity. *J. Exp. Med.*, **138**, 1481–1495.

MacLean, I. H., and Holt, L. B. (1940). Combined immunization with tetanus toxoid and TAB. *Lancet*, **ii**, 581–583.

McGhee, J. R., Farrar, J. J., Michalek, S. M., Mergenhagen, S. E., and Rosenstreich, D. L. (1979). Cellular requirements for lipopolysaccharide adjuvanticity. A role for both T-lymphocytes and macrophage for *in vitro* responses to particulate antigen. *J. Exp. Med.*, **149**, 793–807.

Michael, J. G. (1966). The release of nonspecific bactericidal antibodies by endotoxin. *J. Exp. Med.*, **123**, 205–212.

Mizuguchi, J., Kakiuchi, T., Nariuchi, H., and Matuhasi, T. (1980). Effect of lipopolysaccharide (LPS) on the thymocyte response to PHA: Strain difference. *Immunology*, **41**, 393–398.

Moore, R. N., Steeg, P. S., Männel, D. N., and Mergenhagen, S. E. (1980). Role of lipopolysaccharide in regulating colony-stimulating factor dependent macrophage proliferation *in vitro*. *Infect. Immun.*, **30**, 797–804.

Morrison, D. C., and Ryan, J. L. (1979). Bacterial endotoxins and host immune responses. *Adv. Immunol.*, **28**, 293–439.

Motta, I., Portnoi, D., and Truffa-Bachi, P. (1981). Induction and differentiation of B memory cells by a thymus-independent antigen, trinitrophenylated lipopoly-saccharide. *Cell. Immunol.*, **57**, 327–338.

Muirhead, M. J., Vitetta, E. S., Isakson, P. C., Krolick, K. A., Dees, J. H., and Uhr, J. W. (1981). Increased susceptibility to lethal effect of bacterial lipopolysaccharide in mice with B-cell leukaemia. *J. Natl. Cancer Inst.*, **66**, 745–753.

Munoz, J. (1961). Permeability changes produced in mice by *Bordetella pertussis*. *J. Immunol.*, **86**, 618–626.

Nakano, M., Uhiyama, T., and Saito, K. (1973). Adjuvant effect of endotoxin: Antibody response to sheep erythrocytes in mice after transfer of syngeneic lymphoid cells treated with bacterial lipopolysaccharide *in vitro*. *J. Immunol.*, **110**, 408–413.

Ness, D. B., Smith, S., Talcott, J. A., and Grumet, F. C. (1976). T-cell requirements for the expression of the lipopolysaccharide adjuvant effect *in vivo*: Evidence for a T-dependent and a T-independent mode of action. *Eur. J. Immunol.*, **6**, 650–654.

Neter, E. (1971). Endotoxins and the Immune response. *Curr. Top. Microbiol.*, **47**, 82–124.

Newburger, P. E., Hamaoka, T., and Katz, D. H. (1974). Potentiation of helper T-cell function in IgE antibody response by bacterial lipopolysaccharide (LPS). *J. Immunol.*, **113**, 824–829.

Norcross, M. A., and Smith, R. T. (1977). Regulation of B-cell proliferative responses to lipopolysaccharide by a subclass of thymus T-cell. *J. Exp. Med.*, **145**, 1299–1315.

Nowotny, A. (1969). Molecular aspects of endotoxic reactions. *Bacteriol. Rev.* **33**, 72–106.

Oehler, J. R., Lindsay, L. R., Nunn, M. E., Holden, H. T., and Herberman, R. T. (1978). Natural cell-mediated cytotoxicity in rats. II. *In vivo* augmentation of NK-cell activity. *Int. J. Cancer*, **21**, 210–220.

Oppenheim, J. J., and Gery, I. (1982). Interleukin-1 is more than an interleukin. *Immunol. Today*, **3**, 113–119.

Ortiz-Ortiz, L., and Jaroslow, B. N. (1970). Enhancement by the adjuvant, endotoxin, of an immune response induced *in vitro*. *Immunology*, **19**, 387–399.

Pace, J. L., and Russell, S. W. (1981). Activation of mouse macrophages for tumour cell killing. I. Quantitative analysis of interactions between lymphokine and lipopolysaccharide. *J. Immunol.*, **126**, 1863–1867.

Parks, D. E., Walker, S. M., and Weigle, W. O. (1981). Bacterial lipopolysaccharide (endotoxin) interferes with the induction of tolerance and primes thymus-derived lymphocytes. *J. Immunol.*, **126**, 938–942.

Parr, I., Wheeler, E., and Alexander, P. (1973). Similarities of the anti-tumour actions of endotoxin, lipid A and double-stranded RNA. *Br. J. Cancer*, **27**, 370–389.

Pearlman, D. S., Sayers, J. B., and Talmage, D. W. (1963). The effect of adjuvant amounts of endotoxin on the serum haemolytic complement activity in rabbits. *J. Immunol.*, **91**, 748–756.

Perni, A., and Mota, I. (1973). The production of IgE and IgG1 antibodies in guinea pigs immunized with antigen and bacterial lipopolysaccharides. *Immunology*, **25**, 297–305.

Plescia, O. J., and Braun, W. (1968). *Nucleic Acids in Immunology*. Springer, Berlin, Heidelberg, New York.

Ralph, P., and Nakoinz, I. (1977a). Antibody-dependent killing of erythrocyte and tumour targets by macrophage-related cell lines: Enhancement by PPD and LPS. *J. Immunol.*, **119**, 950–954.

Ralph, P., and Nakoinz, I. (1977b). Direct toxic effects of immunopotentiators on monocytic, myelomonocytic and histiocytic or macrophage tumour cells in culture. *Cancer Res.*, **37**, 546–550.

Ramon, G., and Zoeller, C. (1926). Les 'vaccins associes' par union d'une anatoxine et d'un vaccin microbien (TAB) par melanger d'anatoxines. *C. R. Soc. Biol.*, **94**, 106–109.

Ribi, E. E., Granger, D. L., Milner, K. C., and Strain, S. M. (1975). Tumour regression caused by endotoxins and mycobacterial fractions. *J. Natl. Cancer Inst.*, **55**, 1253–1257.

Rubenstein, H. S., Fine, J., and Coons, A. H. (1962). Localization of endotoxin in the walls of the peripheral vascular system during lethal endotoxaemia. *Proc. Soc. Exp. Biol. Med.*, **111**, 458–467.

Rudbach, J. A. (1971). Molecular immunogenicity of bacterial lipopolysaccharide antigens: Establishing a quantitative system. *J. Immunol.*, **106**, 993–1001.

Schacter, B., Kleinhenz, M. E., Edmonds, K., and Ellner, J. J. (1981). Spontaneous cytotoxicity of human peripheral blood mononuclear cells for the lymphoblastoid cell line CCRF-CEM—Augmentation by bacterial lipopolysaccharide. *Clin. Exp. Immunol.*, **46**, 640–648.

Scheid, M. P., Hoffmann, M. K., Komuro, K., Hammerling, U., Abbott, J., Boyse, E. A., Cohen, G. H., Hooper, J. A., Schulaf, R. S., and Goldstein, A. L. (1973). Differentiation of T-cells induced by preparations from thymus and by nonthymic agents. *J. Exp. Med.*, **138**, 1027–1032.

Schmidtke, J. R., and Dixon, F. J. (1972). Immune response to a hapten coupled to a non-immunogenic carrier. Influence of lipopolysaccharide. *J. Exp. Med.*, **136**, 392–397.

Scibienski, R. J., and Gershwin, M. E. (1977). Immunologic properties of protein-lipopolysaccharide complexes. I. Antibody response of normal, thymectomised and nude mice to a lysozyme–lipopolysaccharide complex. *J. Immunol.*, **119**, 504–509.

Shinohara, N., and Kern, M. (1976). Differentiation of lymphoid cells: B-cells as a direct target and T-cells as a regulator in lipopolysaccharide enhanced induction of immunoglobulin production. *J. Immunol.*, **116**, 1607–1612.

Skidmore, B. J., Chiller, J. M., Morrison, D. C., and Weigle, W. O. (1975). Immunologic properties of bacterial lipopolysaccharide (LPS): Correlation between the mitogenic, adjuvant and immunogenic activities. *J. Immunol.*, **114**, 770–775.

Skidmore, B. J., Chiller, J. M., Weigle, W. O., Riblet, R., and Watson, J. (1976). Immunologic properties of bacterial lipopolysaccharide (LPS). III. Genetic linkage between the *in vitro* mitogenic and *in vivo* adjuvant properties of LPS. *J. Exp. Med.*, **143**, 143–150.

Slowe, A., and Waldmann, H. (1975). The 'intrinsic adjuvanticity' and immunogenicity of trinitrophenylated lipopolysaccharide. *Immunology*, **29**, 825–834.

Solliday, S., Rowley, D. A., and Fitch, F. W. (1967). Adjuvant reversal of antibody suppression of the immune response. *Fed. Proc.*, **26**, 700.

Sultzer, B. M., and Nilsson, B. S. (1972). PPD tuberculin—a B-cell mitogen. *Nature*, **240**, 198–200.

Talmage, D. W., and Pearlman, D. S. (1963). The antibody response: A model based on antagonistic actions of antigen. *J. Theor. Biol.*, **5**, 321–339.

Tracey, D. E., and Adkinson, N. F. (1980). Prostaglandin synthesis inhibitors potentiate BCG-induced augmentation of natural killer cell activity. *J. Immunol.*, **125**, 136–141.

Trenkner, E. (1974). The use of allogeneic T-lymphocyte and bacterial lipopolysaccharides to induce immune responses to monovalent hapten *in vitro*. *J. Immunol.*, **113**, 918–924.

Tsang, R. S. W., Chau, P. Y., Lam, S. K., Labrody, J. T., and Rowley, D. (1981). Antibody response to the lipopolysaccharide and protein antigens of *Salmonella typhi* during typhoid infection. I. Measurement of serum antibodies by radioimmunoassay. *Clin. Exp. Immunol.*, **46**, 508–514.

Uchiyama, T., and Jacobs, D. M. (1978). Modulation of immune response by bacterial lipopolysaccharide (LPS): Cellular basis of stimulatory and inhibitory effects of LPS on the *in vitro* IgM antibody response to a T-independent antigen. *J. Immunol.*, **121**, 2347–2351.

Van Der Loo, W., Gronowicz, E. S., Strober, S., and Herzenberg, L. A. (1979). Cell differentiation in the presence of cytochalasin B: Studies on the 'switch' to IgG secretion after polyclonal B-cell activation. *J. Immunol.*, **122**, 1203–1208.

Ward, P. A., Johnson, A. G., and Abell, M. R. (1959). Studies on the adjuvant action by bacterial endotoxins on antibody formation. *J. Exp. Med.*, **109**, 463–474.

Watson, J., and Riblet, R. (1974). Genetic control of responses to bacterial lipopolysaccharide in mice. I. Evidence for a single gene that influences mitogenic and immunogenic responses to lipopolysaccharide. *J. Exp. Med.*, **140**, 1147–1161.

Watson, J., and Riblet, R. (1975). Genetic control of responses to bacterial lipopolysaccharide in mice. II. A gene that influences a membrane component involved in the activation of bone-marrow derived lymphocytes by lipopolysaccharide. *J. Immunol.*, **114**, 1462–1468.

Watson, J., Trenkner, E., and Cohn, M. (1973). The use of bacterial lipopolysaccharides to show that two signals are required for the induction of antibody synthesis. *J. Exp. Med.*, **138**, 699–714.

Watson, J., Largen, M., and McAdam, K. P. W. J. (1978). Genetic control of endotoxin responses in mice. *J. Exp. Med.*, **147**, 39–49.

Weiner, E., and Levanon, D. (1968). The *in vitro* interaction between bacterial lipopolysaccharide and differentiating monocytes. *Lab. Invest.*, **19**, 584–594.

Weissman, G., and Thomas, L. (1962). Studies on lysosomes. I. *J. Exp. Med.*, **116**, 433–450.

Wetzel, G. D., and Kettman, J. R. (1981). Activation of murine B-cells. II. Dextran sulphate removes the requirement for cellular interaction during lipopolysaccharide-induced mitogenesis. *Cell. Immunol.*, **61**, 176–189.

Immunology of the Bacterial Cell Envelope
Edited by D. E. S. Stewart-Tull and M. Davies
© 1985 John Wiley & Sons Ltd.

CHAPTER 11

Antigens of Type-1 Fimbriae

James P. Duguid

*Bacteriology Department, University of Dundee Medical School,
Ninewells Hospital, Dundee, UK*

I. INTRODUCTION

Fimbriae are filamentous appendages of bacteria, distinguished from flagella by their greater number (e.g. 50–500 per bacillus), much smaller size (e.g. 0.1–1.5 μm in length and 4–10 nm in width), and straight or irregular as opposed to wavy form. They are seen only with the electron microscope and were first clearly described in *Escherichia coli* by Houwink and van Iterson (1950) and Brinton *et al.* (1954), who called them 'filaments', and Duguid *et al.* (1955) who named them 'fimbriae'. Brinton (1959) later introduced the name 'pili', but, as recommended by Ottow (1975) and Jones (1977), this name is better reserved for the very different, scantier filaments associated with bacterial conjugation and DNA transfer, the so-called 'sex pili' of Brinton (1965).

Fimbriae are produced by bacteria of several families, but have been most studied in *Enterobacteriaceae* (Duguid, 1968; Duguid and Old, 1980). The commoner varieties confer adhesive properties on the bacteria, enabling them to adhere to epithelial cells, red blood cells and other solid substrates, and these properties are generally demonstrable by the haemagglutination reactions produced on mixture of the bacteria with red blood cells (Duguid *et al.*, 1955; Duguid and Old, 1980).

Different kinds of fimbriae are formed by different bacteria; those of enterobacteria and pseudomonads were classified into six types by Duguid *et al.* (1966) according to the nature of their adhesive properties. This classification is provisional and will require revision as other types of fimbriae are identified and more is discovered about the composition, stability, antigens, physiology and genetics of the different types.

II. TYPE-1 FIMBRIAE

The fimbriae occurring most widely among the enterobacteria are those classified as type 1. They have been found in many strains of *E. coli, Shigella flexneri, Salmonella* spp., *Klebsiella aerogenes, Citrobacter, Enterobacter, Serratia, Erwinia, Proteus* and *Providencia* (Duguid and Old, 1980). Type-1 fimbriae are defined by (i) their possession of the pattern of adhesive affinities for the red blood cells of different animal species originally observed in the 'group I' strains of *E. coli* by Duguid *et al.* (1955), and (ii) the susceptibility of their adhesive reactivities to complete inhibition in the presence of small concentrations of D-mannose and a few of its analogues (Duguid and Gillies, 1957; Old, 1972).

The adhesive substance of the type-1 fimbriae is termed the mannose-sensitive (MS) adhesin. It reacts strongly with most kinds of animal, plant and fungal cells, including the red blood cells of most animal species, but it is only weakly reactive with human and sheep red blood cells, and unreactive with ox red cells, though strongly reactive with human, sheep and ox leucocytes and epithelial cells. Other types of fimbriae show different patterns of reactivity with different kinds of cells and their adhesiveness is unaffected by the presence of D-mannose, i.e. is mannose-resistant (MR).

Fimbriae are composed of protein. Brinton (1959, 1965) showed that the type-1 fimbriae of *E. coli* consisted of a helical array of identical protein subunits, 17 kDa, with an outer diameter about 7 nm and a hollow core about 2 nm wide. The protein was rich in amino acids with non-polar side-chains and relatively stable to heat and proteolytic enzymes. Recent analyses of the amino acid composition, terminal sequences and other properties of highly purified fimbrial protein have been reported by Korhonen *et al.* (1980), Eshdat *et al.* (1981) and Klemm *et al.* (1982). These studies, however, are still in a preliminary stage and the results so far available do not permit clear conclusions to be drawn about the relation between antigenic character and amino acid composition. Thus, Klemm *et al.* (1982) found that three antigenically distinct varieties, 1A, 1B and 1C, of type 1-like fimbriae of *E. coli* had such minor differences in their *N*-terminal sequences of 16–21 amino acids that their antigenic differences probably reflected greater differences in the composition of other, yet uninvestigated parts of their molecules.

Presumably because of their relative hydrophobicity, type-1 fimbriae have an affinity for air–water interfaces and tend to hold the bacteria at the surface of liquid media. When cultured in aerobic static broth, the fimbriate bacteria tend to grow as a pellicle on the surface of the broth, where their access to atmospheric oxygen for energy production enables them to grow more abundantly than non-fimbriate bacteria confined to the depths of the oxygen-depleted medium (Duguid and Gillies, 1957; Duguid and Wilkinson, 1961; Old *et al.*, 1968).

III. FIMBRIAL PHASE VARIATION

Bacteria genotypically capable of forming fimbriae can readily vary between fimbriate and non-fimbriate phases. The variation may be spontaneous, like flagellar antigen phase variation, or induced by particular environmental conditions. If fimbriate or non-fimbriate bacteria are to be obtained for antigenic studies, it is necessary to apply the conditions of culture that will select or induce the required phase.

Brinton *et al.* (1954) observed a spontaneous variation between fimbriate and non-fimbriate phases in *E. coli* strain B which took place in either direction at the rate of about once per 1000 bacteria per generation, during growth in broth. Apparently similar spontaneous variations were observed in seven 'variable' strains of *E. coli* by Duguid *et al.* (1955) and in all fimbriate strains of *S. flexneri* by Duguid and Gillies (1957). The latter authors found that cultures consisting almost wholly of fimbriate-phase bacteria could be selected by serial culture for 24 or 48 h periods in aerobic static broth and cultures consisting almost wholly of non-fimbriate-phase bacteria by serial aerobic culture on agar plates. The prolonged culture in broth selected the fimbriate phase because the fimbriate bacteria enjoyed enhanced growth in a surface pellicle (Duguid and Gillies, 1957; Duguid and Wilkinson, 1961).

Type-1 fimbriate salmonellae also showed spontaneous variation between fimbriate and non-fimbriate phases, selected, respectively, by serial culture in aerobic static broth and serial culture on agar plates (Duguid *et al.*, 1966). But many strains did not show such clear-cut changes as *S. flexneri*; they still formed a proportion of non-fimbriate bacteria in broth and a proportion of fimbriate bacteria on agar. That the conditions of fimbriae-mediated, pelliculate growth on broth were powerfully selective of the fimbriate phase was confirmed in competitive growth experiments with mixtures of fimbriate and non-fimbriate strains (Old and Duguid, 1970).

Some other cultural conditions associated with a change of fimbrial phase in salmonellae appear to act by directly inducing a change of phenotype rather than by promoting the selective outgrowth of spontaneous phase variants. Thus, the conditions of continued logarithmic growth in plain or glucose broth convert fimbriate cultures to the non-fimbriate phase within a few hours, which is quicker than could be attributed to the selective outgrowth of variants (Duguid *et al.*, 1966), and the synthesis of type-1 fimbriae is subject to catabolite repression by glucose, glycerol, other metabolizable carbohydrates and high concentrations of cyclic AMP (Saier *et al.*, 1978).

IV. ANTIGENICITY OF TYPE-1 FIMBRIAE

As fimbriae are distinct surface structures of bacteria, it appeared likely from the outset that they would bear distinctive antigens capable of reacting in agglutination and other serological tests with intact bacteria. This likelihood was strengthened by the finding that the haemagglutinating activity of fimbriate *E. coli* was diminished by mixture with antiserum to living, fimbriate bacteria, but not by antiserum to bacilli defimbriated by heating for 2.5 h at 100°C (Duguid *et al.*, 1955).

Gillies and Duguid (1958) chose *S. flexneri* as the most suitable bacterium for the first study of fimbrial antigens because it lacked interfering flagellar and capsular antigens and because strains of all O-serovars could be obtained almost wholly in either the fimbriate or the non-fimbriate phase. Over 95% of fimbriate bacteria were obtained in serial subcultures in broth and less than 0.2% in serial subcultures on agar. The degree of fimbriation in the test cultures was assessed either by electron microscopy or, indirectly, by measuring their haemagglutinating power (Duguid and Gillies, 1957).

Fimbriate and non-fimbriate cultures of the same strain were required for the preparation of a 'pure fimbrial antiserum'. A crude fimbrial antiserum was first raised by immunizing a rabbit with injections of a living, fimbriate-phase culture and this serum was freed from antibodies to the O and other non-fimbrial surface antigens by absorption with living bacteria from a non-fimbriate-phase culture.

A. Fimbrial Agglutination

The absorbed fimbrial antiserum agglutinated fimbriate-phase, but not non-fimbriate-phase bacteria of the homologous and heterologous strains of *S. flexneri*. The agglutinating titre of the serum was high, e.g. 15 360, and the clumping rapid and loosely floccular. The latter properties reflected the high proportion of bacteria with long fimbriae in the *S. flexneri* broth cultures. In later, comparable experiments with salmonella cultures, in which the fimbriate bacteria were fewer and the fimbriae shorter, the agglutination by salmonella fimbrial serum was slow and finely granular.

B. Fimbriae and O-inagglutinability

Non-fimbrial antisera raised by immunization with non-fimbriate-phase *S. flexneri* cultures gave compact, somatic-type agglutination with the homologous non-fimbriate bacteria and also, but only at much lower titres, with fimbriate-phase bacteria of the same strains (Gillies and Duguid, 1958). Thus, the profuse, long fimbriae of *S. flexneri* conferred a degree of O-inagglutinability on the bacteria. This effect of fimbriae in masking the O-antigens was slight or absent in fimbrial-phase cultures of salmonellae, in which the fimbriate bacteria were fewer and the fimbriae shorter (Duguid and Campbell, 1969).

C. Immunoelectron Microscopy

The affinity of fimbrial antibodies for fimbriae is demonstrable by electron-microscopic examination of metal-shadowed films (Gillies and Duguid, 1958). Bacteria agglutinated by absorbed fimbrial antiserum show many fimbriae adhering side-by-side to one another and other, separate fimbriae thickened by an irregular deposit of antibody along their edges (Figure 1). Similar bacteria agglutinated by non-fimbrial antiserum show fimbriae radiating separately from one another and unthickened by any surface deposit (Figure 2). The later method of negative staining with phosphotungstic acid demonstrates the binding of antibodies to fimbriae even more clearly and has been used to distinguish antigenically different fimbriae on the same bacterium (e.g. see Ørskov *et al.*, 1980; Adegbola and Old, 1983) (Figure 3).

Figure 1. Fimbriate *Shigella flexneri* agglutinated by homologous fimbrial antiserum. Adjacent fimbriae adhere to one another in bundles of two to six. The bundles and separate fimbriae show an irregular deposit of antibody along their edges. $\times 27\,000$

Figure 2. Fimbriate *Shigella flexneri* agglutinated by antiserum to the non-fimbriate phase of the same strain. The fimbriae radiate separately from the bacteria without adhering to one another and without any deposit of antibody on their edges. $\times 27\,000$

Figures 1 and 2 are electron micrographs of metal-shadowed films. (Reproduced from Gillies and Duguid, 1958, by permission of the Editor of the *Journal of Hygiene*)

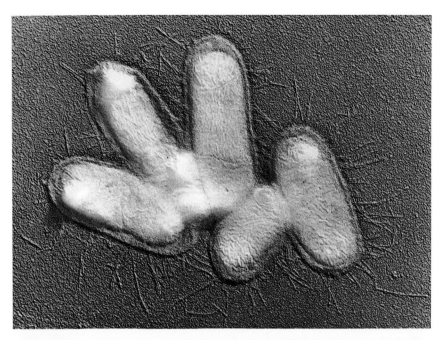

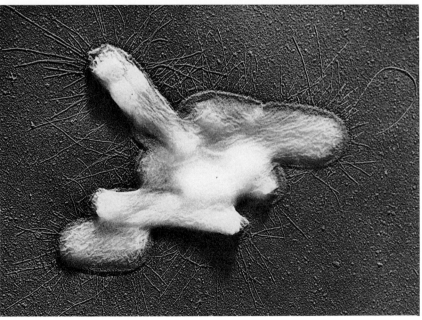

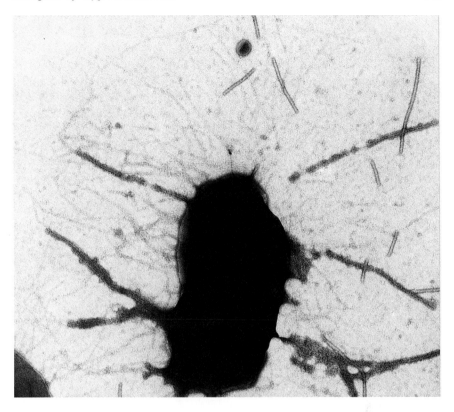

Figure 3. An *Enterobacter aerogenes* bacillus bearing six long and some shorter 'leashes' of type-1 fimbriae heavily coated and matted together with anti-type-1 fimbrial antibody, as well as numerous type-3 fimbriae not coated with the type-1 antibody. A few loose fragments of thicker flagella are also present. Dried film treated with antiserum and stained with uranyl acetate. Electron micrograph, × 60 000. (By courtesy of R. A. Adegbola and D. C. Old)

D. Stability of Fimbrial Antigens

The type-1 fimbriae and fimbrial antigens of *S. flexneri* and *E. coli* are unaffected by heating for 1 h at 60°C, but are detached from the bacteria by heating for 1 h at 90°C or 100°C, when, however, the detached fimbriae are neither disrupted nor rendered non-antigenic (Gillies and Duguid, 1958). After being washed free from the detached fimbriae, the heated bacteria have lost their fimbrial serum agglutinability, fimbrial antibody binding capacity, fimbrial immunogenicity and relative O-inagglutinability. Suspensions of the fimbriae detached at 100°C will precipitate with fimbrial antiserum and in tests with unwashed suspensions of heated bacteria the precipitate may be mistaken for bacterial agglutination. It is only on autoclaving for 20 min at 121°C that the fimbriae are disintegrated and their precipitability by antiserum largely lost.

Holding type-1 fimbriate bacilli in 0.25% (v/v) formaldehyde has no effect on their morphology, haemagglutinating activity, fimbrial serum agglutinability and fimbrial immunogenicity, so that this fixative may be used to kill and preserve vaccines and agglutinable suspensions of fimbriate salmonellae and other organisms (Duguid and Campbell, 1969). Treatment with 0.005 M hydrochloric acid for 5 min at 37°C, as in Duncan's (1935) method for the removal of flagella, does not affect the fimbrial antigens, and treatment with 95% (v/v) ethanol for 30 min at 45°C reduces but does not abolish their reactivity. The relative stability of the fimbrial antigens to these treatments leads to the possibility of their remaining active in heat-killed, alcoholized and formaldehyde-killed vaccines and agglutinable suspensions.

V. FIMBRIAL ANTIGENS IN *S. FLEXNERI* AND *E. COLI*

By cross-agglutination and cross-absorption tests, Gillies and Duguid (1958) showed that the fimbrial antigens were identical in all tested strains of *S. flexneri*. Fimbrial antisera against strains of O-serovars 1a, 2b, 3, 4a and 5 agglutinated fimbriate bacteria of each of these types, and of variants X and Y to the same high titre. Successive absorptions of any serum with fimbriate bacteria of any strain reduced its fimbrial agglutinating titre for all strains to the same extent. Three absorptions removed all activity from each serum for all strains.

A. *Flexneri–coli* Shared Antigens

Although the fimbrial antigens of all strains of *S. flexneri* appeared to be identical, cross-agglutination and absorption tests with type-1 fimbriate *E. coli* bacteria showed that the *flexneri* fimbriae had at least three antigenic determinants (**1, 2** and **3**), one or more of which had shared with all of 26 tested strains of *E. coli*. Table 1 summarizes the distribution of antigens in *S. flexneri* and *E. coli* indicated by the findings of Gillies and Duguid (1958) who, however, did not give the numbers designating the different antigens.

In a typical experiment, an absorbed fimbrial antiserum to a strain of *S. flexneri* serovar 4a, with a titre of 120 000 for the homologous bacteria, agglutinated the type-1 fimbriate bacteria of all of 24 tested strains of *E. coli*. With 16 of the strains (e.g. Nos. 93, 108 and 208, Table 1) the titres were low, 120–960; with eight (51-like and ungrouped A, Table 1), they were higher, 1920–7680, and with one (No. 253) it was 15 360.

The low titres of fimbrial agglutinins for the first 16 *E. coli* strains were reduced or abolished by absorption of the *S. flexneri* serum with the fimbriate bacteria of each representative strain of *E. coli* (Nos. 93, 108, 208, 51 and 253),

Table 1 Antigenic determinants in the type-1 fimbriae of 28 strains of *S. flexneri* and 26 strains of *E. coli*

Strains			Fimbrial antigens*	
Species	Serotype or group	Number	Major	Minor
S. flexneri	1a, 2b, 3, 4a, 5, X, Y	28	**1**	**2, 3**
E. coli	93-like	6	**4**	**2**
	108-like	6	**5**	**2**
	208-like	1	**6**	**2**
	51-like	5	**6**	**2, 3**
	253-like	1	**1**	**2, 3**
	Ungrouped A	3	?	**2, 3**
	Ungrouped B	4	?	**2**

? = indicates that a major fimbrial antigen different from the others may have been present, but was not demonstrable as no serum was raised against these strains.
*Antigens **1**, **2** and **3** are shared between *S. flexneri* and *E. coli*.

presumably, because all 24 strains shared the same minor fimbrial antigen (antigen **2**) with *S. flexneri*. The higher titres of the *S. flexneri* serum against the eight '51-like' and 'ungrouped A' strains were reduced or abolished only by absorption with fimbriate bacteria of strain 51 or strain 253, presumably because all these strains shared a second fimbrial antigen (antigen **3**) with *S. flexneri*. The high titre for strain 253 was reduced and abolished only by absorption with fimbriate bacteria of the same strain, an absorption that also removed all fimbrial agglutinins for the *S. flexneri* bacteria, showing that this one strain of *E. coli* possessed all the fimbrial antigens (**1**, **2** and **3**) present in *S. flexneri*.

B. Major Fimbrial Antigens of *E. coli*

Tests with *E. coli* sera showed that in addition to the *flexneri–coli* shared antigens, different groups of *E. coli* strains possessed major, group-specific fimbrial antigens (e.g. antigens **4**, **5** and **6**, Table 1). The sera were prepared against three 'variable' strains, Nos. 93 (O 9: K ?: H –), No. 108 (O 21: K 4: H 4) and No. 208 (O 55: K 59: H ?), which gave richly fimbriate cultures in broth, used to raise the crude sera, and wholly non-fimbrial-phase cultures on agar, used to absorb the sera free from non-fimbrial antibodies.

In tests against type-1 fimbriate bacteria of 26 strains of *E. coli*, each absorbed serum gave high-titre agglutination with a different group of six strains (93-like; 108-like; 208-like; and 51-like; Table 1) and low titre agglutination with the other *E. coli* strains, and also with *S. flexneri*. The secondary absorption of each serum with fimbriate *S. flexneri* removed the cross-reacting low-titre agglutinins for the heterologous *E. coli* strains, which presumably were directed against the shared antigen **2**, but left unaffected the high-titre agglutinins for the six strains of the group sharing the same major antigen (antigens **4**, **5** or **6**).

Thus, the tests with the *S. flexneri* and three *E. coli* sera revealed the presence of one or other of the major fimbrial antigens (**1**, **4**, **5** and **6**) in 19 of the 26 type-1 fimbriate strains of *E. coli*. If sera had been prepared against some of the remaining seven strains, their reactions might have revealed the presence of further major antigens.

In a later study of different strains of *S. flexneri* and *E. coli*, Cefalù (1960) obtained similar findings to those just described. In further examinations of *E. coli*, Duguid *et al.* (1979) found that type-1 fimbriate bacteria of all of 184 strains from 84 different O-serogroups were agglutinated to high or low titre by fimbrial antisera to strains 93, 108 and 208. Apparently, all strains contained the shared fimbrial antigen **2**. Clegg (1978) tested 147 of the strains with the same three sera after they had been freed from antibodies to the shared antigens by absorption with heterologous bacteria. He found that 51 strains contained the major fimbrial antigen **4**, 23 the antigen **5**, 14 the antigen **6** and 59 none of these three antigens. Antigen **4**, which was the commonest major antigen, was present in several strains of O-serogroup 3. A few strains contained both antigens **4** and **6**, and one strain, C105, contained substantial amounts of all three antigens, **4**, **5** and **6**.

VI. FIMBRIAL ANTIGENS IN SALMONELLAE

Type-1 fimbriae are formed by most strains of most serovars of salmonellae (Duguid *et al.*, 1966), but though they resemble those of *S. flexneri* and *E. coli* in their degree of stability to heat and chemical reagents, their antigenic determinants are entirely distinct.

Duguid and Campbell (1969) prepared 'pure' fimbrial antisera to 24 strains in 19 serovars of salmonella. The absorption of non-fimbrial antibodies from the crude sera was more difficult than for *S. flexneri* sera. Some of the non-fimbrial-phase cultures grown on agar to provide the absorbing bacilli were deficient in flagella and had to be supplemented with flagellate, non-fimbrial-phase bacteria grown for 12 h in 1% (w/v) glucose broth or flagellate bacteria of a different, genotypically non-fimbriate strain.

The absorbed sera were tested for agglutination of live or formaldehyde-killed bacteria of 95 strains in 79 serovars. Other strains could not be tested because their fimbriate-phase cultures contained too few fimbriate bacteria or were autoagglutinable in saline. Each serum agglutinated the fimbriate bacteria of every tested strain and serovar, but not the non-fimbriate-phase bacteria of the same strains grown for 6 h in broth, 12 h in glucose broth or 24 h on agar. Nor did they agglutinate the homologous fimbriate-phase bacteria after these had been defimbriated by heating for 30 min at 90°C or 100°C and washed free from the detached fimbriae. The results suggested that the type-1 fimbriae of all salmonellae share at least one common antigenic determinant (antigen 1).

Cross-absorption tests with the fimbrial sera to strains of 22 serovars and the fimbriate bacteria of the 22 strains showed that 16 strains possessed one or more additional fimbrial antigens (antigens 2–5). The results suggested that only antigen 1 was present in the single strains of *Salmonella arizonae*, *S. bredeney*, *S. montevideo*, *S. paratyphi* C, *S. poona* and *S. saint-paul*; antigens 1 and 2 in *S. aberdeen*, *S. anatum*, *S. cubana*, *S. potsdam*, *S. senftenberg*, *S. thompson* and *S. worthington*; antigens 1, 2 and 3 in *S. heidelberg*, *S. paratyphi* B, *S. stanley* and *S. typhimurium*; antigens 1, 2 and 4 in *S. cholerae-suis* and *S. hvittingfoss*; antigens 1, 2 and 5 in *S. enteritidis*; antigens 1 and 5 in *S. typhi*; and antigens 1, 2, 4 and 5 in *S. newport* (Duguid and Campbell, 1969, and unpublished results). No differences were found in the fimbrial antigens of different strains of the same serovar. Thus, reciprocal absorptions showed that the combination of antigens was identical in all of eight strains of *S. typhimurium*.

A complete absence of cross-agglutination by their fimbrial sera showed there was no sharing of fimbrial antigens between salmonellae on the one hand and *S. flexneri* and *E. coli* on the other. The similarly numbered antigens in the two series were unrelated.

VII. FIMBRIAL ANTIGENS IN OTHER ENTEROBACTERIA

Less is known about the antigens of the type-1 fimbriae in other genera of enterobacteria. In studies of a few strains, Duguid and Campbell (1969) found that the partial sharing of fimbrial antigens between *S. flexneri* and *E. coli* extended to *Klebsiella aerogenes*, and that among the serovars of salmonellae and arizona to *Citrobacter freundii* and *C. ballerupensis*. But there was no sharing between the fimbriae of *Enterobacter cloacae* and those of either the *flexneri–coli–aerogenes* group or the *Salmonella–Arizona–Citrobacter* group.

In a more recent study, Nowotarska and Mulczyk (1977) found that the type-1 fimbrial antigens of *Hafnia*, *Providencia*, *Serratia marcescens* and *Edwardsiella tarda* were distinct in each of these groups and different from those of *E. coli* and salmonellae. A surprising finding was a similarity between the fimbrial antigens of *Klebsiella ozaenae* and those of the *flexneri–coli–aerogenes* organisms, for the only fimbriae found in *K. ozaenae* by Duguid (1968) were type 6, very different in their smaller numbers, greater length and slight haemagglutinating activity from type 1. Yet this similarity has since been confirmed in immunoelectron microscopic studies by Old and Adegbola (1984); the type-6 fimbriae of *K. ozaenae* were heavily coated with antibody raised against the type-1 fimbriae of *K. aerogenes* strain K55.1.

In the studies of Old *et al.* (1983) and Old and Adegbola (1984), type-1 fimbriae were found in 74 out of 132 strains in 11 species and subspecies of *Klebsiella*, 28 out of 49 strains in six species of *Enterobacter*, and 29 out of

56 strains in nine species of *Serratia*. Different major type-1 fimbrial antigens were found in six groups of strains, any one of these antigens being present in all members of the same group and absent from all members of the other five groups. Immunoelectron microscopy did not detect even a minor sharing of type-1 fimbrial antigens between any of the different groups. The six groups were as follows:

(1) *Klebsiella aerogenes*
    K. oxytoca
    K. pneumoniae (sensu stricto)
    K. planticola
    K. terrigena
    K. trevisanii

(2) *Enterobacter cloacae*
    E. amnigenus
    E. sakazakii

(3) *Enterobacter intermedium*

(4) *Enterobacter aerogenes*
    (syn. *Klebsiella mobilis*)

(5) *Serratia marcescens*
    S. ficaria
    S. grimesii
    S. liquefaciens
    S. marinorubra
    S. proteomaculans

(6) *Serratia odorifera*

VIII. RELATION TO OTHER TYPES OF FIMBRIAE

Most studies indicate that the different types of fimbriae classified by Duguid and Old (1980) are antigenically distinct. Thus, the type-MRE fimbriae of *E. coli*, which give mannose-resistant and eluting haemagglutination, were found to be entirely different from the type-1 fimbriae (Duguid *et al.*, 1979; Ørskov *et al.*, 1980; Gaastra and De Graaf, 1982), and the type-3 fimbriae of strains of *K. aerogenes* lacking type-1 fimbriae and the type-4 fimbriae of *Proteus mirabilis* to be different from the type-1 fimbriae of these and other species (Nowotarska and Mulczyk, 1977). Very thin, type-3-like fimbriae, antigenically different from type-1 fimbriae, have been found in some strains of *Salmonella enteritidis* and *S. typhimurium* isolated from pasta (Rohde *et al.*, 1975; Adegbola *et al.*, 1983); this type of fimbria is rare in salmonellae, being absent from the series of Duguid *et al.* (1966), including 21 strains of *S. enteritidis* and 775 of *S. typhimurium*.

There is one clear example of a sharing of antigens between functionally different types of fimbriae. The type-2 fimbriae found in a few strains of salmonellae lacking type-1 fimbriae differ from the latter in being non-adhesive. Yet Old and Payne (1971) found that the type-2 fimbriae of strains of *S. paratyphi* B were antigenically identical with the type-1 fimbriae of other strains of this serovar, for each type of fimbriae could absorb all agglutinins reactive with the other. They suggested that the type-2 fimbriae were a non-functioning mutant form of type-1 fimbriae, which lacked the MS adhesive structure but none of the detectable antigenic determinants of the latter. A mutational origin of the type-2 bacteria was suggested by the finding that they occasionally yielded back-mutants forming type-1 fimbriae.

Klemm *et al.* (1982) have described strains of *E. coli* that form two out of three immunologically different forms of type-1 fimbriae, either 1A and 1B or 1A and 1C, which have nearly homologous N-terminal amino-acid sequences. Whether the 1B and 1C fimbriae lacked the MS adhesiveness of the 1A fimbriae and whether the variation was mutational was unknown.

The recent demonstration of antigenic sharing between the type-1 fimbriae of *Klebsiella aerogenes* and the type-6 fimbriae of *K. ozaenae* by Old and Adegbola (1984) has been described above.

IX. RELATION TO PREVIOUSLY KNOWN ANTIGENS

When in 1955 it was first discovered that fimbriae bore thermolabile antigens reactive in agglutination tests, it was difficult to understand why these had not already been identified among the surface antigens observed in the established schemes for detecting the serovars of *S. flexneri*, *E. coli* and salmonellae. The fimbrial antigens differed from the known O, H and K antigens both in their wider sharing among different organisms and in their different degree of thermolability. They were more thermolabile than the O-antigens, less so than the H-antigens, and different from the L, A and B varieties of K-antigen in Kauffmann's (1947) scheme for *E. coli*. Thus, bacilli retained their fimbrial serum agglutinability but not their L-agglutinability when heated for 1 h at 60°C, and lost their fimbrial agglutinability but not their A-antigens or the agglutinin-binding activity of their B-antigens when heated at 100°C.

Later findings, however, have thrown doubt on the validity of classifying the K-antigens of *E. coli* into L, A and B varieties. Ørskov *et al.* (1977) have proposed that the subdivision of K-antigens should be restricted to two main groups; the polysaccharide K-antigens and the protein K-antigens. The former group includes both thermolabile and thermostable antigens, and the latter group the fimbrial antigens.

To explain the absence of fimbrial antigens from the extant schemes of antigenic analysis of enterobacteria, Gillies and Duguid (1958) suggested that the methods used by serologists to discriminate serovars had been devised in such a way as to avoid cross-reactions due to shared antigens, of which fimbriae are an example. The general use of agar-grown, or young (e.g. 6 h) broth cultures for preparing immunizing vaccines and agglutinable bacterial suspensions would provide bacteria mainly or wholly in the non-fimbriate phase.

X. CROSS-REACTING ANTIGENS OF ENTEROBACTERIA

Some of the early described cross-reacting antigens of enterobacteria may have been fimbrial. The alpha antigen found in some strains of *E. coli*, *K. aerogenes* and *Proteus morgani* by Stamp and Stone (1944) and the beta antigen found in strains of *E. coli*, *S. flexneri* and *Proteus* by Mushin (1949) resembled fimbrial antigens in their degree of stability to heat, ethanol and formaldehyde, their masking of the O-antigens and their tendency to disappear on serial subculture on agar. The beta antigen may have been one of the *flexneri–coli* shared fimbrial antigens, but the alpha antigen differed from these in the failure of alpha bacteria to be agglutinated by 'natural' agglutinins in 40 human sera.

A. X-antigen

An even closer correspondence was noted by Duguid and Campbell (1969) between the fimbrial antigens of salmonellae and the cross-reacting X-antigens found in *Salmonella typhimurium*, *S. newport*, *S. typhi*, *S. paratyphi* B and other salmonellae by Topley and Ayrton (1924), Happold (1928, 1929) and Cruickshank (1939). The X-antigens resembled fimbrial antigens in their thermostability at 60°C, their detachment from bacilli on heating at 100°C, their stability in 0.25% (v/v) formaldehyde, their near absence in young (under 16 h), but abundance in older, cultures in aerobic static broth, and their near absence in glucose broth in which the pH fell to 5.0.

The Mutton strain of *S. typhimurium*, in which the X-antigen was first found, also forms type-1 fimbriae, and the distribution of shared and distinctive fimbrial antigens among salmonellae corresponds with Happold's (1929) observation that the X-antigens included a factor common to different salmonellae but these antigens were not identical in all serovars.

XI. AVOIDANCE OF FIMBRIAL CROSS-REACTIONS IN SEROTYPING

Care must be taken to avoid cross-reactions due to fimbrial antigens and antibodies in agglutination tests for the identification of enterobacteria by their O, H and K antigens. If fimbriate-phase bacteria are used for raising the diagnostic sera and for making the agglutinable bacterial suspensions, the serum to any one serovar of a species may agglutinate live or formaldehyde- or ethanol-killed bacteria of any other serovar.

Agglutinable suspensions for the determination of O-antigens may be prepared from fimbriate-phase cultures by heating the bacteria at 100°C and washing them free from the detached fimbriae. Suspensions for determination of the heat-labile H and K antigens should be made from cultures grown under conditions that select or induce the non-fimbriate phase. Serial culture for 24-h periods on agar plates select the non-fimbriate phase, but such cultures may be deficient in flagella. Richly flagellate, non-fimbriate-phase salmonellae for determination of H-antigens may be obtained by culture for 6 h in plain broth or 12 h in glucose broth seeded from a swarm through semisolid agar.

The few fimbriate bacteria present in cultures grown by methods selective for the non-fimbriate phase may just suffice to induce the production of fimbrial antibodies when injected into an animal. In preparing a diagnostic serum, therefore, it is advantageous to use a genotypically non-fimbriate strain to make the immunizing vaccine.

XIV. FIMBRIAL ANTIBODIES IN HUMAN SERUM

Antibodies to the type-1 fimbriae of *E. coli* and *S. flexneri* are commonly present in human serum. Gillies and Duguid (1958) found that 80 out of 81 sera from adults without dysentery agglutinated fimbriate *S. flexneri* at titres from 30 to 1920. The agglutination was due to fimbrial antibodies, for the titres were not reduced by absorption of the sera with homologous non-fimbriate-phase bacteria. Most of the sera agglutinated fimbriate *E. coli* to about the same titre as *S. flexneri* and it was concluded that the fimbrial antibodies have been formed in response to the uptake of *flexneri–coli* shared antigens from *E. coli* in the intestine.

Antibodies to the fimbrial antigens of salmonellae are found in a smaller proportion of uninfected adults. When present, however, they may cause false-positive reactions in Widal tests made with suspensions containing fimbriate bacteria. Such antibodies were found in the sera of 13 out of 100 patients with fever or diarrhoea by Duguid and Wright (see Duguid and Campbell, 1969). The positive sera agglutinated fimbriate *S. typhimurium* at titres of 120–1920, but not alcoholized (O) or formolized (H) suspensions of non-fimbriate *S. typhimurium*. They also agglutinated the fimbriate bacteria of salmonellae not sharing O or H antigens with *S. typhimurium* and were freed from the *S. typhimurium* agglutinins by absorption with these heterologous bacteria.

Later sera from the patients possessing the fimbrial antibodies did not show a rise of titre, and cultures from their faeces did not yield salmonellae. Production of the antibodies therefore did not seem to be due to recent salmonella infection. In some cases it was probably the result of typhoid–paratyphoid (TAB) vaccination, for the two patients with the highest titres had been vaccinated recently and potent fimbrial antigens were demonstrated in each of three tested batches of commercial vaccine.

Similar observations were made by Cruickshank (1939) on antibodies to the X-antigens, now presumed to be fimbrial. The serum of a patient with brucellosis strongly agglutinated an alcoholized suspension of *S. paratyphi* B in a Widal test, but the reaction was shown to be false, due to the presence of X-antibodies in the serum and X-antigens in the suspension. Similar X-antibody was found at titres of 20 or greater in the sera of 25% of 'normal' persons, 19% of typhoid and paratyphoid patients, and 5 of 12 persons given TAB vaccine.

In a larger study, Brodie (1977) found salmonella fimbrial antibodies at titres of 25–800 in 64% 300 typhoid patients in an outbreak due to a type-1 fimbriate strain of *S. typhi* phage-type 34. He also found such antibodies at titres of 25–1600 in 65% of laboratory staff immunized with a phenolized TAB vaccine and 95% of nurses immunized with an alcoholized one.

There is now substantial evidence, reviewed by Gaastra and De Graaf (1982), that antibodies to some types of adhesive fimbriae other than type 1, e.g. the K88 and K99 fimbriae of *E. coli*, are protective against intestinal infection in animals. They inhibit bacterial adhesion to the intestinal epithelium, promote phagocytosis of the bacteria and bring about replacement of the fimbriate bacteria by a population of phenotypically non-fimbriate variant bacteria. Vaccination of a dam with purified K88 fimbriae gives her offspring a colostrum-transmitted passive immunity against infection with a K88-positive pathogen.

Evidence for a comparable protective action by antibodies to type-1 fimbriae is less convincing. *In vitro*, certainly, such antibodies, or their Fab fragments, inhibit the adhesion of type-1 fimbriate bacteria to erythrocytes (Gillies and Duguid, 1958), porcine intestinal epithelial cells (Isaacson *et al.*, 1978) and human urinary and buccal epithelial cells (Korhonen *et al.*, 1981) and greatly enhance the stimulation of phagocytic granulocytes by type-1 fimbriate bacteria (Perry *et al.*, 1983). These activities of the antibodies might be protective against infection, but such protection has not yet been demonstrated *in vivo*.

It seems unlikely that antibodies to the type-1 fimbriae can have a major role in conferring resistance to salmonella infections, for genotypically non-fimbriate salmonellae are nearly as infective as comparable fimbriate strains, showing that the fimbrial adhesin is unnecessary for infection (Duguid *et al.*, 1976). The finding, moreover, that many patients infected with genotypically fimbriate typhoid or paratyphoid bacteria fail to form fimbrial antibodies suggests that the bacteria multiply in the body mainly in their non-fimbriate phase, against which the fimbrial antibodies can hardly be protective. For similar reasons, it seems unlikely that antibodies to the fimbriae of *S. flexneri* confer any resistance to that organism, but evidence is still lacking to show whether or not antibodies to the type-1 fimbriae of other pathogens have a protective role.

REFERENCES

Adegbola, R. A., and Old, D. C. (1983). Fimbrial haemagglutinins in *Enterobacter* species. *J. Gen. Microbiol.*, **129**, 2175–2180.

Adegbola, R. A., Old, D. C., and Aleksic, S. (1983). Rare MR/K-like haemagglutinins (and type 3-like fimbriae) of *Salmonella* strains. *FEMS Microbiol. Lett.*, **19**, 233–238.

Brinton, C. C. (1959). Non-flagellar appendages of bacteria. *Nature*, **183**, 782–786.

Brinton, C. C. (1965). The structure, function, synthesis and genetic control of bacterial pili and a molecular model for DNA and RNA transport in gram-negative bacteria. *Trans. N. Y. Acad. Sci.*, **27**, 1003–1054.

Brinton, C. C., Buzzell, A., and Lauffer, M. A. (1954). Electrophoresis and phage susceptibility studies on a filament-forming variant of the *E. coli* B bacterium. *Biochim. Biophys. Acta*, **15**, 533–542.

Brodie, J. (1977). Antibodies and the Aberdeen typhoid outbreak in 1964. II. Coombs', complement fixation and fimbrial agglutination tests. *J. Hyg.*, **79**, 181–192.

Cefalù, M. (1960). Le fimbrie in *Shigella flexneri* ed *Escherichia coli* con particolare riguardo alle proprietà antigeniche. *Riv. Inst. Sierter. Ital.*, **35**, 13–37.

Clegg, S. (1978). The adhesive and antigenic properties of enterobacterial haemagglutinins. *Ph.D. Thesis*, University of Dundee.

Cruickshank, J. C. (1939). Somatic and 'X' agglutinins to the *Salmonella* group. *J. Hyg.*, **39**, 224–237.

Duguid, J. P. (1968). The function of bacterial fimbriae. *Arch. Immunol. Ther. Exp.*, **16**, 173–188.

Duguid, J. P., and Campbell, I. (1969). Antigens of the type-1 fimbriae of salmonellae and other enterobacteria. *J. Med. Microbiol.*, **2**, 535–553.

Duguid, J. P., and Gillies, R. R. (1957). Fimbriae and adhesive properties in dysentery bacilli. *J. Pathol. Bacteriol.*, **74**, 397–411.

Duguid, J. P., and Old, D. C. (1980). Adhesive properties of Enterobacteriaceae. In *Bacterial Adherence (Receptors and Recognition, Series B*, Vol. 6) (Ed. E. H. Beachey), pp.187–217. Chapman and Hall, London.

Duguid, J. P., and Wilkinson, J. F. (1961). Environmentally induced changes in bacterial morphology. In *Microbial Reaction to Environment, Symposia of the Society for General Microbiology*, No. XI (Eds. G. G. Meynell and H. Gooder), pp.69–99. Cambridge University Press, UK.

Duguid, J. P., Smith, I. W., Dempster, G., and Edmunds, P. N. (1955). Non-flagellar filamentous appendages ('fimbriae') and haemagglutinating activity in *Bacterium coli*. *J. Pathol. Bacteriol.*, **70**, 335–348.

Duguid, J. P., Anderson, E. S., and Campbell, I. (1966). Fimbriae and adhesive properties in salmonellae. *J. Pathol. Bacteriol.*, **92**, 107–138.

Duguid, J. P., Darekar, M. R., and Wheater, D. W. F. (1976). Fimbriae and infectivity in *Salmonella typhimurium*. *J. Med. Microbiol.*, **9**, 459–473.

Duguid, J. P., Clegg, S., and Wilson, M. I. (1979). The fimbrial and non-fimbrial haemagglutinins of *Escherichia coli*. *J. Med. Microbiol.*, **12**, 213–227.

Duncan, J. T. (1935). Inactivation of the 'H' antigen by dilute mineral acid. *Br. J. Exp. Pathol.*, **16**, 405–410.

Eshdat, Y., Silverblatt, F. J., and Sharon, N. (1981). Dissociation and reassembly of *Escherichia coli* type 1 pili. *J. Bacteriol.*, **148**, 308–314.

Gaastra, W., and De Graaf, F. K. (1982). Host-specific fimbrial adhesins of noninvasive enterotoxigenic *Escherichia coli* strains. Microbiol. Rev., **46**, 129–161.

Gillies, R. R., and Duguid, J. P. (1958). The fimbrial antigens of *Shigella flexneri*. *J. Hyg.*, **56**, 303–318.

Happold, F. C. (1928). A precipitinogen obtained from cultures of *B. aertryke* Mutton *(Salmonellae aertryke)*. *J. Pathol. Bacteriol.*, **31**, 237–247.

Happold, F. C. (1929). The effect of cultural variation on the antigenic development of *B. aertryke* Mutton. *Br. J. Exp. Pathol.*, **10**, 263–272.

Houwink, A. L., and van Iterson, W. (1950). Electron microscopical observations on bacterial cytology. ii. A study of flagellation. *Biochim. Biophys. Acta*, **5**, 10–11.

Isaacson, R. E., Fusco, P. C., Brinton, C. C., and Moon, H. W. (1978). *In vitro* adhesion of *Escherichia coli* to porcine small intestinal epithelial cells: pili as adhesive factors. *Infect. Immun.*, **21**, 392–397.

Jones, G. W. (1977). The attachment of bacteria to the surfaces of animal cells. In *Microbial Interactions (Receptors and Recognition, Series B,* Vol. 3*)* (Ed. J. L. Reissig), pp.141–176. Chapman and Hall, London.

Kauffmann, F. (1947). The serology of the coli group. *J. Immunol.*, **57**, 71–100.

Klemm, P., Ørskov, I., and Ørskov, F. (1982). F7 and type 1-like fimbriae from three *Escherichia coli* strains isolated from urinary tract infections: protein, chemical and immunological aspects. *Infect. Immun.*, **36**, 462–468.

Korhonen, T. K., Nurmiaho, E.-L., Ranta, H., and Svanborg Edén, C. (1980). New method for isolation of immunologically pure pili from *Escherichia coli. Infect. Immun.*, **27**, 569–575.

Korhonen, T. K., Leffler, H., and Svanborg-Eden, C. (1981). Binding specificity of piliated strains of *Escherichia coli* and *Salmonella typhimurium* to epithelial cells, *Saccharomyces cerevisiae* cells and erythrocytes. *Infect. Immun.*, **32**, 796–804.

Mushin, R. (1949). A new antigenic relationship among faecal bacilli due to a common β antigen. *J. Hyg.*, **47**, 227–235.

Nowotarska, M., and Mulczyk, M. (1977). Serologic relationship of fimbriae among *Enterobacteriaceae. Arch. Immunol. Ther. Exp.*, **25**, 7–16.

Old, D. C. (1972). Inhibition of the interaction between fimbrial haemagglutinins and erythrocytes by D-mannose and other carbohydrates. *J. Gen. Microbiol.*, **71**, 149–157.

Old, D. C., and Adegbola, R. A. (1984). A comparative immunoelectronmicroscopical study of fimbriae of *Enterobacter* and *Klebsiella. Syst. Appl. Microbiol.*, **5**, 157–168.

Old, D. C., Corneil, I., Gibson, L. F., Thomson, A. D., and Duguid, J. P. (1968). Fimbriation, pellicle formation and the amount of growth of salmonellas in broth. *J. Gen. Microbiol.*, **51**, 1–16.

Old, D. C., and Duguid, J. P. (1970). Selective outgrowth of fimbriate bacteria in static liquid medium. *J. Bacteriol.*, **103**, 447–456.

Old, D. C., and Payne, S. B. (1971). Antigens of the type-2 fimbriae of salmonellae: 'cross-reacting material' (CRM) of type-1 fimbriae. *J. Med. Microbiol.*, **4**, 215–225.

Old, D. C., Adegbola, R., and Scott, S. S. (1983). Multiple fimbrial haemagglutinins in *Serratia* species. *Med. Microbiol. Immunol.*, **172**, 107–115.

Ørskov, I., Ørskov, F., Jann, B., and Jann, K. (1977). Serology, chemistry and genetics of O and K antigens of *Escherichia coli. Bacteriol. Rev.*, **41**, 667–710.

Ørskov, I., Ørskov, F., and Birch-Andersen, A. (1980). Comparison of *Escherichia coli* fimbrial antigen F7 with type 1 fimbriae. *Infect. Immun.*, **27**, 657–666.

Ottow, J. C. G. (1975). Ecology, physiology and genetics of fimbriae and pili. *Annu. Rev. Microbiol.*, **29**, 79–108.

Perry, A., Ofek, I., and Silverblatt, F. J. (1983). Enhancement of mannose-mediated stimulation of human granulocytes by type 1 fimbriae aggregated with antibodies on *Escherichia coli* surfaces. *Infect. Immun.*, **39**, 1334–1345.

Rohde, R., Aleksic, S., Müller, G., Plasvic, S., and Aleksic, V. (1975). Profuse fimbriae conferring O-inagglutinability to several strains of *S. typhimurium* and *S. enteritidis* isolated from pasta products: Cultural, morphological, and serological experiments. *Zentralbl. Bakteriol. Hyg. Abt. Orig. A*, **230**, 38–50.

Saier, M. H., Schmidt, M. R., and Leibowitz, M. (1978). Cyclic AMP-dependent synthesis of fimbriae in *Salmonella typhimurium*: effects of *cys* and *pts* mutations. *J. Bacteriol.*, **134**, 356–358.

Stamp, Lord, and Stone, D. M. (1944). An agglutinogen common to certain species of lactose and non-lactose-fermenting coliform bacilli. *J. Hyg.*, **43**, 266–272.

Topley, W. W. C., and Ayrton, J. (1924). 'Further investigations into the biological characteristics of *B. enteritidis (aertryke). J. Hyg.*, **23**, 198–222.

Immunology of the Bacterial Cell Envelope
Edited by D. E. S. Stewart-Tull and M. Davies
© 1985 John Wiley & Sons Ltd.

CHAPTER 12

Antigenic and Functional Properties of Enterobacterial Fimbriae

Timo K. Korhonen, Mikael Rhen, Vuokko Väisänen-Rhen and Auli Pere
*Department of General Microbiology, University of Helsinki,
Mannerheimintie 172, SF-00280, Helsinki 28, Finland*

I. INTRODUCTION

In nature, most bacteria probably live attached to some kind of a surface. The importance of bacterial adhesion was first discovered by marine microbiologists who noticed that marine bacteria live attached to interfaces that give them access to nutrients (ZoBell and Allen, 1935). In soil, microbial activity is highest on the surfaces of mineral particles and plant roots (Marshall, 1971). Recent interest in bacterial adhesion has focused on pathogenic bacteria, and it is now evident that the first step in many infectious diseases is bacterial adhesion to host tissue at the site of infection. However, in mammals bacterial adhesion probably also has a role in the stabilization of the normal bacterial flora, e.g. in human intestine and mouth (Ørskov *et al.*, 1980; Gibbons and van Houte, 1980). Bacterial adhesion also involves bacterium–bacterium interaction, which is essential in conjugation (Manning and Achtman, 1979), in pellicle formation on static liquid surfaces (Old and Duguid, 1970), and in the formation of dental plaque (Gibbons and van Houte, 1980). Adherence is therefore of fundamental importance in both bacterial ecology and pathogenicity.

In enteric bacteria, the adhesive properties are associated with the presence of fimbriae on the bacterial cell. Fimbriae are non-flagellar protein filaments occurring on the surface of bacteria (Duguid *et al.*, 1955). It is generally believed that the filament is composed of a single type of subunit, with molecular weights of 17 000 to 29 500. Fimbriae were first described as distinct organelles by Houvink and van Iterson (1950), and subsequently were detected in several, mostly gram-negative, bacterial species. The terms 'fimbria' and 'pilus' were used synonymously, but in this chapter we follow the suggestions of Ottow (1975) and Jones (1977): 'fimbria' is used for the filament that functions in bacterial adhesion; 'pilus' is reserved for the filament involved in the conjugative transfer of nucleic acids.

Duguid *et al.* (1955) were the first to demonstrate that the presence of fimbriae on *Escherichia coli* was associated with haemagglutinative and adhesive properties of the bacterium. Since then several types of fimbriae on enteric bacteria have been differentiated by their haemagglutination properties and natural sources. A complex picture is emerging and it is evident that one bacterial species, e.g. *E. coli*, is able to synthesize various types of fimbriae which are associated with different clinical situations. The complexity of the phenomenon is further increased by the recent findings that one strain, and perhaps even one cell, of *E. coli* may possess many distinct fimbriae, the synthesis of which undergoes very rapid phase variation (Duguid and Old, 1980; Ørskov *et al.*, 1980; Rhen *et al.*, 1983c,d).

Ideally, fimbriae should be classified according to their binding specificities and serological properties. This type of classification, however, is not possible at present since only a few fimbrial receptors are known at the molecular level. Serological properties have been used in the classification of *E. coli* fimbriae (Ørskov and Ørskov, 1983), but this may lead to an underestimation of the functional properties of fimbriae. The number of chemically and serologically well-characterized fimbrial proteins is still rather small, and no systematic serological comparison has been done between the existing antigenic types. Even less informative is the classification based on morphology (cf. Ottow, 1975) since differences in fimbrial morphology are too small to be of practical value, and some fimbriae, e.g. type 1 and P, with unrelated binding properties are morphologically indistinguishable (Korhonen *et al.*, 1982). Fimbriae on *E. coli* have also been classified according to the haemagglutination patterns obtained with various erythrocytes (Duguid *et al.*, 1979; Evans *et al.*, 1979a). This classification does not take into account the fact that one strain may have many different fimbriae and such a scheme is therefore hard to interpret.

It is customary to divide *E. coli* fimbriae into two groups: common mannose-binding type-1 fimbriae (MS fimbriae), and haemagglutinins that cause mannose-resistant haemagglutination (MR fimbriae). This crude classification should be abandoned since it is obvious that the MR fimbriae are a heterogeneous group with different binding specificities, some of which have already been characterized on the molecular level (Korhonen *et al.*, 1982; Väisänen *et al.*, 1982, Väisänen-Rhen *et al.*, 1983; Parkkinen *et al.*, 1983). The receptor structures for the major types of enterobacterial fimbriae will no doubt be resolved in the near future and a classification based on receptor specificity will become possible.

A summary of the 'major types' of *E. coli* fimbriae is given in Table 1. These types have been differentiated mainly by their haemagglutination properties (or receptor specificities when known), by their serological properties, and by their natural sources, i.e. by the serovars of the strains carrying the fimbriae and by the clinical situation in which they occur. As will be discussed below, many of the 'major types' possess antigenic variants, and a number of other fimbriae may function on organisms in similar clinical situations. This chapter reviews recent findings on the immunological and functional properties of enterobacterial fimbriae. Our emphasis is on *E. coli* fimbriae; for previous reviews and for reviews on other enterobacterial fimbriae the reader is referred to the literature (Brinton, 1965; Ottow, 1975; Jones, 1977, 1980; Duguid and Old, 1980; Beachey, 1981; Gaastra and de Graaf, 1982).

II. PURIFICATION OF FIMBRIAE

The first step is the detachment of fimbriae from the cell surface, either by mechanical agitation in a homogenizer (Novotny *et al.*, 1969), or by heating the cell suspension to 60°C (Stirm *et al.*, 1967), or by passing the cell suspension through a flattened needle (Rhen *et al.*, 1983c). Heat reportedly denatures the P fimbriae of *E. coli* (Svanborg Edén and Hansson, 1978) so it may not be applicable to all fimbrial types. Following detachment, the fimbriae are concentrated, usually by one of the following methods; ammonium sulphate or isoelectric precipitation (Brinton, 1965), membrane filtration (Beard *et al.*, 1972), or polyethylene glycol precipitation (Helmuth and Achtman, 1978).

Brinton (1965) was the first to isolate type-1 fimbriae from *E. coli* by repeated isoelectric and magnesium chloride precipitations. Salit and Gotschlich (1977a) purified these fimbriae further by isopycnic ultracentrifugation in a caesium chloride gradient, but the preparation was still contaminated by outer membrane protein. This was probably due to the hydrophobic nature of the fimbrial filaments and their tendency to aggregate in aqueous solutions with themselves and with cell wall material. Isoelectric precipitation and ultracentrifugation have been used to prepare K88 antigen (Stirm *et al.*, 1967) and colonization factor antigen (CFA) (Evans *et al.*, 1978a). The resulting K88 antigen contained considerable amounts of lipopolysaccharide (LPS). Gel filtration first in 2.0 M

Table 1 Types of fimbriae on *E. coli*

Fimbria	Haemagglutination		Occurrence	Reference
	Type of erythrocyte	Sensitivity		
Type 1	Horse Guinea pig Chicken	αD-Mannosides	Most strains	Duguid *et al.*, 1955 Old, 1972 Salit and Gotschlich, 1977a
P	Human P$_1$, P$_2$ P$_1^k$ or P$_2^k$	αD-Gal(1→4)βD-Gal	Human pyelonephritogenic strains	Källenius *et al.*, 1980 Leffler and Svanborg Edén, 1980 Korhonen *et al.*, 1982 Väisänen-Rhen *et al.*, 1984
M	Human blood group M	Glycophorin A	Some human pathogenic strains	Väisänen *et al.*, 1982 Jokinen *et al.*, 1985
S	Human	Neuraminyl α(2→3) galactosides	O18acK1H7 strains from neonatal meningitis	Parkkinen *et al.*, 1983 Korhonen *et al.*, 1984
K88	Guinea pig Chicken	?	ETEC strains in pigs	Jones and Rutter, 1974 Parry and Porter, 1978
K99	Horse Sheep	?	ETEC strains in calves, lambs and pigs	Isaacson, 1978 de Graaf *et al.*, 1981 de Graaf and Roorda, 1982
CFA/I CFA/II	Human Bovine	?	ETEC strains in humans	Evans *et al.*, 1975 Evans and Evans, 1978
987P	None	—	ETEC strains in pigs	Nagy *et al.*, 1977 Isaacson and Richter, 1981
F41	Human Guinea pig	?	ETEC strains in calves and lambs	Morris *et al.*, 1980 de Graaf and Roorda, 1982

CFA, colonization factor antigen; ETEC, enterotoxigenic *E. coli*.

urea buffer and then in 6.0 M guanidium chloride buffer was used by Mooi and de Graaf (1979) to purify K88 antigens. It is apparent that the fimbriae so obtained were partially fragmented. Ion-exchange chromatography was used to isolate K99 (Isaacson, 1977) and CFA/I antigen (Evans *et al.*, 1979b).

Amino acid analysis of purified fimbrial proteins (e.g. Brinton, 1965; Salit and Gotschlich, 1977a) and hydrophobic interaction chromatography of fimbriated bacterial cells (Smyth *et al.*, 1978; Öhman *et al.*, 1982) have shown that fimbriae are very hydrophobic proteins. It is our experience that fimbriae are difficult to separate from contaminating outer membrane components by methods designed for water-soluble proteins because they have a strong tendency to aggregate in detergent-free medium. A purification procedure that takes advantage of the hydrophobicity and the stability of fimbrial filaments was developed in the authors' laboratory (Korhonen *et al.*, 1980c). In this procedure, detached fimbriae are treated with 0.5% (w/v) deoxycholate (DOC) to disaggregate fimbriae and to dissolve LPS. Outer membrane proteins are not solubilized by DOC, so fimbriae can be separated from these components by ultracentrifugation in a 10–60% (w/v) sucrose gradient in the presence of DOC. The fimbrial preparation is then passed through a Sepharose column with 6.0 M urea as eluate. Urea dissociates flagellae into subunits but the fimbrial filaments remain intact and can be separated from flagellins by gel filtration in urea. Stability in concentrated urea and DOC indicates strong interaction between fimbrial subunits, and strong treatment is indeed required to dissociate type-1 fimbrial filaments into subunits (McMichael and Ou, 1979; Eshdat *et al.*, 1981). The method has been used to purify fimbriae from flagellated strains, and with modifications in some instances, to purify type 1, P, M, S, and F41 fimbriae and K99 antigen from *E. coli* (Korhonen *et al.*, 1982, 1984; de Graaf and Roorda, 1982), type-1 fimbriae from *Salmonella typhimurium* (Korhonen *et al.*, 1980b) and *Klebsiella pneumoniae* (Fader *et al.*, 1982) as well as type-3 fimbriae of *K. aerogenes* (Korhonen *et al.*, 1983). Thus it seems that stability in the presence of mild detergents and concentrated urea is a property common to many enterobacterial fimbriae.

Only one biospecific purification procedure has been reported. Deneke *et al.* (1979) isolated fimbriae from a human enterotoxigenic *E. coli* strain by adsorption onto guinea pig erythrocytes in the presence of mannose (to exclude type-1 fimbriae) and elution at 37°C. The preparation gave two bands in sodium dodecyl sulphate–polyacrylamide electrophoresis (SDS–PAGE), indicating that it contained two aggregated fimbriae. Because of fimbrial aggregation the applicability of biospecific purification methods is probably limited. Moreover, after detachment from cells some fimbriae, e.g. CFA/I and P (Evans *et al.*, 1979b, Korhonen *et al.*, 1982), bind poorly to erythrocytes. Affinity purification of fimbriae should be performed in the presence of detergents (for disaggregation) and is probably limited to those fimbriae that possess strong binding properties (e.g. type 1 and M).

An additional problem encountered in purification of fimbriae is the fact that one strain may have many different fimbriae, which are difficult to separate. This is a problem met with pyelonephritogenic *E. coli* strains, which may have two or three other fimbriae in addition to those of type 1 (Korhonen *et al.*, 1982; Ørskov and Ørskov, 1983). We have recently developed a method for the fractionation of fimbriae from a single strain. While analyzing cross-reactions between various P fimbriae by immune blotting we noticed that some proteins in the preparations did not cross-react (Rhen *et al.*, 1983d). This allowed the opportunity to fractionate fimbriae by immune precipitation (Figure 1). When grown on CFA agar plates the *E. coli* KS71 model strain had three types of fimbriae, A, B and C (lane g in Figure 1). Fractionation was carried out in two steps: the first precipitations (lanes a–c in Figure 1) were done with cross-reacting antisera to remove superfluous fimbrial antigens, then the supernates were precipitated with antiserum to the unfractionated KS71 fimbriae (anti-A + B + C) lanes d–f). All precipitations were performed in 0.1% DOC to prevent fimbrial aggregation. Anti-A + B + C precipitated all fimbriae in a single step (lanes a and d). The P-fimbrial antiserum used in lane b had a low avidity for the KS71A fimbriae and left a fraction in solution (precipitated in lane e). This allowed the chance to isolate the KS71A fimbriae from the other two. The antiserum used in lane c did not precipitate the KS71C fimbriae and this enabled their

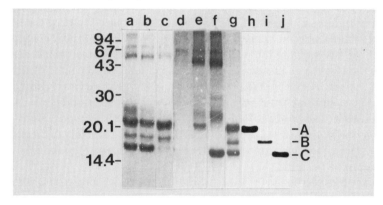

Figure 1. Fractionation of *E. coli* KS71 fimbriae by immune precipitation (lanes a–f) and by cloning of the structural genes (lanes h–j); lane g shows the purified KS71 fimbriae. Lanes a–c show SDS–PAGE analysis of the first precipitation (see text), lanes d–f are from second precipitation with antiserum to purified KS71ABC fimbriae (d was obtained from a, e from b, and f from c). Anti-fimbrial sera used in the first precipitation were (a) anti-KS71ABC, (b) anti-*E coli* ER2, and (c) anti-*E. coli* IH11002. The positions of the standard proteins (in kDa) are indicated on the left. The 50 kDa and 24 kDa peptides seen in several lanes are the heavy and light chains, respectively, of the rabbit immunoglobulin G molecule. Lanes h–j show fimbriae purified from recombinant strains that had received structural genes for the A, the B or the C fimbriae, respectively. (Modified from Rhen *et al.* (1983b,d) by permission of the Federation of European Microbiological Societies.)

purification (lane f). The fimbriae–antibody immune complexes were effectively dissociated with 1.0 M propionic acid and the fimbriae were separated from antibodies by sedimentation ultracentrifugation (Rhen *et al.*, 1983d). When grown in static broth the strain *E. coli* KS71 forms type-1 fimbriae also (here named KS71D fimbriae), which were purified by immune precipitation with an antiserum specific for type-1 fimbriae (Rhen *et al.*, 1983d).

When viewed in an electron microscope, KS71A and KS71C fimbriae were morphologically similar to type-1 (KS71D) fimbriae (Rhen *et al.*, 1983d). Fractionation confirmed that the multiple peptides seen in many fimbrial preparations (Jann *et al.*, 1981; Korhonen *et al.*, 1982) were derived from distinct filaments. Thus the tenet that each fimbrial filament is composed of only one type of subunit was upheld. In this context it should also be noted that a fimbrial preparation showing only one peptide band in SDS–PAGE can be composed of two antigenically unrelated fimbriae of equal apparent molecular weight (Rhen *et al.*, 1983a,d). Therefore observation of a single peptide band in SDS–PAGE should not be interpreted as an absolute proof of homogeneity and purity of a fimbrial preparation.

The immune precipitation method has proved to be very efficient in the fractionation of fimbriae on pyelonephritogenic *E. coli* strains but is naturally limited to fimbriae that are not cross-reactive serologically. For example, KS71B fimbriae could not be purified by immune precipitation since they cross-react with KS71A fimbriae (Rhen *et al.*, 1983a,d). Purification of KS71B fimbriae was possible when the structural genes for the fimbriae were cloned into a non-fimbriated *E. coli* strain (Rhen *et al.*, 1983b). Thus, a combination of immune precipitation and recombinant DNA technology makes it possible to separate all fimbriae from a single strain, as exemplified for *E. coli* KS71 (Figure 1, lanes h–j). Besides preparative purposes, the immune precipitation assay can be used for rapid screening and serological analysis of *E. coli* fimbriae.

III. TYPE-1 FIMBRIAE

Type-1 fimbriae, sometimes called MS fimbriae, cause mannose-sensitive haemagglutination. Because most enterobacterial species have these fimbriae and fresh isolates usually synthesize them, they are sometimes referred to as the common fimbriae. Their properties have been reviewed by Duguid and Old (1980) (see also Chapter 11).

Type-1 fimbriae have been purified from *E. coli* (Brinton, 1965; Salit and Gotschlich, 1977a; Korhonen *et al.*, 1980c), *S. typhimurium* (Korhonen *et al.*, 1980b), *K. pneumoniae* (Fader *et al.*, 1982), *K. aerogenes* and *Enterobacter agglomerans* (Korhonen *et al.*, 1983). In these species type-1 fimbriae are morphologically identical: about 7 nm in diameter and usually about 2 μm in length. The type-1 fimbrillins seem to differ in apparent molecular weights ranging from 21 000–21 500 from *S. typhimurium* and *K. pneumoniae* to

17 000–19 000 from other enteric bacteria. Type-1 fimbrillins from *E. coli, S. typhimurium* and *K. pneumoniae* have quite similar amino acid compositions, with a high proportion (about 40%) of hydrophobic amino acids.

The N-terminal amino acid sequences of type-1 fimbrillins from *E. coli, K. pneumoniae* and *S. typhimurium*, together with those for some other *E. coli* fimbrillins, are shown in Figure 2. The N-terminal sequences of type-1 fimbrillins are almost identical. Interestingly, all fimbrial sequences besides CFA/I show common invariant residues, i.e. glycine at positions 11 and 17, and some common features (residues at positions 13, 15 and 19–22 and charged or polar residues linking glycine at position 17). Glycine is generally thought to be an important amino acid for protein conformation because its small size allows folding of polypeptide chains. The sequence of the KS71C fimbria is almost identical to that of the *E. coli* type-1 fimbrillin; however, the KS71C has no mannose-binding properties and is serologically unrelated to the type-1 fimbriae (Rhen *et al.*, 1983a,d). The KS71C fimbria corresponds to the so-called type-1C, or pseudotype-1, fimbria described by Klemm *et al.* (1982). The KS71C and type-1C fimbriae are related to type-1 fimbriae also in their amino acid compositions. The lack of common functional or serological properties in fimbrial proteins having identical or similar N-terminal amino acid sequences suggests that the N-terminus is not involved in receptor binding but represents a common structural requirement in the filament.

Despite similar chemical and functional properties, type-1 fimbriae from different enterobacterial species show low serological cross-reactions. It is generally believed that type-1 fimbriae are serologically related within an individual species (Duguid and Campbell, 1969; Nowotarska and Mulczyk, 1977). Duguid and Campbell studied cross-reactions by agglutinating bacteria with anti-fimbrial antibodies obtained from whole-cell antisera absorbed with non-fimbrial variants. They found type-1 fimbriae serologically related in *Shigella flexneri, E. coli* and *K. aerogenes* as well as in *Salmonella, Citrobacter* and *Arizona* (see p.311). No cross-reaction was observed in enzyme-linked immunosorbent assay (ELISA) by Korhonen *et al.* (1981, 1983) between type-1 fimbriae from *E. coli* and S. typhimurium, whereas type-1 fimbriae from a *K. aerogenes* strain showed a low (1.0–5.0%) cross-reaction with both *E. coli* and *S. typhimurium* type-1 fimbriae.

In *E. coli* and *S. typhimurium* the synthesis of type-1 fimbriae is coded by chromosomal genes (Brinton, 1965). A culture of *E. coli* or *S. typhimurium* may undergo a reversible transition from a fimbriated phase to a non-fimbriated phase; the former phase is favoured in a static liquid culture (Old and Duguid, 1970). Using operon fusing techniques, Eisenstein (1981) recently showed that the on/off switch in type-1 fimbrial synthesis is controlled at transcriptional level.

The presence of type-1 fimbriae on various enterobacterial species was associated with mannose-sensitive haemagglutination (Duguid *et al.*, 1955; Old 1972); guinea pig, horse and fowl erythrocytes were strongly agglutinated. The

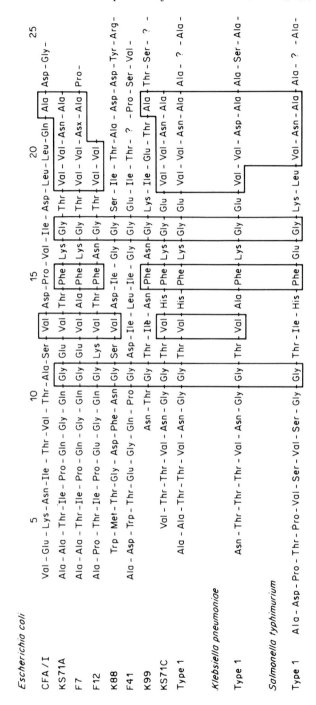

Figure 2. N-terminal amino acid sequences of enterobacterial fimbrillins. The data are from Klemm (1982), Rhen *et al.* (1983a), Klemm *et al.* (1982, 1983), de Graaf and Roorda (1982), Gaastra *et al.* (1979), Hermodson *et al.* (1978), Fader *et al.* (1982), Waalen *et al.* (1983)

role of type-1 fimbriae as mannose-sensitive haemagglutinins was confirmed with purified fimbriae, which agglutinated erythrocytes at a concentration of about 10 μg/ml (Salit and Gotschlich, 1977a; Korhonen *et al.*, 1980b). Work with purified *E. coli* and *S. typhimurium* type-1 fimbriae showed that *Saccharomyces cerevisiae* was agglutinated by fimbriae at a lower concentration than that for horse erythrocytes (Korhonen, 1979; Korhonen *et al.*, 1980b). Yeast cells are covered by phosphomannan complexes containing receptors for type-1 fimbriae. While studying the agglutination properties of 453 *E. coli* strains, Hagberg *et al.* (1981) found that some strains caused mannose-resistant haemagglutination of guinea pig erythrocytes (the most commonly used cells in screening procedures for the presence of type-1 fimbriae), whereas yeast cell agglutination was always mannose-sensitive. Yeast cells offer a convenient and sensitive means to test for the presence of type-1 fimbriae on enterobacterial cells.

The binding specificity of type-1 fimbriae was first studied by Old (1972) in *S. typhimurium* and *Shigella flexneri*. He showed that haemagglutination by strains carrying type-1 fimbriae was specifically inhibited by β-D-mannosides. Unmodified hydroxyl groups at positions C-2, C-3, C-4 and C-6 in the D-mannopyranosyl molecule were necessary for maximum inhibition. The binding properties of type-1 fimbriae are therefore more specific than those of concanavalin A, which also binds to glucose (Smith and Goldstein, 1967). The sugar specificities were confirmed with purified type-1 fimbriae by inhibition of haemagglutination, yeast cell agglutination, and monkey kidney cell adhesion (Salit and Gotschlich, 1977a,b; Korhonen, 1979; Korhonen *et al.*, 1980b). These studies showed that β-methyl-D-mannoside was more potent than D-mannose as an inhibitor; fructose was about 20 times less active. Studies with mannose-containing oligosaccharides led Firon *et al.* (1982) to conclude that in *E. coli* type-1 fimbriae the size of the binding site corresponds to the size of a trisaccharide. Information on the number and the location of the binding sites on the filament is scarce. Eshdat *et al.* (1981) dissociated type-1 fimbriae into subunits and found that about 25% of the subunits retained mannose-binding properties. This result does not favour either a terminal or a lateral location for the binding sites.

Although type-1 fimbriae are involved in numerous adhesion processes (Duguid *et al.*, 1966; Ofek *et al.*, 1977; Salit and Gotschlich, 1977b) their physiological functions are still somewhat unclear. Their presence is not correlated with bacterial virulence in any human disease, and about 80% of all *E. coli* isolates are usually able to synthesize them (Hagberg *et al.*, 1981). Although mannosides prevent colonization by *E. coli* in orally infected mice (Aronson *et al.*, 1979), *S. typhimurium* strains that carry type-1 fimbriae are only slightly more virulent than non-fimbriated variants (Duguid *et al.*, 1976). Type-1 fimbriae mediate enterobacterial adherence to rat urinary tract and bladder epithelial cells (Fader and Davis, 1980; Korhonen *et al.*, 1981) and may increase enterobacterial virulence in rats, but there has been no clear demonstration for a pathogenic function in human beings. It should be noted that rat and human urinary tract cells differ in their glycosphingolipids and are therefore susceptible to different *E. coli* fimbriae (Korhonen *et al.*, 1981). Van den Bosch *et al.* (1980) reported that some pyelonephritogenic *E. coli* strains adhere to human urinary tract epithelial cells in a mannose-sensitive manner, i.e. by their type-1 fimbriae. However, several research groups have excluded type-1 fimbriae from human uroepithelial adhesion (Svanborg Edén and Hansson, 1978; Källenius and Möllby, 1979; Ørskov *et al.*, 1980; Korhonen *et al.*, 1981). Adhesion to urinary slime (or Tamm–Horsfall protein), which easily contaminates urinary tract epithelial cells, may be responsible for the observed mannose sensitivity. Ørskov *et al.* (1980) proposed that adhesion to slime in the large intestine is the normal physiological function of type-1 fimbriae and that they function as colonization factor of the normal flora. This would explain their common occurrence and lack of correlation with virulence in human beings. Binding to mucus may prevent bacterial adhesion to underlying epithelial cells and lead to elimination of the bacteria, e.g. from the urinary tract. The role of mucus in defence against bacterial attachment to epithelial cells has recently been reviewed by Gibbons (1982).

A pathogenic role for type-1 fimbriae is made even less probable by the finding that enteric bacteria associate with and are phagocytosed by human white blood cells or rat and mouse peritoneal macrophages in the absence of serum opsonins. These associations are inhibited by mannosides and it seems that phagocytes have on their surfaces mannose-containing structures that bind type-1 fimbriae. Silverblatt *et al.* (1979) demonstrated that the extent of type-1 fimbriation affects the susceptibility of *E. coli* to phagocytosis and killing by human polymorphonuclear leucocytes. Recently Leunk and Moon (1982) showed that a type-1 fimbriated strain of *S. typhimurium*, when injected intravenously into mice, was cleared more rapidly than a non-fimbriated variant of the strain. The clearance rate of the fimbriated bacteria was greatly reduced by mannosides, and it was shown that the liver selectively traps type-1 fimbriated bacteria and that this trapping involves bacterial adhesion to both endothelial and Kupffer cells. The authors concluded that type-1 fimbriae were a major factor in the hepatic clearance of *S. typhimurium*. Also mouse and rat peritoneal macrophages are known to contain receptors for type-1 fimbriae (Bar-Shavit *et al.*, 1980; Blumenstock and Jann, 1982). Taken together, these results strongly suggest that type-1 fimbriae decrease enterobacterial virulence in human beings by enhancing phagocytosis and adhesion to mucin.

The molecular nature of the receptor for type-1 fimbriae on epithelial cells and phagocytes is not known; mannose-containing glycolipids have been proposed for rat bladder (Davis *et al.*, 1981). Evidence for the glycolipid nature of the receptor came from studies showing that lipase treatment of epithelial cells reduced adhesion of a type-1 fimbriated *E. coli* strain.

IV. FIMBRIAE ON HUMAN UROPATHOGENIC *E. COLI* STRAINS

E. coli is the main causative agent in human childhood urinary tract infections (UTI). Interest in the adhesion of *E. coli* to human uroepithelial cells was aroused when Svanborg Edén *et al.* (1976) found a correlation between bacterial adhesion to urinary tract epithelial cells *in vitro* and virulence *in vivo*. They compared the adherence properties of 48 *E. coli* strains and found that strains isolated from the urine of patients with acute pyelonephritis adhere to human uroepithelial cells better than strains associated with cystitis or asymptomatic bacteriuria (ABU). Electron microscopy revealed that the adhering strains were fimbriated, but the adhesion was found to be unaffected by mannose (Svanborg Edén and Hansson, 1978). This was the first piece of evidence of uroepithelial adhesion being mediated by fimbriae other than type-1 fimbriae. Such fimbriae are termed 'P fimbriae' after pyelonephritis and P antigen recognition.

The first observation on the receptor structure for P fimbriae was the finding that adhesion to human uroepithelial cells was directly related to MR haemagglutination of human erythrocytes (Källenius and Möllby, 1979; Hagberg *et al.*, 1981) which suggested a common receptor on the two cells. The receptor structure was resolved by two approaches. Leffler and Svanborg Edén (1980, 1981) found that the total glycolipid fraction extracted from human urinary tract epithelial cells inhibited adhesion and that the inhibitory effect was associated with the glycosphingolipid part of the fraction. Further chemical purification showed that globoside (βD-GalNac(1→3)αD-Gal(1→4)βD-Gal–(1→4)βD-Glc–Cer) was an effective inhibitor. Thus, in these studies the receptor was isolated from target cells. Källenius *et al.* (1980, 1981b) found that erythrocytes from the rare human blood group p̄ were not agglutinated by pyelonephritogenic *E. coli* strains. These erythrocytes lack the P blood group antigens, namely globoside (P antigen), trihexocyl ceramide (P^k antigen; αD-Gal(1→4)βD-Gal(1→4)βD-Glc–Cer) and P_1 antigen (βD-Gal(1→4)βD-Gal(1→4)–βD-GalNAc(1→3)βD-Gal(1→4)βD-Glc–Cer). Initially it was proposed that trihexocyl ceramide was the active receptor, but later studies showed that both globoside and trihexocyl ceramide were able to function as receptors (Väisänen *et al.*, 1981). The minimal structure recognized by the bacteria is αD-Gal(1→4)βD-Gal disaccharide moiety of the blood group antigens, and while this structure is terminal in trihexocyl ceramide and the P_1 antigen (the bacteria probably recognize the latter too) it is subterminal in globoside. Studies of the absolute configuration of globoside showed that the terminal GalNAc is out of plane leaving the αD-Gal(1→4)βD-Gal stretch exposed and therefore accessible to P fimbriae (Svenson *et al.*, 1983). Based on these studies a receptor-specific particle agglutination test for rapid identification of P-fimbriated *E. coli* was developed by Svenson *et al.* (1982).

P-fimbriated bacteria do not adhere to rat urinary tract epithelial cells and rat erythrocytes are not agglutinated by the bacteria (Korhonen *et al.*, 1981).

Since the linkage between the two galactose units in rat globoside is $\alpha(1\rightarrow3)$ (Siddiqui *et al.*, 1972), it seems that the P-fimbrial binding is specific for the $\alpha(1\rightarrow4)$ linkage. It is therefore essential to choose the right animals for challenge studies related to human UTI; monkeys have proved suitable since they have the receptor and lack significant renal reflux (Roberts *et al.*, 1984). P blood-group-specific glycosphingolipids are known to occur in many tissues (Mårtenson, 1969), and recent evidence has suggested that P_1 antigen may also occur in glycoproteins on human erythrocytes (Haselberger and Schenkel-Brunner, 1982).

The blood group p̄ is very rare and many of the individuals with this phenotype live in Umeå district in Sweden. It is interesting to note that these persons have no recorded histories of UTI nor do pyelonephritogenic *E. coli* strains adhere to their urinary tract epithelial cells (Källenius *et al.*, 1981b). This is an example of genetic resistance to infectious disease. It has been claimed that persons with the blood group P_1, due to the higher receptor density on their epithelial cells, are more prone than other people to UTI (Lomberg *et al.*, 1981). No direct measurements of the receptor densities on epithelial cells have been made and therefore this argument needs confirmation. However, receptor density on urinary tract epithelial cells may determine the susceptibility of certain individuals to UTI. Källenius and Winberg (1978) found that adherence of one *E. coli* strain to uroepithelial cells was significantly lower with healthy girls than with girls who suffered from repeated urinary tract infections (UTI-prone). This was confirmed by Svanborg Edén and Jodal (1979) on a larger material. Thus, it seems that epithelial cells from UTI-prone persons are more susceptible to *E. coli* adhesion than cells from healthy persons. So far this is the only well-documented factor that explains the susceptibility to UTI of some individuals who lack reflux or other predisposing factors.

About 10% of the *E. coli* strains from patients with pyelonephritis possess MR fimbriae other than P (Väisänen *et al.*, 1981; Väisänen-Rhen *et al.*, 1984) and agglutinate p̄ erythrocytes in a MR manner; this binding specificity has been provisionally termed X. X fimbriae may occur alone or together with P fimbriae (and naturally with type-1 fimbriae) on a single strain. X fimbriae are frequent on O2, O75 and O18 strains and represent a heterogeneous class of haemagglutinins. We have recently shown that one of these X strains shows blood-group-M-specific haemagglutination and binds to glycophorin A (Väisänen *et al.*, 1982). The strain binds to glycophorin A from solubilized erythrocyte membranes of MM but not of NN persons. M and N glycophorins differ in their N-terminal amino acid sequences, and the terminal serine residue in glycophorin M is evidently part of the receptor (Jokinen *et al.*, 1985). Glycophorin is the major sialic-acid-containing glycoprotein in the erythrocyte membrane, but sialic acids do not seem to be involved in the binding since neurominidase treatment of native or SDS-denatured glycophorin A does not abolish the binding activity. Our present studies have shown that this agglutinin is a fimbrial protein termed 'M'

M fimbriae are unique in the sense that they recognize an amino acid, in this case a terminal serine residue, hence demonstrating that not all fimbriae necessarily bind to carbohydrates. Another binding specificity was found in some X strains with serotype O18K1H7 or O2K1 (Parkkinen *et al.*, 1983). The haemagglutination by these strains was abolished after neuraminidase treatment of p̄ erythrocytes, and inhibition studies with glycoproteins and oligosaccharides showed that the strains had fimbriae with binding specificities for sialyl $\alpha(2\rightarrow3)$ galactosides (Korhonen *et al.*, 1984). This S fimbria is more frequent among strains from neonatal sepsis and meningitis than among UTI strains, but its clinical significance is still unknown. Thus, in human pyelonephritogenic *E. coli* strains MR haemagglutination of human erythrocytes may be caused by at least four types of haemagglutinins. Although P antigen recognition is by far the most frequent MR haemagglutinin in these strains, the results cited above stress the importance of defining the term 'MR' in precise molecular terms.

It is well documented that P fimbriae mediate P antigen recognition and uroepithelial adhesion of *E. coli* (Svanborg Edén and Hansson, 1978; Korhonen *et al.*, 1980a, 1981, 1982; Rhen *et al.*, 1983a,b). P fimbriae occur more frequently on pyelonephritogenic than on cystitic or ABU or faecal *E. coli* strains (Källenius *et al.*, 1981a; Leffler and Svanborg Edén, 1981; Väisänen-Rhen *et al.*, 1984), and this explains the better average adhesion shown by the pyelonephritogenic strains. The frequency of P fimbriae is 70–90% on pyelonephritogenic strains but only about 10% on faecal strains. When the physiological functions of P fimbriae are being studied, it is very important to consider the clinical status of the patient from when the strain was isolated, i.e. to differentiate between pyelonephritis and other types of UTI, and to exclude patients who have obstructive anomalies or reflux. Failure to do so may lead to an underestimation of the role of P fimbriae as virulence factors (Harber *et al.*, 1982).

P fimbriae occur frequently in *E. coli* strains of serovars O1K1H7, O4K12H5, O6K2H1, O16K1H6 and O18acK5H7 (Väisänen-Rhen *et al.*, 1984) which account for about half of the pyelonephritogenic *E. coli* strains isolated in Finland. Besides P fimbriae, the strains within the serovars have other common properties, e.g. presence or absence of other fimbriae and of haemolytic activity, similar outer membrane protein patterns and equal mean numbers of plasmids per strain. These strains probably represent groups that have a common evolutionary origin and have adapted to virulence. The clonal distribution of virulent *E. coli* strains was recently documented by Achtman *et al.* (1983) for capsulated K1 bacteria, and P fimbriation seems to follow the clonality established by Achtman *et al.* The concept of clonality has made possible an evaluation of different virulence factors of human UTI (Väisänen-Rhen *et al.*, 1984). It seems that the major virulence factor in childhood pyelonephritis is P fimbriation; other factors are haemolytic activity and acidic capsules. Most pyelonephritis strains had either K1 or K5 or K12 capsular antigens. Haemolytic activity was associated with virulence in the 250 UTI and faecal strains studied, although some of the clones, which were highly capable of causing pyelonephritis, lacked haemolysins. Haemolysins may increase virulence by causing tissue damage or by increasing the amount of available iron (Cavalieri and Snyder, 1982; Linggood and Ingram, 1982). High nutritional iron status increases the susceptibility of rats to experimental pyelonephritis (Hart *et al.*, 1982). Acidic capsules present on most of the pyelonephritogenic *E. coli* strains increased bacterial resistance to phagocytosis and to the bactericidal activity of serum (Gemski *et al.*, 1980; Horwitz, 1982).

A P fimbrial preparation is an ideal candidate for a vaccine against human UTI so the extent of their cross-reactivity in different *E. coli* serovars is relevant. A problem encountered in their serological analysis is the fact that most pyelonephritogenic *E. coli* strains express many fimbriae when grown on agar plates (Korhonen *et al.*, 1982). Few P fimbriae have been purified to apparent purity in SDS–PAGE. They include KS71A and KS71B fimbriae (Rhen *et al.*, 1983a,b,c) and F7 and F12 fimbriae studied by Klemm *et al.* (1982, 1983). The latter are MR fimbriae from pyelonephritogenic strains and so probably P fimbriae. These fimbriae have apparent molecular weights in the mass range of 18 200–22 000.

It is evident that one *E. coli* may have two different P fimbriae when grown on CFA agar plates. Our model strain *E. coli* KS71 (serovar O4K12) has three different fimbriae: A, B and C (Figure 1). That KS71A and KS71B fimbriae both mediate P antigen recognition is evident from the findings of Rhen *et al.* (1983a,b,d): (i) anti-KS71A cross-reacts with KS71B fimbriae; (ii) Fab fragments from anti-KS71A serum inhibit uroepithelial adhesion and haemagglutination of *E. coli* KS71 but not of the P-fimbriated *E. coli* ER2 (however, the latter is inhibited by anti-KS71ABC Fab fragments); (iii) anti-KS71C Fab fragments have no effect on haemagglutination or adhesion of *E. coli* KS71 and ER2; (iv) after cloning of structural genes for KS71A, KS71B or KS71C fimbriae separately into a non-fimbriated and non-haemagglutinative *E. coli* K12 strain, the recipients of KS71A or KS71B genes haemagglutinate in a P-specific manner, whereas recipients of KS71C structural genes are non-haemagglutinative. No binding properties have been demonstrated for KS71C fimbriae so far.

The apparent molecular weight of F7 (isolated from an *E. coli* O6K2H1 strain) is equal to that of KS71A, and although the N-terminal amino acid sequences of the two proteins are almost identical (Figure 2), their amino acid compositions are slightly different (Rhen *et al.*, 1983a). Hence KS71A and F7 probably are closely related but not identical P fimbriae. F7 was later reported (Ørskov and Ørskov, 1983) to give two lines in crossed immunoelectrophoresis and to be composed of two antigens, $F7_1$ and $F7_2$. It is reasonable to assume that KS71A and KS71B correspond to $F7_1$ and $F7_2$. F12 was isolated from an O16K1H6 strain of *E. coli* and the preparation showed only one peptide band in SDS–PAGE with an apparent molecular weight of 18 200. However, the preparation gave two precipitation lines against anti-fimbrial serum in crossed immunoelectrophoresis. The N-terminal amino acid sequence of F12 is shown in Figure 2; it is very similar to KS71A and F7. Klemm *et al.* (1983) concluded that F12 was probably composed of two highly homologous fimbrial proteins having identical size and N-terminal amino acid sequence. This emphasizes the need to judge the homogeneity of a fimbrial preparation on more rigorous criteria than observation of a single peptide band in SDS–PAGE.

It is evident from the above that the immunochemistry of P fimbriae is very complex. Total fimbrial fractions from several P-fimbriated bacteria (each containing two or three different fimbrial antigens) cross-react with each other but not with type-1 fimbriae (Korhonen *et al.*, 1982). We have recently begun to estimate the frequencies of fimbrial antigens in pyelonephritogenic *E. coli* strains by means of the immune precipitation technique described above (Figure 1). It is our experience that immune precipitation and subsequent analysis in SDS–PAGE does not detect cross-reactions of less than about 5% of the homologous reaction estimated in ELISA. About 60% of the P-fimbriated strains tested (representing all the important serovars causing UTI) showed immunoprecipitation with anti-KS71B, whereas the frequency of anti-KS71A-positive strains was only about 40%. These cross-reactions seem to be correlated with the serovars of the strains: most O4 and O6 strains reacted strongly with anti-KS71A and anti-KS71B, whereas only some of the O2, O16 and O18 strains showed reaction. *E. coli* O7 strains reacted only weakly with the two P-fimbrial antisera. Thus there is significant antigenic variation among *E. coli* P fimbriae.

A slightly different approach by Ørskov and Ørskov (1983) analysed fimbrial extracts in crossed immunoelectrophoresis with anti-fimbrial sera obtained by absorption of whole-cell antisera with non-fimbriated variants of the same serovar. Their results were similar to our own: the frequencies of F7 and KS71A followed the same distribution and a number of fimbrial antigenic types were identified on *E. coli* strains from human UTI. The number of antigenic types needed in constructing a P-fimbrial vaccine against human UTI is not yet clear.

Genetic analysis of P fimbriae has only begun. Hull *et al.* (1981) cloned type-1 and MR (apparently P) fimbriae separately to *E. coli* K12 and presented evidence suggesting chromosomal location for the structural genes of the two fimbriae. We recently cloned the structural genes for KS71A, KS71B and KS71C fimbriae separately into *E. coli* K12 (see Figure 1) and showed that they are chromosomally coded (Rhen *et al.*, 1983b). Their separate cloning was the ultimate proof of their separateness as fimbrial antigens and shows that they are located on different sites on the chromosome. An intriguing feature of KS71 fimbrial antigens is their rapid phase variation (Rhen *et al.*, 1983c). Our original observation was that precipitation of bacteria with either anti-KS71A or anti-KS71C could separate the cells into distinct populations. In agar-grown *E. coli* KS71, about half of the cells were devoid of fimbriae, one quarter had only KS71C fimbriae and one quarter had KS71A-B fimbriae (the latter cannot be differentiated at present). Thus, the different fimbriae apparently do not exist on a single cell, but the bacterial population in a single colony consists of heterogeneous cells expressing different fimbriae. After subculture on agar plates each of the separated populations gave colonies expressing each of the three KS71 fimbriae. The switch in fimbrial synthesis (either from A–B to C or vice versa or from a non-fimbriated phase to A–B or C or vice versa) is reversible and very rapid. We have thus demonstrated phase variation, i.e. alternative synthesis of different proteins, in the fimbrial antigens of *E. coli* KS71 (Rhen *et al.*, 1983c). This may have significance in bacterial virulence since by phase variation of fimbrial antigens the bacterium may escape host defence.

V. FIMBRIAE ON PORCINE ENTEROTOXIGENIC *E. COLI* STRAINS

The K88 antigens are fimbriae found on *E. coli* strains, mostly of O serovars 8 and 149, that produce diarrhoea in piglets (Ørskov *et al.*, 1964; Smith and Linggood, 1971; Söderlind and Möllby, 1979). K88b, K88ac, K88ad and K88ad(e) are the four immunologically distinct but cross-reacting types that have been distinguished for the K88 antigen (Ørskov *et al.*, 1964; Mooi and de Graaf, 1979; Gaastra *et al.*, 1979). The filaments are composed of subunits of 23 500–26 000 molecular weight. The four variants differ slightly in their amino acid composition, but have identical N- and C-terminal amino acid sequences (Figure 2). Cyanogen bromide cleavage yielded four peptides from K88ab and K88ac fimbrillins and five peptides from K88ad and K88ad(e) fimbrillins, and this would indicate that the fimbrillins differed in their methionine content, despite the contradictory findings of amino acid analysis. The N-terminal sequences were identical in three of the cyanogen bromide fragments. These results suggested that the antigenic determinants that give rise to the variants (b, c, d or e) must be located on the middle part of the subunits. The sequencing of K88ab antigen (Klemm, 1981) allowed Klemm and Mikkelsen (1982) by computerized algorithms to predict the location of antigenic determinants on the K88ab fimbrillin. Nine peptide fragments, composed of 6–9 amino acid residues and scattered along the fimbrillin, were found to be potential antigenic determinants. Interestingly, some of the known differences in K88ab and K88ad amino acid sequences were located on sites with high antigenic potential. As more sequences of the K88 antigens become available it will be possible to determine the antigenic determinants on these fimbrial proteins at the secondary structural level.

The *E. coli* strains that bear K88 antigens cause MR and temperature-sensitive agglutination of guinea pig erythrocytes (Jones and Rutter, 1974). A partially purified K88ab and K88ac preparation agglutinated chicken and guinea pig erythrocytes, while a K88ab preparation only agglutinated the latter (Parry and Porter, 1978). Gibbons *et al.* (1975) tried to identify the receptor for K88 antigens by haemagglutination inhibition with different glycoproteins. In some cases the

presence of a terminal βD-galactosyl structure in a heterosaccharide side-
chain of a glycoprotein correlated with inhibitory activity. Preliminary work
of Kearns and Gibbons (1979) suggested that the intestinal receptor for the K88
antigen is a glycolipid. Recently Anderson *et al.* (1980) suggested that *N*-
acetylhexosamines may have a role in attachment after testing various saccharides
and glycoproteins for their ability to inhibit the binding of ^{125}I-labelled K88
to isolated porcine intestinal brush border membranes *in vitro*. *N*-
Acetylhexosamines inhibited the binding of cell-free K88 to the membranes.
However, this was not repeated with bacterial cells carrying K88 antigens, so
the receptor must be considered as incompletely resolved.

   The *E. coli* strains that cause diarrhoea in piglets proliferate in the small
intestine and colonize the anterior small intestine (Smith and Jones, 1963). The
rapid proliferation of *E. coli* in the small intestine is attributable to the ability
of the bacteria to attach to the intestinal epithelium (Arbuckle, 1970). Clinical
disease is caused by the production of enterotoxins, and the K88-positive strains
produce either heat-labile or heat-stable enterotoxins or both. Smith and
Linggood (1971) elegantly showed that both the production of enterotoxins and
the K88 antigen are needed for *E. coli* to cause diarrhoea in piglets. Further,
it is now well established that *E. coli* strains that bear K88 antigens bind to
pig intestine *in vitro* whereas K88-negative strains do not (Jones and Rutter,
1972; Wilson and Hohman, 1974; Sellwood *et al.* 1975).

   However, K88-positive bacteria do not cause diarrhoea and do not adhere
to intestinal tissue in all piglets (Rutter *et al.*, 1975; Sellwood *et al.*, 1975).
Two pig phenotypes were products of two alleles at a single locus inherited in
a simple Mendelian manner and have been designated 'adhesive' and 'non-
adhesive'. The brush borders of the non-adhesive piglets did not bind
K88-positive bacteria and the piglets were resistant to this particular form of
diarrhoea. Comparison of glycolipids from adhesive and non-adhesive piglet
intestinal epithelia showed differences between the two phenotypes (Kearns and
Gibbons, 1979). The non-adhesive piglets may represent individuals that are
genetically resistant to K88-associated diarrhoea due to lack of bacterial
receptors. This may be analogous to the genetic resistance to human UTI
observed in p̄ persons who lack receptors for P fimbriae. Recently Bijlsma *et
al.* (1982) divided pigs into five phenctypes (A–E) by their susceptibility to
adherence by ab, ac and ad variants of K88. The non-adhesive phenotype of
Sellwood *et al.* (1975) included the phenotypes D and E of Bijlsma *et al.* The
phenotype D bound the K88ad variants and was found in older pigs. It is thus
apparent that age-related changes on brush border epithelium affect
K88-mediated adhesion. The phenotype A was susceptible to all the three K88
variants, and phenotypes B and C were susceptible to two of the K88 variants
(either ab + ac or ab + ad). Although inhibition studies with isolated K88 fimbriae
did not clearly show whether the K88 variants recognized different receptors,
these results suggest that antigenic variation (i.e. blood-group-like antigens) on

the surface of porcine brush borders may render the piglets susceptible to different K88 variants.

Besides K88 antigens, porcine ETEC strains may have other types of fimbriae to mediate their attachment to pig intestinal epithelium. One such fimbria, termed 987P (Nagy *et al.*, 1977), was recently purified by Isaacson and Richter (1981) and found to be composed of a 20 000 molecular weight fimbrillin. 987P is morphologically identical to type-1 fimbriae and may occur simultaneously with K88 on a single strain (Schneider and To, 1982). Interestingly, no haemagglutinating activity was found in 987P fimbriae, indicating that the receptor recognized by these fimbriae does not occur on erythrocytes. Also K99-positive *E. coli* strains bind to porcine small intestinal epithelium (Isaacson *et al.*, 1978). Moreover, Awad-Masalmekh *et al.* (1982) found strains that were capable of causing diarrhoea in piglets and adhered to piglet intestine but lacked K88, K99, or 987P antigens. No fimbriae were found on these strains by electron microscopy, but it could also be possible that the strains possess fimbrial antigens (such as F41) with a morphology that is difficult to visualize in an electron microscope.

VI. K99 AND F41 ANTIGENS

The K99 antigen was first described by Smith and Linggood (1972) as the 'common K antigen' on *E. coli* strains enteropathogenic for calves and lambs. The term K99 was introduced by Ørskov *et al.* (1975). The antigen was present on most *E. coli* strains that caused diarrhoea in calves (Guinée *et al.*, 1976). These strains were mostly of O serovars 8, 9, 20 and 101 (Myers and Guinée, 1976). The K99 antigen occurred also on some *E. coli* strains of O serovars 8, 9, 64, 101 and 140, which caused diarrhoea in piglets (Moon *et al.*, 1977; Smyth *et al.*, 1981). The possession of K99 in these strains is correlated with the possession of heat-stable enterotoxin, which is responsible for the clinical symptoms.

Slightly conflicting results were reported on the morphology of the K99 antigen. According to Isaacson (1977) the filament has a diameter of 8 nm, whereas van Embden *et al.* (1980) reported a very thin filament, about 2–4 nm in diameter with irregular zigzag form. The K99 antigen was purified by two groups (Isaacson, 1978; Isaacson *et al.*, 1981; de Graaf *et al.*, 1981), and both have reported the fimbrillin molecular weight to be about 18 500 although the two preparations differed considerably in their amino acid composition. The N-terminal amino acid sequence of K99 is shown in Figure 2. A characteristic feature of K99 is its isoelectric point of about 10.0; all other fimbrial proteins studied so far have acidic isoelectric points. Purified K99 agglutinated sheep and horse erythrocytes in a MR manner but the receptor structure on these erythrocytes is still unknown (Isaacson, 1978; de Graaf and Roorda, 1982).

K99-positive strains of O serovars 9 and 101 may carry another, anionic fimbrial antigen termed F41 (Morris *et al.*, 1980), which was recently purified by de Graaf and Roorda (1982). F41 had 29 500 molecular weight subunits and an isoelectric point of 4.6. K99 and F41 antigens differ in their amino acid composition and are not serologically cross-reative. The N-terminal amino acid sequence of F41 shows limited homology with that of K99 and K88 (Figure 2). The purified F41 has a filamentous structure with a diameter of 3.2 nm and it agglutinates guinea pig and human erythrocytes. Adhesion to calf intestinal epithelium of bacterial cells carrying F41 was inhibited by purified F41, indicating involvement of F41 in bacterial adherence to calf epithelium. However, adhesion was much higher with strains having K99 either alone or in combination with F41 suggesting that K99 could be the principal adhesin in calf enterotoxigenic *E. coli* strains.

The role of K99 in the adhesion of *E. coli* to calf intestinal epithelium has been documented reasonably well. In contrast to the K99-positive parent strain, K99-negative strains prepared by curing with acridine orange cannot produce diarrhoea in lambs and do not proliferate in lamb small intestine (Smith and Linggood, 1972). After transfer of the K99 plasmid into *E. coli* K12 the recipients were able to attach to calf brush border preparations, and the attachment was inhibited by purified K99 fimbriae (de Graaf and Roorda, 1982). K99-positive ETEC strains also adhered to porcine small intestine (Isaacson *et al.*, 1978; Moon *et al.*, 1977).

Runnels *et al.* (1980) noticed that calves, pigs and mice may develop with age resistance to the adhesion of K99-positive bacterial. They found that intestinal epithelial cells from 6-week-old pigs, 2-week-old calves and adult mice took up significantly fewer K99-positive *E. coli* than did epithelial cells from neonates. It should be noted that 2-day-old calves and lambs are known to have become resistant to experimental challenge with K99-positive ETEC (Smith and Halls, 1967), and this could be due in part to changes in their epithelial cell surface structure. However, as noted above, the receptor structure for K99 is not known.

De Graaf *et al.* (1980) found that alanine repressed the production of K99, a finding which explained the observation that K99 was produced poorly in complex media. These authors also proposed that repression of K99 synthesis by alanine could partly explain why K99-positive ETEC induced diarrhoea in animals only in the first few postnatal days when metabolic reactions in the intestine had not developed to produce enough alanine to repress the production of K99 antigen.

VII. FIMBRIAE ON HUMAN ENTEROTOXIGENIC *E. COLI* STRAINS

Colonization factor antigens (CFA) are fimbriae found on human enterotoxigenic *E. coli* strains (Evans *et al.*, 1975). Two variants were described:

CFA/I, which occurs on ETEC strains of O serovars 15, 25, 63 and 78 (Ørskov *et al.*, 1976; Evans *et al.*, 1978a), and CFA/II, which occurs on ETEC strains of O serovars 6 and 8 (Evans and Evans, 1978; Smyth *et al.*, 1979). The variants differ immunologically and are distinguishable by their haemaglutination patterns: CFA/I-positive strains cause MR- and temperature-sensitive haemagglutination of human, bovine and chicken erythrocytes, whereas CFA/II-positive strains do not haemagglutinate human erythrocytes. Evans *et al.* (1978a) found CFA/I in 86% of the *E. coli* strains causing diarrhoea in Mexico, whereas significantly lower frequencies (about 20%) were reported by other workers (Cravioto *et al.*, 1979, 1982; Bergman *et al.*, 1981). CFA/II seems to have a frequency similar to that of CFA/I.

Morphologically CFA/I resembles the type-1 fimbria. Two different chemical characterizations were reported: the subunits were 23 800 (Evans *et al.*, 1979b) or 14 500 molecular weight (Klemm, 1979). Differences were also seen in their amino acid compositions. It should be noted that both studies were made on the same *E. coli* strain. The value reported by Evans *et al.* is probably that of a dimer (Wevers *et al.*, 1980). Klemm (1982) has recently determined the complete amino acid sequence of CFA/I and confirmed the 15 000 subunit. The N-terminal amino acid sequence of the CFA/I fimbrillin is not homologous with that of the other fimbrillins (Figure 2). The complete sequence allowed Klemm and Mikkelsen (1982) to identify the probable antigenic determinants on the CFA/I fimbrillin. They proposed that these were six peptide fragments (consisting of 5–6 amino acids each) located at different sites on the fimbrillin. These findings can be used in designing synthetic peptide vaccines against enteric organisms.

A MR haemagglutination of human, bovine and chicken erythrocytes is exhibited by the purified CFA/I fimbriae, but only after attachment to latex microbeads (Evans *et al.*, 1979b). It was reported that 1% (w/v) *N*-acetylneuraminic acid inhibited the haemagglutination, but later it was suggested that this was due to pH changes induced by sialic acid (Lindahl *et al.*, 1982). Farris *et al.* (1980) found that high concentrations of GM_2-like gangliosides inhibited the haemagglutination by CFA/I-positive strains. The receptor was proposed to be a terminal $\alpha(2\rightarrow8)$-bound *N*-acetylneuraminic acid (Lindahl *et al.*, 1982). These studies were done on one strain only and therefore need to be confirmed on a larger material.

In contrast to a CFA-positive parent strain, a strain lacking CFA does not produce diarrhoea and is not able to proliferate in the infant rabbit (Evans *et al.*, 1975). Also, in contrast to CFA-positive strains, CFA-negative ETEC do not adhere to infant rabbit intestine (Evans *et al.*, 1977, 1978b), and a cell-free CFA/I preparation binds to the intestinal mucosa of an infant rabbit, as demonstrated by indirect immunofluorescence. In human volunteers CFA-positive *E. coli* caused diarrhoea and showed an extended excretion pattern (Evans *et al.*, 1978b). These results suggest that CFAs mediate the adherence of human ETEC strains to human intestinal epithelium, and thus function in a similar manner to K88 and K99 antigens.

Human ETEC strains have other types of fimbrial antigen in addition to CFAs. Deneke *et al.* (1979) isolated from a human ETEC strain fimbriae which bound to buccal cells in a MR manner and showed two peptides in SDS–PAGE. Thus, the strain apparently had two distinct fimbriae. The adhesin of a human ETEC strain of O serovars 26 binding to human foetal small intestine is coded by a 56 000 molecular weight colicinogenic plasmid (Williams *et al.*, 1978); the morphological properties of this adhesin were not reported. Wevers *et al.* (1980) isolated from an enterotoxigenic O18ac *E. coli* strain fimbriae with an apparent subunit of 21 000. These fimbriae were unrelated to CFA/I or type-1 fimbriae both serologically and in amino acid composition. Smyth (1982) reported that fimbrial extracts from O6K15 strains (which agglutinated bovine erythrocytes and presumably possessed CFA/II) gave multiple peptides in SDS–PAGE and hence probably contained many fimbrial proteins. Finally, Czirók *et al.* (1982) reported that non-enterotoxigenic *E. coli* strains, isolated from cases of infant diarrhoea, had many of the fimbrial antiens associated with strains from human UTI. Taken together, these results emphasize the multiplicity of fimbrial antigens on *E. coli* strains associated with a given clinical condition.

VIII. ENTEROBACTERIAL FIMBRIAE AS VACCINES

The realization that fimbriae-mediated adhesion is a prerequisite for many bacterial infections has focused much interest on the use of purified fimbriae as vaccines. Fimbriae would be ideal candidates for making vaccines: they are (1) large highly antigenic polymers, (2) located on the outer surfaces of bacteria, and (3) not covered by capsular antigens. Those binding to the same receptor should have common antigenic determinants, the receptor binding domains. However, the number of serological comparisons within a functional type, except type 1 and K88, of *E. coli* fimbriae are too scarce to allow conclusions on cross-reactivity. The goal with fimbrial vaccines is to produce antibodies that would enhance phagocytosis of the infecting organisms and prevent bacterial adhesion at the infection site. Inhibition of bacterial adhesion by anti-fimbrial antibodies has been successful *in vitro* in most of the adhesion systems discussed above.

A number of *E. coli* frimbriae have been tested as vaccines (Table 2) (reviewed by Korhonen and Rhen, 1982). A fimbrial vaccine was tested by Rutter and Jones (1973) and Rutter *et al.* (1976). They injected 15 mg of purified K88 antigen into the posterior mammary gland of four sows three months before parturition and gave a booster dose of 30 mg subcutaneously in the flank 10 days before parturition. Piglets were challenged orally with 1×10^{10} CFU K88-positive bacteria at birth before suckling. In the four litters from the control gilts, 20/29 piglets died within three days, whereas only 4/31 piglets from the vaccinated gilts died of diarrhoea. All piglets showed clinical signs of diarrhoea, but the

Table 2 Enterobacterial fimbriae tested as vaccine

Fimbrial antigen	Immunization in	Protection against	Reference
K88	Pig	Diarrhoea	Rutter and Jones, 1973 Rutter et al., 1976
K99	Lamb	Diarrhoea	Sojka et al., 1978
K99	Cow	Diarrhoea	Acres et al., 1979 Nagy, 1980 Snodgrass et al., 1978
K99	Pig	Diarrhoea	Morgan et al., 1978
987P	Pig	Diarrhoea	Morgan et al., 1978 Nagy et al., 1978 Isaacson et al., 1980
CFA/I	Rabbit	Diarrhoea	Evans et al., 1982
CFA/I and CFA/II	Rabbit	Diarrhoea	Åhren and Svennerholm, 1982
Type 1	Rat	Ascending pyelonephritis	Silverblatt and Cohen, 1979
Type 1	Man	Diarrhoea	Levine et al., 1982
P fimbriae	Monkey	Ascending pyelonephritis	Roberts et al., 1984

symptoms in the piglets from vaccinated gilts were less severe. Serum, colostrum and milk from the vaccinated sows contained anti-K88 antibodies (mostly IgG) that inhibited adhesion of the challenge strain. The bactericidal and bacteriostatic activities in the serum and mammary secretions from both groups of sows were similar. It was concluded that inhibition of adhesion by K88 antibodies in the colostrum and milk was responsible for the observed protection. These studies were the first to demonstrate that anti-fimbrial antibodies, transmitted in the colostrum to the small intestine of a suckling piglet, efficiently protected the animal from diarrhoea during the period when it was most susceptible to the disease.

There have now been several reports of similar experiments in which isolated K99 or 987P fimbriae have protected piglets, lambs or calves against experimental diarrhoea (Table 2). CFA/I and CFA/II have been shown to protect rabbits against intestinal loop challenge with homologous bacteria. However, in some of these studies impure fimbrial preparations were used and the protective effect of anti-O antibodies has not always been ruled out. In a study of Åhren and Svennerholm (1982) it was shown also that Fab fragments to CFA/I were protective, and this strongly suggested that protection was due to an inhibition of bacterial adhesion. Interestingly, there was a synergistic protective effect of antibodies against CFA/I or CFA/II and enterotoxin. This was judged to be due to the action of antibodies at different stages in the pathogenic process, i.e. bacterial adhesion and binding of enterotoxin.

Purified type-1 fimbriae of *E. coli* have been tested as vaccine against ascending pyelonephritis in rats and against human diarrhoea. Fewer challenge bacteria were found in the kidneys in rats immunized with the fimbriae than in control rats (Silverblatt and Cohen, 1979). It should be kept in mind that owing to the differences in their surface glycosphingolipid, rat and human urinary tract epithelial cells are susceptible to different fimbriae of *E. coli* (Korhonen *et al.*, 1981). Levine *et al.* (1982) showed that parenterally inoculated type-1-fimbrial vaccine was safe and immunogenic and did not adversely affect intestinal functions in human beings. However, protection against challenge by a homologous strain having both type-1 and CFA/I fimbriae was seen only with the highest dose of vaccine (about 1.8 mg per person). A significant rise in the antibody titre to the O antigen of the test strain was also found, and such antibodies may have had a protective role. Interestingly, the vaccine did not alter the prevalence of type-1 fimbriated *E. coli* in the normal colonic flora. P fimbriae are now being tested for protection against provoked pyelonephritis in monkeys (Roberts *et al.*, 1984). Preliminary trials have shown that immunization does provide protection against a heterologous strain. Protection was correlated with high levels of anti-P-fimbriae antibodies in the serum, and electron microscopy provided evidence for anti-P-fimbriae antibodies in the kidneys.

Surprisingly little is known about the levels of anti-fimbriae antibodies in healthy and infected human beings and animals. It is our experience that most laboratory animals have low antibody levels to type-1 fimbriae of *E. coli*. Svanborg Edén *et al.* (1979) found anti-type-1-fimbriae antibodies of the IgA class in human milk. Similar antibodies were found against type-1 fimbriae of *K. pneumoniae* (Davis *et al.*, 1982). It is interesting to note that the non-immunoglobulin fraction of human milk contains substances (presumably receptor analogues) that inhibited haemagglutination by CFA/I-, CFA/II- and K88-fimbriated *E. coli* (Holmgren *et al.*, 1981). No inhibition was found for type-1 fimbriae.

Local and systemic antibody responses after pyelonephritis have been evaluated in human beings and rabbits. Rene and Silverblatt (1982) found antibody responses to type-1 fimbriae in the serum of four adult human males with pyelonephritis. The levels and type of antibody were grossly dependent on the detection method used (either ELISA or immunoelectron microscopy), but apparently, the serum antibodies were mostly of the IgG class; no antibodies were found in the urine. Later Rene *et al.* (1982) studied the antibody responses to the fimbriae of the infecting strain in adult females with cystitis. The fimbriae used as antigens were purified from bacteria grown in broth so most of them must have been of type 1. The serum levels of anti-fimbriae IgG and IgM were higher in the patients than in control persons, but no antibodies were found in the patients' urines or vaginal secretions. In contrast, Svanborg Edén *et al.* (1982b) found an antibody response to MR (probably P) fimbriae in both the urine and serum of a child with pyelonephritis. These antibodies were of IgG, IgM and IgA classes, and the urine IgG and IgA levels were at a maximum seven days after the onset of infection. Antibodies to type-1 fimbriae were found in the urine of only 3/11 patients analysed. Thus, it appears that a local antibody response to P but not type-1 fimbriae takes place after pyelonephritis in human beings. This is to be expected since P fimbriae are needed for bacterial adhesion to human urinary tract epithelium and are probably expressed at the onset of infection. Smith *et al.* (1981) found both serum and local (intrarenal) anti-type-1-fimbriae antibodies in rabbits after an experimental *E. coli* pyelonephritis. Local anti-fimbriae antibodies were of the IgG class; none of IgA and IgM were found. The onset of local and systemic responses to fimbriae was delayed, since anti-type-1-fimbriae IgG could be detected in urine 20 days after infection, whereas anti-O antibodies were detectable by day 11. These results, taken together, suggest that local antibodies to fimbriae are formed after pyelonephritis; whether they are enough to prevent adhesion at the site of infection remains to be established.

IX. CONCLUSIONS

Vaccination trials seem to indicate that fimbriae-based vaccines can prevent infectious disease at the first stage of the process, i.e. adhesion to epithelial cells, before the bacteria have established themselves in the host. Indeed, commercially available K88 and K99 vaccines have proved effective in preventing diarrhoea in animals. Some of these vaccines have resulted from recombinant DNA technology aimed at improving the yields of a given fimbrial antigen. The fimbriae associated with human diseases have not yet been adequately tested as vaccines. Trials with type-1 fimbriae in human beings and with P fimbriae in monkeys have shown that the proteins are safe and immunogenic, and vaccination with P fimbriae protects against experimental pyelonephritis. The remaining problem with fimbrial vaccines is the lack of knowledge on the extent of cross-reactivity among fimbrial antigens. It is obvious that many fimbrial antigenic types function in human diarrhoea and pyelonephritis. Development of fimbrial vaccines therefore requires a thorough serological comparison of the fimbriae functioning in those diseases.

An intriguing possibility for the development of fimbrial vaccine is the use of synthetic peptides based on antigenic determinants identified on the subunits. Such peptides could be designed by comparison of the amino acid sequences of the antigenic variants of a fimbrial type and, perhaps more effectively, by recognition of the sequences responsible for binding to receptor molecules. Obviously, the design of this type of vaccine requires knowledge of the chemical properties of fimbrial proteins.

The work on cloned K88 fimbrial genes (Gaastra and de Graaf, 1982) has given valuable information of the mechanisms of fimbrial synthesis. This knowledge is largely lacking for fimbriae functioning in human diseases. Clarification of the biosynthetic mechanisms is not of theoretical value alone, since mutants, e.g. those secreting fimbriae into growth medium, can be extremely helpful in the production of fimbrial vaccines. It is quite probable that fimbrial antigens for vaccines will be produced by such mutants constructed after cloning of the fimbrial antigens that stimulate the production of cross-reactive antibodies.

Although many fimbrial antigens have been identified on *E. coli*, their receptors are known only in a few cases. Once these structures are known they can be utilized in the prevention of infectious disease by inhibiting bacterial adhesion at the infection site. This approach has proved to be effective in preventing colonization of orally infected mice (Aronson *et al.*, 1979) and in preventing experimental pyelonephritis in mice (Svanborg Edén *et al.*, 1982a) and, more relevantly, in monkeys (Roberts *et al.*, 1984) by P-fimbriated *E. coli*.

A problem that may be encountered with fimbrial vaccines is antigenic drift resulting from vaccination. Söderlind *et al.* (1982) studied *E. coli* strains isolated from K88-vaccinated and unvaccinated piglets suffering from diarrhoea and found that both the serological and enterotoxigenic spectra of *E. coli* strains were greatly changed by vaccination with a multicomponent whole-cell vaccine. Notably, the diarrhoeal piglets in the vaccination group had a high incidence of K99-positive bacteria known to adhere to pig intestine. This indicated that vaccination with K88, although protective against diarrhoea by K88-positive

E. coli, may lead to the selection of ETEC strains with other fimbrial antigens. Thus, the antigenic composition of fimbrial vaccines should be designed so that protection is also given against less frequently occurring antigenic types.

ACKNOWLEDGEMENT

This work was supported by the Yrjö Jahnsson Foundation.

REFERENCES

Achtman, M., Mercer, A., Kusecek, B., Pohl, A., Heuzenroeder, M., Aaronson, W., Sutton, A., and Silver, R. P. (1983). Six widespread bacterial clones among *Escherichia coli* K1 isolates. *Infect. Immun.,* **39**, 315–335.

Acres, S. D., Isaacson, R. E., Babiuk, L. A., and Kapitany, R. A. (1979). Immunization of calves against enterotoxigenic colibacillosis by vaccinating dams with purified K99 antigen and whole cell bacterins. *Infect. Immun.,* **25**, 121–126.

Åhren, C. M., and Svennerholm, A. L. (1982). Synergistic protective effect of antibodies against *E. coli* enterotoxin and colonization factor antigens. *Infect. Immun.,* **38**, 74–79.

Anderson, M. J., Whitehead, J. S. and Kim, Y. s. (1980). Interaction of *Escherichia coli* K88 antigen with porcine intestinal brush border membranes. *Infect. Immun.,* **29**, 897–901.

Arbuckle, J. B. R. (1970). The location of *Escherichia coli* in the pig intestine. *J. Med. Microbiol.,* **3**, 333–340.

Aronson, M., Medalia, O., Schori, L., Mirelman, D., Sharon, N., and Ofek, I. (1979). Prevention of colonization of the urinary tract of mice with *Escherichia coli* by blocking adherence with methyl αD-mannopyranoside. *J. Infect. Dis.,* **139**, 329–332.

Awad-Masalmeth, M., Moon, H. W., Runnels, P. L., and Schneider, R. A. (1982). Pilus production, haemagglutination and adhesion by porcine strains of enterotoxigenic *Escherichia coli* lacking K88, K99 and 987P antigens. *Infect. Immun.,* **35**, 305–313.

Bar-Shavit, Z., Goldman, R., Ofek, I., Sharon, N., and Mirelman, D. (1980). Mannose-binding activity of *Escherichia coli*: a determinant of attachment and ingestion of the bacteria by macrophages. *Infect. Immun.,* **29**, 417–424.

Beachey, E. H. (1981). Bacterial adherence: adhesin–receptor interactions mediating the attachment of bacteria to mucosal surfaces. *J. Infect. Dis.,* **143**, 325–345.

Beard, J. P., Howe, T. G. B., and Richmond, M. H. (1972). Purification of sex pili from *Escherichia coli* carrying a derepressed F-like factor. *J. Bacteriol.,* **111**, 814–820.

Bergman, M. J., Updike, W. S., Wood, S. J., Brown, S. E., III, and Guerrant, R. L. (1981). Attachment factors among enterotoxigenic *Escherichia coli* from patients with acute diarrhoea from diverse geographic area. *Infect. Immun.,* **32**, 881–888.

Bijlsma, I. G. W., de Nijs, A., van der Meer, C., and Frik, J. F. (1982). Different pig phenotypes affect adherence of *Escherichia coli* to jejunal brush borders by K88ab, K88ac or K88ad antigen. *Infect. Immun.,* **37**, 891–894.

Blumenstock, E., and Jann, K. (1982). Adhesion of piliated *Escherichia coli* strains to phagocytes: differences between bacteria with mannose-sensitive pili and those with mannose-resistant pili. *Infect. Immun.,* **35**, 264–269.

Brinton, C. C. Jr. (1965). The structure, function, synthesis and genetic control of bacterial pili and a molecular mechanism for DNA and RNA transport in Gram-negative bacteria. *Trans. N.Y. Acad. Sci.*, **27**, 1003–1054.

Cavalieri, S. J., and Snyder, I. S. (1982). Cytotoxic activity of partially purified *Escherichia coli* alpha haemolysin. *J. Med. Microbiol.*, **15**, 11–21.

Cravioto, A., Gross, R. J., Scotland, S. M., and Rowe, B. (1979). Mannose-resistant haemagglutination of human erythrocytes by strains of *Escherichia coli* from extraintestinal sources: lack of correlation with colonization factor antigen (CFA/I). *FEMS Microbiol. Lett.*, **6**, 41–44.

Cravioto, A., Scotland, S. M., and Rowe, B. (1982). Haemagglutination activity and colonization factor antigens I and II in enterotoxigenic and non-enterotoxigenic strains of *Escherichia coli* isolated from humans. *Infect. Immun.*, **36**, 189–197.

Czirók, É., Ørskov, I., and Ørskov, F. (1982). O:K:H:F serotypes of fimbriated *Escherichia coli* strains isolated from infants with diarrhoea. *Infect. Immun.*, **37**, 519–525.

Davis, C. P., Avots-Avotins, A. E., and Fader, R. C. (1981). Evidence for a bladder cell glycolipid receptor for *Escherichia coli* and effect of neuraminic acid and colominic acid on adherence. *Infect. Immun.*, **34**, 944–948.

Davis, C. P., Houston, C. W., Fader, R. C., Goldblum, R. M., Weaver, E. A., and Goldman, A. S. (1982). Immunoglobulin A and secretory immunoglobulin A antibodies to purified type-1 *Klebsiella pneumoniae* pili in human colostrum. *Infect. Immun.*, **38**, 496–501.

de Graaf, F. K., and Roorda, I. (1982). Production, purification and characterization of the fimbrial adhesive antigen F41 isolated from the calf enteropathogenic *Escherichia coli* strain B41. *Infect. Immun.*, **36**, 751–753.

de Graaf, F. K., Klaasen-Boor, P., and van Hees, J. E. (1980). Biosynthesis of the K99 surface-antigen is repressed by alanine. *Infect. Immun.*, **30**, 125–128.

de Graaf, F. K., Klemm, P., and Gaastra, W. (1981). Purification, characterization and partial covalent structure of the adhesive antigen K99 of *Escherichia coli*. *Infect. Immun.*, **33**, 877–883.

Deneke, C. F., Thorne, G. M., and Gorbach, S. K. (1979). Attachment pili from enterotoxigenic *Escherichia coli* pathogenic for humans. *Infect. Immun.*, **26**, 362–368.

Duguid, J. P., and Campbell, I. (1969). Antigens of the type-1 fimbriae of *Salmonellae* and other enterobacteria. *J. Med. Microbiol.*, **2**, 535–553.

Duguid, J. P., and Old, D. C. (1980). Adhesive properties of Enterobacteriaceae. In *Bacterial Adherence.* (*Receptors and Recognition, Ser B*, Vol. 6) (Ed. E. H. Beachey), pp.185–217. Chapman and Hall, London.

Duguid, J. P., Smith, I. W., Demster, G., and Edmunds, P. N. (1955). Non-flagellar filamentous appendages ('fimbriae') and haemagglutinating activity in *Bacterium coli*. *J. Pathol. Bacteriol.*, **70**, 335–348.

Duguid, J. P., Anderson, E. S., and Campbell, I. (1966). Fimbriae and adhesive properties in *Salmonellae*. *J. Pathol. Bacteriol.*, **92**, 107–138.

Duguid, J. P., Darekar, M. R., and Wheater, D. W. F. (1976). Fimbriae and infectivity in *Salmonella typhimurium*. *J. Med. Microbiol.*, **9**, 459–473.

Duguid, J. P., Clegg, S., and Wilson, M. I. (1979). The fimbrial and non-fimbrial haemagglutinins of *Escherichia coli*. *J. Med. Microbiol.*, **12**, 213–227.

Eisenstein, B. (1981). Phase variation of type-1 fimbriae in *Escherichia coli* is under transcriptional control. *Science*, **214**, 337–339.

Eshdat, Y., Silverblatt, F. J., and Sharon, N. (1981). Dissociation and reassembly of *Escherichia coli* type-1 pili. *J. Bacteriol.*, **148**, 308–314.

Evans, D. G., and Evans, D. J., Jr. (1978). New surface-associated heat-labile colonization factor antigen (CFA/II) produced by enterotoxigenic *Escherichia coli* of serogroups O6 and O8. *Infect. Immun.*, **21**, 638–647.

Evans, D. G., Silver, R. P., Evans, D. J., Jr., Chase, D. G., and Gorbach, S. L. (1975). Plasmid-controlled colonization factor associated with virulence in *Escherichia coli* enterotoxigenic for humans. *Infect. Immun.*, **12**, 656–667.

Evans, D. G., Evans, D. J., Jr., and Tjoa, W. (1977). Haemagglutination of human group A erythrocytes by enterotoxigenic *Escherichia coli* isolated from adults with diarrhoea: correlation with colonization factor. *Infect. Immun.*, **18**, 330–337.

Evans, D. G., Evans, D. J., Jr., Tjoa, W., and DuPont, H. L. (1978a). Detection and characterization of colonization factor of enterotoxigenic *Escherichia coli* isolated from adults with diarrhoea. *Infect. Immun.*, **19**, 727–736.

Evans, D. G., Satterwhite, T. K., Evans, D. J., Jr., and DuPont, H. L. (1978b). Difference in serological responses and excretion patterns of volunteers challenged with enterotoxigenic *Escherichia coli* with and without the colonization factor antigen. *Infect. Immun.*, **19**, 883–888.

Evans, D. J., Jr., Evans, D. G., and DuPont, H. L. (1979a). Haemagglutination patterns of enterotoxigenic and enteropathogenic *Echerichia coli* determined with human, bovine, chicken and guinea pig erythrocytes in the presence and absence of mannose. *Infect. Immun.*, **23**, 336–346.

Evans, D. G., Evans, D. J. Jr., Clegg, S., and Pauley, J. A. (1979b). Purification and characterization of the CFA/I antigen of enterotoxigenic *Escherichia coli*. *Infect. Immun.*, **25**, 738–748.

Evans, D. G., de la Cabada, F. J., and Evans, D. J., Jr. (1982). Correlation between intestinal immune response to colonization factor antigen/I and acquired resistance to enterotoxigenic *Escherichia coli* diarrhoea in adult rabbit model *Eur. J. Clin. Microbiol.*, **1**, 178–185.

Fader, R. C., and Davis, C. P. (1980). Effect of piliation of *Klebsiella pneumoniae* infection in rat bladders. *Infect. Immun.*, **30**, 554–561.

Fader, R. C., Duffy, L. K., Davis, C. P., and Kurosky, A. (1982). Purification and chemical characterization of type-1 pili isolated from *Klebsiella pneumoniae*. *J. Biol. Chem.*, **257**, 3301–3305.

Farris, A., Lindahl, H., and Wadström, T. (1980). GM_2-like glycoconjugate as possible receptor for the CFA/I and K99 haemagglutinins of enterotoxigenic *Escherichia coli*. *FEMS Microbiol. Lett.*, **7**, 265–269.

Firon, N., Ofek, I., and Sharon, N. (1982). Interaction of mannose-containing oligosaccharides with the fimbrial lectin of *Escherichia coli*. *Biochem. Biophys. Res. Commun.*, **105**, 1426–1432.

Gaastra, W., and de Graaf, F. K. (1982). Host-specific fimbrial adhesins of noninvasive enterotoxigenic *Escherichia coli* strains. *Microbiol. Rev.*, **46**, 129–161.

Gaastra, W., Klemm, P., Walker, J. M., and de Graaf, F. K. (1979). K88 fimbrial proteins: amino- and carboxy-terminal sequences of intact proteins and cyanogen bromide fragments. *FEMS Microbiol. Lett.*, **6**, 15–18.

Gemski, P., Cross, A. S., and Sadoff, J. C. (1980). K1-antigen-associated resistance to the bactericidal activity of serum. *FEMS Microbiol. Lett.*, **9**, 193–197.

Gibbons, R. A., Jones, G. W., and Sellwood, R. (1975). An attempt to identify the intestinal receptor for the K88 adhesin by means of haemagglutination inhibition test using glycoproteins and fractions from sow colostrum. *J. Gen. Microbiol.*, **86**, 228–240.

Gibbons, R. J. (1982). Review and discussion of role of mucus in mucosal defence. In *Recent Advances in Mucosal Immunity* (Eds. W. Strober, L. Å. Hanson and K. W. Sell), pp.345–351. Raven Press, New York.

Gibbons, R. J., and van Houte, J. (1980). Bacterial adherence and the formation of dental plaques. In *Bacterial Adherence (Receptors and Recognition, Ser. B*, Vol. 6) (Ed. E. H. Beachey), pp.61–104. Chapman and Hall, London.

Guinée, P. A. M., Jansen, W. H., and Agterberg, C. M. (1976). Detection of the K99 antigen by means of agglutination and immunoelectrophoresis in *Escherichia coli* isolates from calves and its correlation with enterotoxigenicity. *Infect. Immun.*, **13**, 1369–1377.

Hagberg, L., Jodal, U., Korhonen, T. K., Lidin-Janson, G., Lindberg, U., and Svanborg, Edén, C. (1981). Adhesion, haemagglutination and virulence of *Escherichia coli* causing urinary tract infections. *Infect. Immun.*, **31**, 564–570.

Harber, M. J., Chick, S., MacKenzie, R., and Asscher, A. W. (1982). Lack of adherence to epithelial cells by freshly isolated urinary pathogens. *Lancet*, **i**, 586–588.

Hart, R. C., Kadis, S., and Chapman, W. L. (1982). Nutritional iron status and susceptibility to *Proteus mirabilis* pyelonephritis in the rat. *Can. J. Microbiol.*, **28**, 713–717.

Haselberger, C. G., and Schenkel-Brunner, H. (1982). Evidence for erythrocyte membrane glycoproteins being carriers of blood-group P_1 determinants. *FEBS Lett.*, **149**, 126–128.

Helmuth, R., and Achtman, M. (1978). Cell–cell interactions in conjugating *Escherichia coli:* purification of F pili with biological activity. *Proc. Natl. Acad. Sci.*, USA, **75**, 1237–1241.

Hermodson, M. A., Chen, K. C. S., and Buchanan, T. M. (1978). *Neisseria* pili proteins: amino-terminal sequence and identification of an unusual amino acid. *Biochemistry*, **17**, 442–445.

Holmgren, J., Svennerholm, A.-M. and Åhren, C. (1981). Nonimmunoglobulin fraction of human milk inhibits bacterial adhesion (haemagglutination) and enterotoxin binding of *Escherichia coli* and *Vibrio cholerae. Infect. Immun.*, **33**, 136–141.

Horwitz, M. A. (1982). Phagocytosis of microorganisms. *Rev. Infect. Dis.*, **4**, 104–123.

Houvink, A. L., and van Iterson, W. (1950). Electron microscopical observations on bacterial cytology. II. A study on flagellation. *Biochem. Biophys. Acta*, **5**, 10–44.

Hull, R. A., Gill, R. E., Hsu, P., Minshew, B. H., and Falkow, S. (1981). Construction and expression of recombinant plasmids encoding type-1 or D-mannose-resistant pili from urinary tract infection *Escherichia coli* isolate. *Infect. Immun.*, **33**, 933–938.

Isaacson, R. E. (1977). K99 surface antigen of *Escherichia coli:* purification and partial characterization. *Infect. Immun.*, **15**, 272–279.

Isaacson, R. E. (1978). K99 surface antigen of *Escherichia coli:* antigenic characterization. *Infect. Immun.*, **22**, 555–559.

Isaacson, R. E., and Richter, P. (1981). *Escherichia coli* 987P pilus: purification and partial characterization. *J. Bacteriol.*, **146**, 784–789.

Isaacson, R. E., Fusco, P. C., Brinton, C. C., and Moon, H. W. (1978). *In vitro* adhesion of *Escherichia coli* to porcine small intestinal epithelial cells: pili as adhesive factors. *Infect. Immun.*, **21**, 392–397.

Isaacson, R. E., Dean, E. A., Morgan, R. L., and Moon, H. W. (1980). Immunization of suckling pigs against enterotoxigenic *Escherichia coli* induced diarrheal disease by vaccinating dams with purified K99 or 987P pili: antibody production in response to vaccination. *Infect. Immun.*, **29**, 824–826.

Isaacson, R. E., Colmenero, J., and Richter, P. (1981). *Escherichia coli* K99 pili are composed of one subunit species. *FEMS Microbiol. Lett.*, **12**, 229–232.

Jann, K., Jann, B., and Schmidt, G. (1981). SDS polyacrylamide gel electrophoresis and serological analysis of pili from *Escherichia coli* of different pathogenic origin. *FEMS Microbiol. Lett.*, **11**, 21–25.

Jokinen, M., Ehnholm, C., Väisänen-Rhen, V., Korhonen, T. K., Pipkorn, R., Kalkkinen, N., and Gahmberg, C. G. (1985). Identification of the major human red cell sialoglycoprotein, glycophorin A^M, as the receptor for *Escherichia coli* 1H11165 and characterization of the receptor site. *Eur. J. Biochem.*, in press.

Jones, G. W. (1977). The attachment of bacteria to the surfaces of animal cells. In *Microbial Interactions (Receptors and Recognition, Ser. B*, Vol. 3), (Ed. J. L. Reissig), pp.140–176. Chapman and Hall, London.

Jones, G. W. (1980). The adhesive properties of *Vibrio cholerae* and other *Vibrio* species. In *Bacterial Adherence (Receptors and Recognition, Ser. B*, Vol. 6) (Ed. E. H. Beachey), pp.219–243. Chapman and Hall, London.

Jones, G. W., and Rutter, J. M. (1972). Role of the K88 antigen in the pathogenesis of neonatal diarrhoea caused by *Escherichia coli* in piglets. *Infect. Immun.*, **6**, 918–927.

Jones, G. W., and Rutter, J. M. (1974). The association of K88 antigen with haemagglutinating activity in porcine strains of *Escherichia coli*. *J. Gen. Microbial.*, **84**, 135–144.

Källenius, G., and Möllby, R. (1979). Adhesion of *Escherichia coli* to human periurethral cells correlated to mannose-resistat agglutination of human erythrocytes. *FEMS Microbiol. Lett.*, **5**, 295–299.

Källenius, G., and Winberg, J. (1978). Bacterial adherence to periurethral epithelial cells in girls prone to urinary tract infection. *Lancet*, **ii**, 540–543.

Källenius, G., Möllby, R., Svenson, S. B., Winberg, J., Lundblad, A., and Svenson, S. (1980). The P^k antigen as receptor of pyelonephritogenic *Escherichia coli*. *FEMS Microbiol. Lett.*, **7**, 297–302.

Källenius, G., Möllby, R., Svenson, S. B, Helin, H. B., Hultberg, H., Cedergren, C., and Winberg, J. (1981a). Occurrence of P-fimbriated *Escherichia coli* in urinary tract infections. *Lancet*, **ii**, 1369–1372.

Källenius, G., Svenson, S. B., Möllby, R., Cedergren, B., Hultberg, H., and Winberg, J. (1981b). Structure of carbohydrate part of receptor on human uroepithelial cells for pyelonephritogenic *Escherichia coli*. *Lancet*, **ii**, 604–606.

Kearns, M. J., and Gibbons, R. A. (1979). The possible nature of the pig intestinal receptor for the K88 antigen of *Escherichia coli*. *FEMS Microbiol. Lett.*, **6**, 165–168.

Klemm, P. (1979). Fimbrial colonization factor CFA/I protein from human enteropathogenic *Escherichia coli* strain. *FEBS Lett.*, **108**, 107–110.

Klemm, P. (1981). The complete amino acid sequence of the K88 antigen, a fimbrial protein from *Escherichia coli*. *Eur. J. Biochem.*, **117**, 617–627.

Klemm, P. (1982). Primary structure of the CFA/I fimbrial protein from human enterotoxigenic *Escherichia coli* strains. *Eur. J. Biochem*, **124**, 339–348.

Klemm, P., and Mikkelsen, L. (1982). Prediction of antigenic determinants and secondary structures of the K88 and CFA1 fimbrial proteins from enteropathogenic *Escherichia coli*. *Infect. Immun.*, **38**, 41–45.

Klemm, P., Ørskov, I., and Ørskov, F. (1982). F7 and type-1-like fimbriae from three *Escherichia coli* strains isolated from urinary tract infections. *Infect. Immun.*, **36**, 462–468.

Klemm, P., Ørskov, I., and Ørskov, F. (1983). Isolation and characterization of the F12 adhesive fimbrial antigens from uropathogenic *Escherichia coli* strains. *Infect. Immun.*, **40**, 91–96.

Korhonen, T. K. (1979). Yeast cell agglutination by purified enterobacterial pili. *FEMS Microbiol. Lett.*, **6**, 421–425.

Korhonen, T. K., and Rhen, M. (1982). Bacterial fimbriae as vaccines. *Ann. Clin. Res.*, **14**, 272–277.

Korhonen, T. K., Edén, S., and Svanborg Edén, C. (1980a). Binding of purified *Escherichia coli* pili to human urinary tract epithelial cells. *FEMS Microbiol. Lett.*, **7**, 237–240.

Korhonen, T. K., Lounatmaa, K., Ranta, H., and Kuusi, N. (1980b). Characterization of type-1 pili of *Salmonella typhimurium* LT2. *J. Bacteriol.*, **144**, 800–805.

Korhonen, T. K., Nurmiaho, E.-L., Ranta, H., and Svanborg Edén, C. (1980c). New method for isolation of immunologically pure pili from *Escherichia coli*. *Infect. Immun.*, **27**, 569–575.

Korhonen, T. K., Leffler, H., and Svanborg Edén, C. (1981). Binding specificity of piliated strains of *Escherichia coli* and *Salmonella typhimurium* to epithelial cells, *Saccharomyces cerevisiae* cells, and erythrocytes. *Infect. Immun.*, **32**, 796–804.

Korhonen, T. K., Väisänen, V., Saxén, H., Hultberg, H., and Svenson, S. B. (1982). P-antigen-recognizing fimbriae from human uropathogenic *Escherichia coli* strains. *Infect. Immun.*, **37**, 286–291.

Korhonen, T. K., Tarkka, E., Ranta, H., and Haahtela, H. (1983). Type-3 fimbriae of *Klebsiella*: molecular characterization and role in bacterial adhesion to plant roots. *J. Bacteriol.*, **155**, 860–865.

Korhonen, T. K. Väisänen-Rhen, V., Rhen, M., Pere, A., Parkkinen, J., and Finne, J. (1984). *Escherichia coli* fimbriae binding to sialyl galactosides. *J. Bacteriol.*, **159**, 762–766

Leffler, H., and Svanborg Edén, C. (1980). Chemical identification of a glycosphingolipid receptor for *Escherichia coli* attaching to human urinary tract epithelial cells and haemagglutinating human erythrocytes. *FEMS Microbiol. Lett.*, **8**, 127–134.

Leffler, H., and Svanborg, Edén, C. (1981). Glycolipid receptors for uropathogenic *Escherichia coli* on human erythrocytes and uroepithelial cells. *Infect. Immun.*, **34**, 920–929.

Leunk, R. D., and Moon, R. J. (1982). Association of type-1 pili with the ability of livers to clear *Salmonella typhimurium*. *Infect. Immun.*, **36**, 1168–1174.

Levine, M. M., Black, R. E., Brinton, C. C., Jr., Clements, M. L., Fusco, P., Hughes, T. P., O'Donnel, S., Robins-Browne, R., Wood, S., and Young, C. R. (1982). Reactogenicity, immunogenicity and efficacy studies of *Escherichia coli* type 1 somatic pili parenteral vaccine in man. *Scand. J. Infect. Dis. Suppl.*, **33**, 83–95.

Lindahl, M., Faris, A., and Wadström, T. (1982). Colonization factor antigen on enterotoxigenic *Escherichia coli* is a sialic-specific lectin. *Lancet*, **i**, 280.

Lindahl, M. A., and Ingram, P. L. (1982). The role of alpha haemolysin in the virulence of *Escherichia coli* for mice. *J. Med. Microbiol.*, **15**, 23–30.

Linggood, M. A., and Ingram, P. L. (1982). The role of alpha haemolysin in the virulence of *Escherichia coli* for mice. *J. med. Microbiol.*, **15**, 23–30.

Lomberg, H., Jodal, U., Svanborg Edén, C., Leffler, H., and Samuelsson, B. (1981). P_1 blood group and urinary tract infection. *Lancet*, **i**, 551–552.

Manning, P. A., and Achtman, A. (1979). Cell-to-cell interactions in conjugating *Escherichia coli*: the involvement of the cell envelope. In *Bacterial Outer Membranes* (Ed. M. Inouye), pp.409–447. John Wiley, New York.

Marshall, K. C. (1971). Sorptive interactions between soil particles and microorganisms. In *Soil Biochemistry* (Ed. A. D. McLaren and J. Skujins), pp.409–445. Marcel Dekker, New York.

Mårtenson, E. (1969). Glycosphingolipids of animal tissue. In *Progress in the Chemistry of Fats and Other Lipids*, Vol. X, Part 4, pp.367–407. Pergamon, New York.

McMichael, J. C., and Ou, J. T. (1979). Structure of common pili from *Escherichia coli*. *J. Bacteriol.*, **138**, 969–975.

Mooi, F. R., and de Graaf, F. K. (1979). Isolation and characterization of K88 antigens. *FEMS Microbiol. Lett.*, **5**, 17–20.

Moon, H. W., Nagy, B., Isaacson, R. E., and Ørskov, I. (1977). Occurrence of K99 antigen on *Escherichia coli* isolated from pigs and colonization of pig ileum by K99[+] enterotoxigenic *E. coli* from calves and pigs. *Infect. Immun.*, **15**, 614–620.

Morgan, R. I., Isaacson, R. E., Moon, H. W., Brinton, C. C., and To, C. C. (1978). Immunization of suckling pigs against enterotoxigenic *Escherichia coli* induced diarrheal disease by vaccinating dams with purified 987 or K99 pili: protection correlates with pilus homology of vaccine and challenge. *Infect. Immun.*, **22**, 771–777.

Morris, J. A., Thorne, C. J., and Sojka, W. J. (1980). Evidence for two adhesive antigens on the K99 reference strain *Escherichia coli* B41. *J. Gen. Microbiol.*, **118**, 107–113.

Myers, L. L., and Guinée, P. A. M. (1976). Occurrence and characteristics of enterotoxigenic *Escherichia coli* isolated from calves with diarrhea. *Infect. Immun.*, **13**, 1117–1119.

Nagy, B. (1980). Vaccination of cows with a K99 extract to protect newborn calves against experimental enterotoxic colibacillosis. *Infect. Immun.*, **27**, 21–24.

Nagy, B., Moon, H. W., and Isaacson, R. E. (1977). Colonization of porcine intestine by enterotoxigenic *Escherichia coli*: selection of piliated forms *in vivo*, adhesion of piliated forms to epithelial cells *in vitro*, and incidence of a pilus antigen among enteropathogenic *E. coli*. *Infect. Immun.*, **16**, 344–352.

Nagy, B., Moon, H. W., Isaacson, R. E., To, C. C., and Brinton, C. C. (1978). Immunization of suckling pigs against enterotoxigenic *Escherichia coli* infection by vaccinating dams with purified pili. *Infect. Immun.*, **21**, 269–274.

Nowotarska, M., and Mulckzyk, M. (1977). Serological relationship of fimbriae among *Enterobacteriaceae*. *Arch. Immunol. Ther. Exp.*, **25**, 7–46.

Novotny, C., Carnahan, J., and Brinton, C. C., Jr. (1969). Mechanical removal of F pili, type 1 pili and flagella from Hfr and RTF donor cells and the kinetics of their reappearance. *J. Bacteriol.*, **98**, 1294–1306.

Ofek, I., Mirelman, D., and Sharon, N. (1977). Adherence of *Escherichia coli* to human mucosal cells mediated by mannose receptors. *Nature*, **265**, 623–625.

Öhman, L., Magnusson, K.-E., and Stendahl, O. (1982). The mannose-specific lectin activity of *Escherichia coli* type 1 fimbriae assayed by agglutination of glycolipid-containing liposomes, erythrocytes and yeast cells and hydrophobic interaction chromatography. *FEMS Microbiol. Lett.*, **14**, 149–153.

Old, D. C. (1972). Inhibition of the interaction between fimbrial haemagglutinins and erythrocytes by D-mannose and other carbohydrates. *J. Gen. Microbiol.*, **71**, 149–157.

Old, D. C., and Duguid, J. P. (1970). Selective outgrowth of fimbriae bacteria in static liquid medium. *J. Bacteriol.*, **103**, 447–456.

Ørskov, I., and Ørskov, F. (1983). Serology of *Escherichia coli* fimbriae. *Prog. Allergy*, **33**, 80–105.

Ørskov, I., Ørskov, F., Sojka, W. J., and Wittig, W. (1964). K antigens K88ab(L) and K88ac(L) in *E. coli*. *Acta. Path. Microbiol. Scand.*, **62**, 439–447.

Ørskov, I., Ørskov, F., Smith, H. W., and Sojka, W. J. (1975). The establishment of K99, a thermolabile transmissible *Escherichia coli* K antigen, previously called 'Kco', possessed by calf and lamb enteropathogenic strains. *Acta Pathol. Microbiol. Scand.*, **83**, 31–36.

Ørskov, I., Ørskov, F., Evans, D. J., Jr., Sack, R. B., and Wadström, T. (1976). Special *Escherichia coli* serotypes among enterotoigenic strains from diarrheoa in adults and children. *Med. Microbiol. Immunol.*, **162**, 73–80.

Ørskov, I., Ørskov, F., and Birch-Andersen, A. (1980). Comparison of *Escherichia coli* fimbrial antigen F7 with type 1 fimbriae. *Infect. Immun.*, **27**, 657–666.

Ottow, J. C. G. (1975). Ecology, physiology and genetics of fimbriae and pili. *Annu. Rev. Microbiol.*, **29**, 79–108.

Parkkinen, J., Finne, J., Achtman, M., Väisänen, V., and Korhonen, T. K. (1983). *Escherichia coli* strains binding neuraminyl α2–3 galactosides. *Biochem. Biophys. Res. Commun.*, **111**, 456–461.

Parry, S. H., and Porter, P. (1978). Immunological aspects of cell membrane adhesion demonstrated by porcine enteropathogenic *Escherichia coli*. *Immunology*, **34**, 41–49.

Rene, P., and Silverblatt, F. J. (1982). Serological response to *Escherichia coli* pili in pyelonephritis. *Infect. Immun.*, **37**, 749–754.

Rene, P., Dinolfo, M., and Silverblatt, F, J. (1982). Serum and antibody responses to *Escherichia coli* pili in cystitis. *Infect. Immun.*, **38**, 542–547.

Rhen, M., Klemm, P., Wahlström, E., Svenson, S. B., Källenius, G., and Korhonen, T. K. (1983a). P fimbriae of *Escherichia coli:* immuno- and protein chemical characterization of fimbriae from two pyelonephritogenic strains. *FEMS Microbiol. Lett.*, **18**, 233–238.

Rhen, M., Knowles, J., Penttinen, M., Sarvas, M., and Korhonen, T. K. (1983b). P fimbriae of *Escherichia coli*: molecular cloning of DNA fragments containing the structural genes. *FEMS Microbiol. Lett.*, **19**, 119–123.

Rhen, M., Mäkelä, P. H., and Korhonen, T. K. (1983c). P fimbriae of *Escherichia coli* are subject to phase variation. *FEMS Microbiol. Lett.*, **19**, 267–271.

Rhen, M., Wahlström, E., and Korhonen, T. K. (1983d). P fimbriae of *Escherichia coli*: fractionation by immune precipitation. *FEMS Microbiol. Lett.*, **18**, 227–232.

Roberts, J. A., Hardaway, K., Kaack, B., Fussell, E. N., and Baskin, G. (1984). Prevention of pyelonephritis by immunization with P fimbriae. *J. Urol.*, **131**, 602–607.

Runnels, P. L., Moon, H. W., and Schneider, R. A. (1980). Development of resistance with host age to adhesion of K99$^+$ *Escherichia coli* to isolated intestinal epithelial cells. *Infect. Immun.*, **28**, 298–300.

Rutter, J. M., and Jones, G. W. (1973). Protection against enteric disease caused by *Escherichia coli*—a model for vaccination with a virulence determinant. *Nature*, **257**, 135–136.

Rutter, J. M., Burrows, M. R., Sellwood, R., and Gibbons, R. A. (1975). A genetic basis for resistance to enteric disease caused by *Escherichia coli*. *Nature*, **257**, 135–136.

Rutter, J. M., Jones, G. W., Brown, G. T. H., Burrows, M. R. and Luther, P. D. (1976). Antibacterial activity in colostrum and milk associated with protection against enteric disease caused by K88-positive *Escherichia coli*. *Infect. Immun.*, **13**, 667–676.

Salit, I. E., and Gotschlich, E. C. (1977a). Hemagglutination by purified type 1 *Escherichia coli* pili. *J. Exp. Med.*, **146**, 1169–1181.

Salit, I. E., and Gotschlich, E. C. (1977b). Type 1 *Escherichia coli* pili: characterization of binding to monkey kidney cells. *J. Exp. Med.*, **146**, 1182–1194.

Schneider, R. A., and To, S. C. M. (1982). Enterotoxigenic *Escherichia coli* strains that express K88 and 987P pilus antigens. *Infect. Immun.*, **36**, 417–418.

Sellwood, R., Gibbons, R. A., Jones, G. W., and Rutter, J. M. (1975). Adhesion of enteropathogenic *Escherichia coli* to pig intestinal brush borders: the existence of two pig phenotypes. *J. Med. Microbiol.*, **8**, 405–411.

Siddiqui, B., Kawanami, J., Li, Y.-T., and Hakomori, S. (1972). Structures of ceramide tetrasaccharides from various sources: uniqueness of rat kidney ceramide tetrasaccharide. *J. Lipid Res.*, **13**, 657–662.

Silverblatt, F. J., and Cohen, L. S. (1979). Antipili antibody affords protection against experimental pyelonephritis. *J. Clin. Invest.*, **64**, 333–336.

Silverblatt, F. J., Dreyer, J. S., and Schauer, S. (1979). Effect of pili on susceptibility of *Escherichia coli* to phagocytosis. *Infect. Immun.*, **24**, 218–223.

Smith, E. E., and Goldstein, I. J. (1967). Protein–carbohydrate interaction. V. Further inhibition studies directed toward defining the stereochemical requirements of the reaction sites of concanavalin A. *Arch. Biochem. Biophys.*, **121**, 88–95.

Smith, H. W., and Halls, S. (1967). The transmissible nature of the genetic factor in *Escherichia coli* that controls haemolysin production. *J. Gen. Microbiol.*, **47**, 153–161.

Smith, H. W., and Jones, J. E. T. (1963). Observations on the alimentary tract and its bacterial flora in healthy and diseased pigs. *J. Pathol. Bacteriol.*, **86**, 387–346.

Smith, H. W., and Linggood, M. A. (1971). Observations on the pathogenic properties of the K88, hly and ent plasmids of *Escherichia coli* with particular reference to porcine diarrhoea. *J. Med. Microbiol*, **4**, 467–485.

Smith, H. W., and Linggood, M. A. (1972). Further observations on *Escherichia coli* enterotoxins with particular regard to those produced by atypical piglet strains and by calf and lamb strains: the transmissible nature of these enterotoxins and of a K antigen possessed by calf and lamb strains. *J. Med. Microbiol.*, **5**, 243–250.

Smith, J. W., Wagner, S., and Swenson, R. M. (1981). Local immune response to *Escherichia coli* pili in experimental pyelonephritis. *Infect. Immun.*, **31**, 17–20.

Smyth, C. J. (1982). Two mannose-resistant haemagglutinins on enterotoxigenic *Escherichia coli* of serotype O6:K15:H16 or H – isolated from travellers' and infantile diarrhoea. *J. Gen. Microbiol.*, **128**, 2081–2096.

Smyth, C. J., Jonsson, P., Olsson, E., Söderlind, O., Rosengren, J., Hjertén, S., and Wadström, T. (1978). Differences in hydrophobic surface characteristics of porcine enteropathogenic *Escherichia coli* with or without K88 antigen as revealed by hydrophobic interaction chromatography. *Infect. Immun.*, **22**, 462–472.

Smyth, C. J., Kajser, B., Bäck, E., Faris, Möllby, R., Söderlind, O., Stintzing, G., and Wadström, T. (1979). Occurrence of adhesins causing mannose-resistant haemagglutination of bovine erythrocytes in enterotoxigenic *Escherichia coli*. *FEMS Microbiol. Lett.*, **5**, 85–90.

Smyth, C. J., Olsson, E., Moncalvo, C., Söderlind, O., Ørskov, F., and Ørskov, I. (1981). K99 antigen-positive enterotoxigenic *Escherichia coli* from piglets with diarrhea in Sweden. *Infect. Immun.*, **13**, 252–257.

Snodgrass, D. R., Nagy, L. K., Sherwood, D., and Campbell, I. (1982). Passive immunity in calf diarrhea: vaccination with K99 antigen of enterotoxigenic *Escherichia coli* and rotavirus. *Infect. Immun.*, **37**, 586–591.

Söderlind, O., and Möllby, R. (1979). Enterotoxins, O-groups and K88 antigen in *Escherichia coli* from neonatal piglets with and without diarrhea. *Infect. Immun.*, **24**, 611–616.

Söderlind, O., Olsson, E., Smyth, C. J., and Möllby, R. (1982). Effect of parenteral vaccination of dams on intestinal *Escherichia coli* in piglets with diarrhea. *Infect. Immun.*, **36**, 900–906.

Sojka, W. J., Wray, C., and Morris, J. A. (1978). Passive protection of lambs against experimental enteric colibacillosis by colostral transer of antibodies from K99 vaccinated ewes. *J. Med. Microbiol.*, **11**, 493–499.

Stirm, S., Ørskov, F., Ørskov, I., and Mansa, B. (1967). Episome-carried surface antigen K88 of *Escherichia coli*. II. Isolation and chemical analysis. *J. Bacteriol.*, **93**, 731–739.

Svanborg Edén, C., and Hansson, H. A. (1978). *Escherichia coli* pili as mediators of attachment to human urinary tract epithelial cells. *Infect. Immun.*, **21**, 229–237.

Svanborg Edén, C., and Jodal, U. (1979). Attachment of *Escherichia coli* to urinary sediment epithelial cells from urinary tract infection-prone and healthy children. *Infect. Immun.*, **26**, 837–840.

Svanborg Edén, C., Hanson, L. Å. Jodal, U., Lindberg, U., and Sohl-Åkerlund, A. (1976). Variable adhesion to normal urinary tract epithelial cells of *Escherichia coli* strains associated with various forms of urinary tract infection. *Lancet*, **ii**, 490–492.

Svanborg Edén, C., Carlsson, B., Hanson, L. Å., Jann, B., Jann, K., Korhonen, T., and Wadström, T. (1979). Anti-pili antibodies in breast milk. *Lancet*, **ii**, 1235.

Svanborg Edén, C., Preter, R., Hagverg, L., Hull, R., Hull, S., Leffler, H., and Schoolnik, G. (1982a). Inhibition of experimental ascending urinary tract infection by an epithelial cell-surface receptor analogue. *Nature*, **298**, 560–562.

Svanborg Edén, C., Hanson, L. Å., Jodal, U., Leffler, H., Mårild, S., Korhonen, T., Brinton, C., Jann, B., Jann, K., and Silverblatt, F. (1982b). Receptor analogues and antipili antibodies as inhibitors of attachment of uropathogenic *Escherichia coli*. In *Recent Advances in Mucosal Immunity* (Eds. W. Strober, L. Å. Hanson and K. W. Sell), pp.355–369. Raven Press, New York.

Svenson, S. B., Källenius, G., Möllby, R., Hultberg, H., and Winberg, J. (1982). Rapid identification of P-fimbriated *Escherichia coli* by a receptor-specific particle agglutination test. *Infection*, **10**, 209–214.

Svenson, S. B., Hultberg, H., Källenius, G., Korhonen, T. K., Möllby, R., and Winberg, J. (1983). P fimbriae of pyelonephritogenic *Escherichia coli*: identification and chemical characterization of receptors. *Infection*, **11**, 61–67.

Väisänen, V., Elo, J., Tallgren, L. G., Siitonen, A., Mäkelä, P. H., Svanborg Edén, C., Källenius, G., Svenson, S. B., Hultberg, H., and Korhonen, T. (1981). Mannose-resistant haemagglutination and P antigen recognition are characteristic of *Escherichia coli* causing primary pyelonephritis. *Lancet*, **11**, 1366–1369.

Väisänen-Rhen, V., Korhonen, T. K., Jokinen, M., Gahmberg, C. G., and Enhnolm, C. (1982). Blood group M specific haemagglutinin in pyelonephritogenic *Escherichia coli*. *Lancet*, **i**, 1192.

Väisänen-Rhen, V., Korhonen, T. K., and Finne, J. (1983). Novel cell-binding activity specific for *N*-acetyl–D-glucosamine in an *Escherichia coli* strain. *FEBS Lett.*, **159**, 233–236.

Väisänen-Rhen, V., Elo, J., Väisänen, E., Siitonen, A., Ørskov, I., Ørskov, F., Svenson, S. B., Mäkelä, P. H., and Korhonen, T. K. (1984). P-fimbriated clones among uropathogenic *Escherichia coli* strains. *Infect. Immun.*, **43**, 149–155.

van den Bosch, J. F., Verboom-Sohmer, U., Postma, P., de Graaf, J., and MacLaren, D. (1980). Mannose-sensitive and mannose-resistant adherence to human uroepithelial cells and urinary virulence of *Escherichia coli*. *Infect. Immun.*, **29**, 226–233.

van Embden, J. D. A., de Graaf, F. K., Schouls, L. M., and Teppema, J. S. (1980). Cloning and expression of deoxyribonucleic acid fragment that encodes for the adhesive antigen K99. *Infect. Immun.*, **29**, 1125–1133.

Waalen, K., Sletten, K., Frøholm, L. O., Väisänen, V., and Korhonen, T. K., (1983). The N-terminal amino acid sequence of type 1 fimbria (pili) of *Salmonella typhimurium* LT2. *FEMS Microbiol. Lett.*, **16**, 149–151.

Wevers, P., Picken, R., Schmidt, G., Jann, B., Jann, K., Goleck, J. R., and Kist, M. (1980). Characterization of pili associated with *Escherichia coli* O18ac. *Infect. Immun.*, **29**, 685–691.

Williams, P. H., Sedgwick, M. I. Evans, N., Turner, P. J., George, R. H., and McNeish, A. S. (1978). Adherence of an enteropathogenic strain of *Escherichia coli* to human intestinal mucosa is mediated by a colicinogenic conjugative plasmid. *Infect. Immun.*, **22**, 393–402.

Wilson, M. R., and Hohman, A. W. (1974). Immunity to *Escherichia coli* in pigs: adhesion of enteropathogenic *Escherichia coli* to isolated intestinal epithelial cells. *Infect. Immun.*, **10**, 776–782.

ZoBell, C. E., and Allen, E. C. (1935). The significance of marine bacteria in the fouling of submerged surfaces. *J. Bacteriol*, **29**, 239–251.

Immunology of the Bacterial Cell Envelope
Edited by D. E. S. Stewart-Tull and M. Davies
© 1985 John Wiley & Sons Ltd.

CHAPTER 13

Illustrated Guide to the Anatomy of the Bacterial Cell Envelope

John H. Freer

*Department of Microbiology, Alexander Stone Building, University of Glasgow,
Garscube Estate, Bearsden, Glasgow G61 1QH, UK*

I. PREAMBLE

The bacterial surface presents a bewildering array of immunogenic components, and the precise composition of this antigenic mosaic often depends on the conditions of cultivation of the organism as well as its genetic potential. For example, (a) whether or not capsular material is present may depend on the carbon:nitrogen ratio in the growth medium, and (b) the presence of teichoic acids on the available phosphorus. Also, such structures as fimbriae are expressed only at appropriate temperatures and their production may be specifically inhibited by certain metabolites. Examples of such effects are the inhibition of colonization factor antigen expression at 18°C or the inhibition of K99 synthesis by L-alanine.

Some outer membrane proteins in gram-negative bacteria are inducible, e.g. the siderophore receptors, the elaboration of which may reflect low levels of available iron. Many of these influences are even more significant *in vivo* than in laboratory-grown cultures.

The point about the cell surface that I am making is that it is not a static, well-defined chemical entity for any organism, but that its composition is a reflection of the conditions under which the organism finds itself at any particular time. In addition, host factors may also be adsorbed at the bacterial cell surface, adding further to its physical complexity, yet possibly masking foreign antigens in the host.

Here, in these few pages, I will illustrate in very broad terms (1) what we might find in the surface layers of the bacterial cell, (2) what these layers look like, and (3) what kind of structures we might find associated with the cell surface, yet not strictly speaking part of the cell walls. This is by no means a comprehensive catalogue of bacterial surface structures, but is more a summary of the main types present and discussed in this book. There are two further points which are relevant to the following discussion. First, it may seem obvious, but is worth emphasizing, that the methods used to visualize bacterial structures are usually those which utilize the various preparative techniques of electron microscopy. These involve the generation of predictable artifacts which are recognized as corresponding to the various chemical entities which make up the cell structures. Secondly, although the differences between the surface layers of gram-positive and gram-negative bacteria are often emphasized, both groups share many common structures such as capsules and other extracellular polymeric carbohydrates, fimbriae and flagella. Although the detailed structure of the basal body of the flagellum differs slightly in the two groups, the organelles are thought to share common functional design principles, the structural differences simply reflecting additional anchorage apparatus in the case of the gram-negative bacteria. Here, these extramural components will be considered without regard to their specific origins.

II. FINE STRUCTURE OF SURFACE COMPONENTS OF GRAM-POSITIVE AND GRAM-NEGATIVE BACTERIA

The plasma membrane is usually protected against swelling and environmental stress in the form of mechanical shear by the cell wall layers. In gram-positive organisms, these are seen in thin-section electron micrographs or in freeze-fracture replicas as relatively thick, amorphous structures, usually without discernible layering across their thickness. Figure 1 illustrates diagrammatically, the arrangement of components which may be present in the surface layers of gram-positive bacteria. The cell wall consists largely of a covalent complex of peptidoglycan (PG) and wall teichoic acids (TA) or teichuronic acids (TUA) as the principal polymers, usually with a glycerol lipoteichoic acid (LTA) anchored in the plasma membrane (PM) but exposed at the cell surface. In addition, there may be protein or carbohydrate components exposed at the cell surface as part of the cell wall matrix, and, if present, these are usually immunodominant and play an important role in virulence. Examples are the M protein (Mp) in group A streptococci and the group specific C carbohydrate (C) in this genus. Under appropriate conditions, gram-positive organisms may be

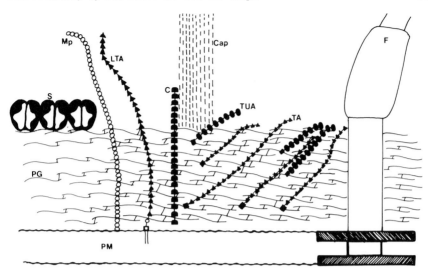

Figure 1

encapsulated (Cap), with acidic polysaccharides occurring most frequently, but occasionally more complex polymers may be found as in the pneumococci, or polypeptide may replace polysaccharide as in the gamma-glutamyl capsules of some bacilli. Such structures are frequently expressed *in vivo* and, by virtue of their antiphagocytic activity, act as important virulence determinants. In addition, highly ordered protein subunits may make up an additional layer on the outer surface of the cell wall proper. This layer, the S layer (S), differs in molecular detail from species to species. It is evidently a non-essential structure, since its absence does not affect viability. Flagella (F) may also be present in gram-positive bacteria and these are usually of similar overall appearance to those of gram-negative species (however, see below).

The gram-negative cell surface is somewhat more complex in appearance, usually consisting of a distinctly layered envelope around the cell (Figure 2). The outer membrane (OM) composed of lipopolysaccharide (LPS), phospholipids (pl), glycolipid such as enterobacterial common antigen (eca) and proteins, many of which have pore-forming capacities (pore), surrounds the rigid or R layer (PG), which is structurally analogous to the wall of the gram-positive bacterium. These two layers are often closely apposed and in most species linked by lipoprotein molecules, a fraction of which is covalently attached to the rigid layer and at the same time anchored by a diglyceride moiety in the outer membrane (lp). The outer membrane is separated from the plasma membrane over most of its length by a compartment, the periplasmic space. This may be a misnomer, since the so-called space apparently contains a variety of proteins (pp) involved in diverse functions such as transport of nutrients,

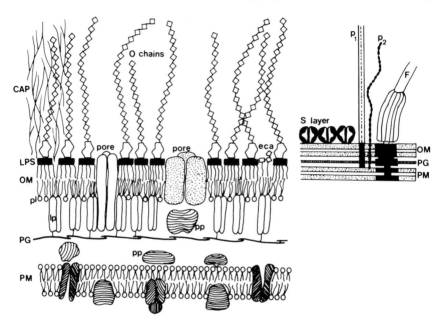

Figure 2

cleavage of substrates, environmental sensing, etc. At several sites in the envelope
however, the plasma membrane (PM) is intimately and firmly associated with
the outer two layers (R layer and OM) forming areas (Bayer's patches or
junctions) where physical continuity between the outer membrane and the plasma
membrane exists, allowing exchange of phospholipids between the two
membranes. However, proteins and lipopolysaccharides are strictly localized
in their respective membranes. Gram-negative bacteria also synthesize acidic
polysaccharide capsules (CAP), which may vary in the tightness with which they
are associated with the cell surface. Many are loosely adherent and others form
considerable accumulations of cell-free slime or gum in the surrounding medium.
Fimbriae are widespread in this group whereas they are much more restricted
in the gram-positive genera. Structurally, there are two types of arrangement
of subunits which yield either beaded strands of subunits (approx. 3 nm in
diameter) found in **K**88 and **K**99 pili (p_2), or the arrangement of subunits in
a helical fashion to form a hollow tube about 7 nm in diameter, as found in
type-1 and CFA fimbriae (p_1). Flagella (F) are similar to those found in gram-
positive species, apart from an additional pair of anchoring rings being present
in the basal body. In some genera of gram-negative organisms, a continuation
of the outer membrane surrounds the flagellar filament, giving rise to the so-
called sheathed flagella in genera such as *Vibrio* and *Pseudomonas*. In these
instances, the apparent diameter of the filament is increased to about 35 nm

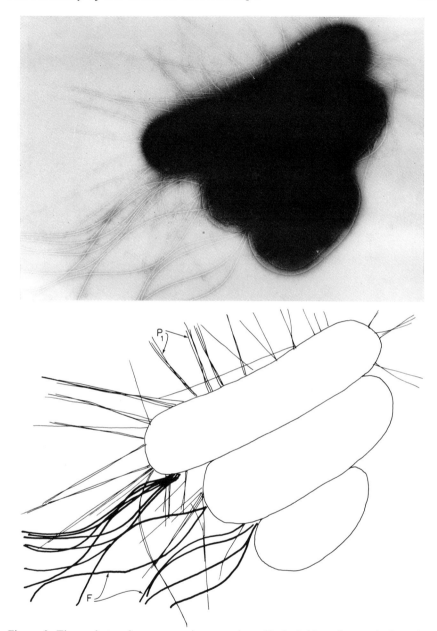

Figure 3. The archetypal gram-negative organism, *Escherichia coli*, negatively stained to show peritrichous flagella (F) with filaments of characteristic wavelength and numerous common or type-1 fimbriae approximately 7 nm in diameter (P_1). Note the fimbriae often adhere to each other in a fasiculate manner, giving a twisted ribbon-like appearance.
× 21 725

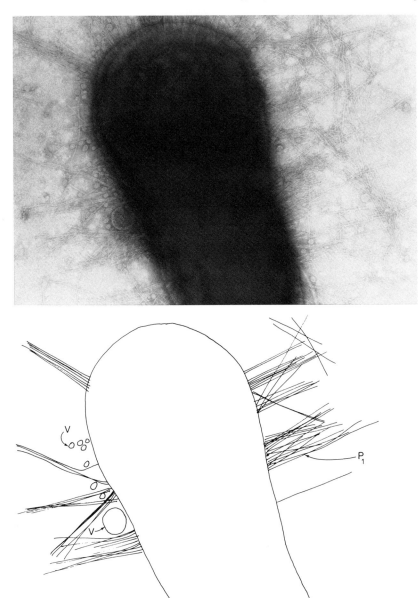

Figure 4. A micrograph of a negatively-stained cell of *E. coli* showing more detail of the fimbriae (P₁) with diameters of approximately 7 nm. The hollow core of the tubular structures can be seen filled with stain. In this strain, the cell releases relatively large amounts of outer membrane in the form of small vesicles (V) rich in lipopolysaccharide. × 49 115

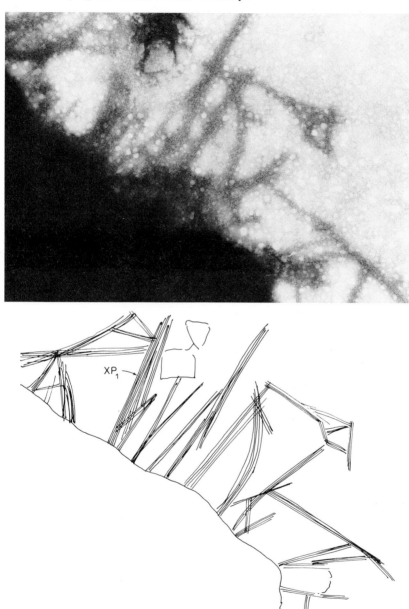

Figure 5. A negatively stained cell of *E. coli* with the fimbriae 'stained' by reaction with anti-fimbrial IgG, which can be seen cross-linking adjacent fimbriae (xP$_1$) ×46 365

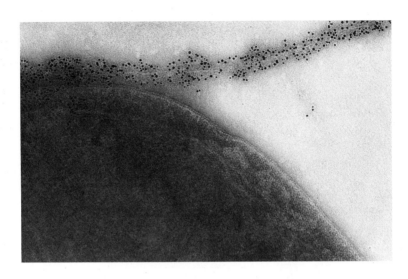

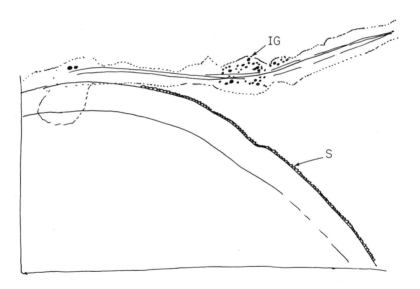

Figure 6. Specific anti-fimbrial IgG can be conjugated to colloidal gold to give a specific immunological labelling reagent (Immunogold label). The fimbriae in this specimen of *Bacteroides nodosus* are labelled with such a reagent, and the label appears as small (5 nm) electron-dense spheres (IG) specifically associated with the fimbriae. Note also the structured layer (S) on the outer surface of the cell. The specimen was negatively stained after reaction with the labelling reagent. × 109 500

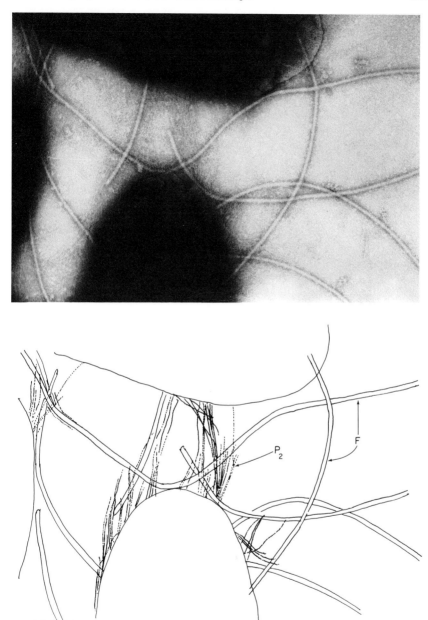

Figure 7. Two negatively stained cells of *E. coli* K12 which carry on their surface K88 antigen (pili). This appears as beaded strands approximately 3 nm in diameter (P$_2$) stretching out from the cell surfaces. Detached flagella filaments are also evident in this preparation (F). ×63 800

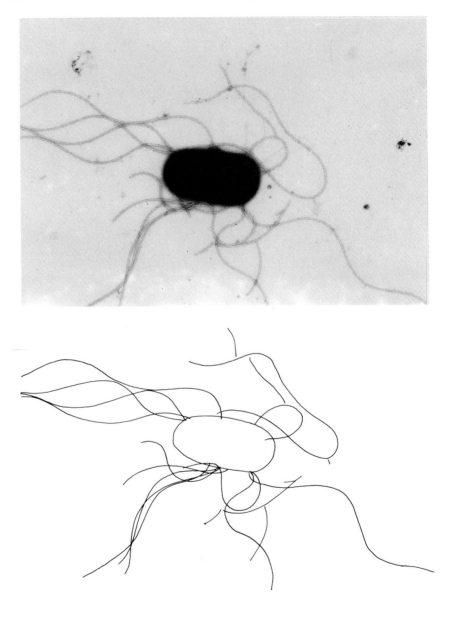

Figure 8. Experimentally observed immune stimulatory activities of immunopotentiators in humoral, cell-mediated and autoimmune responses. IL-1, Interleukin 1; IL-2, Interleukin 2; BCDF, B-cell differentiation factor; BCGF, B-cell growth factor.

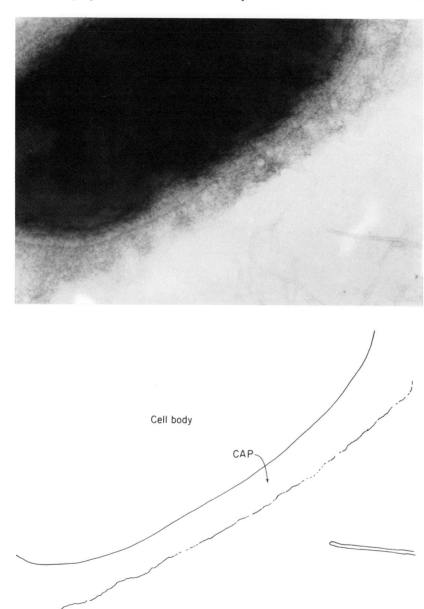

Figure 9. A capsulated gram-negative coliform, negatively stained to show the fibrous nature of the gel which forms a well defined, cell-associated capsule (CAP). ×49 115

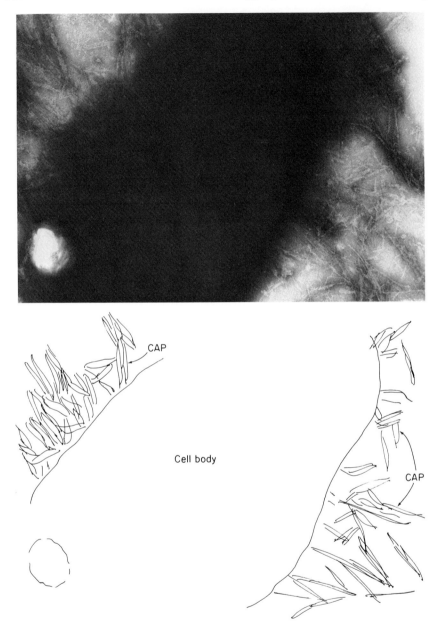

Figure 10. Another gram-negative coliform organism negatively stained to show large amounts of loosely adhering capsular material (CAP) which, in this case, is more noticeably fibrous. Much of this material is released from the cell and appears as aggregates free in the culture medium. × 49 115

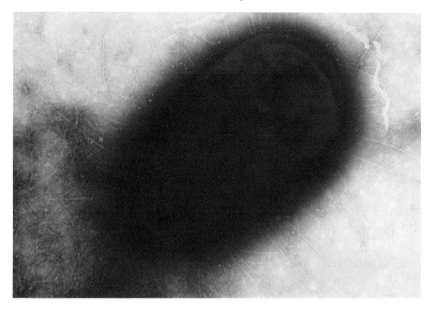

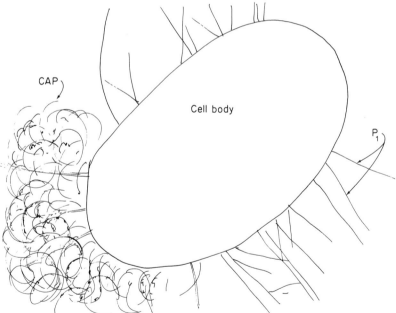

Figure 11. Yet another coliform organism, negatively stained and showing more finely fibrous, curly strands of capsular material localized at one pole of the cell (CAP). Also present are tubular fimbriae (P_1). $\times 30\,965$

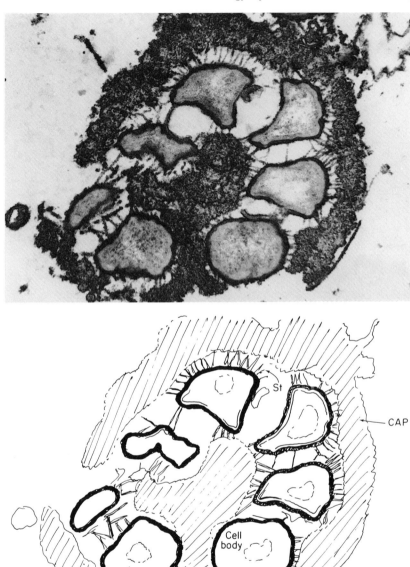

Figure 12. Gram-negative organisms from the solid phase of rumen contents in the form of a microcolony embedded in a considerable accumulation of capsular material. This preparation is a thin section stained with ruthenium red to show acidic polysaccharide as electron-dense material. The strands (St) which apparently connect the bacterial cells to the mass of capsular material (CAP) are probably artifacts caused by shrinkage of the organisms away from the capsular mass during specimen preparation. × 37 840

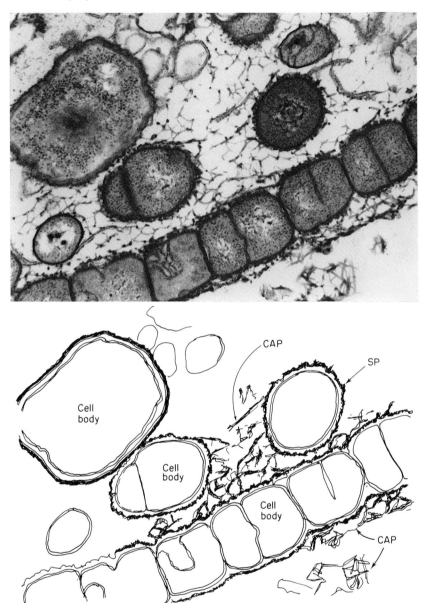

Figure 13. The predominance of capsular material in specimens of rumen contents is clearly seen in this thin section stained by ruthenium red. All the organisms seen are embedded in a mass of acidic polysaccharide, which has condensed into strands (CAP) of darkly stained material associated with the various cell surfaces. Note also that the outer layers of the cell envelopes are also stained darkly, showing closely associated acidic polysaccharides (SP). ×30 965

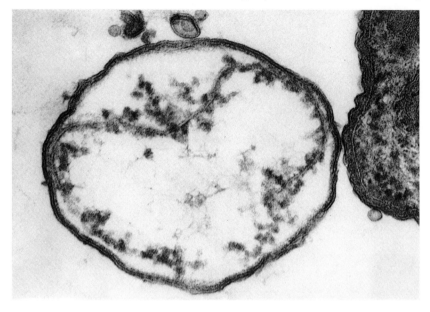

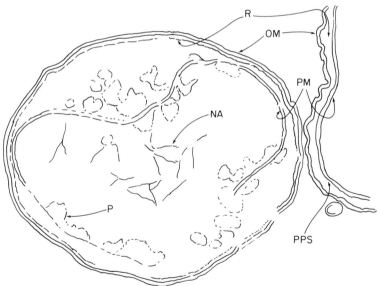

Figure 14. Thin section of a lysed cell of *Pseudomonas aeruginosa* showing the various layers of the cell envelope. In this cell, most of the cytoplasmic contents have been released, apart from a few polysomes (P) and threads of DNA (NA). The outer membrane profile can be seen as a triple-tracked structure (OM), with the associated rigid layer (R) lying immediately beneath it, and still closely apposed. The plasma membrane (PM) has peeled away and is present in several large fragments. An envelope profile of an intact cell is seen alongside the lysed cell and shows the relationships of the various envelope layers to one another in the viable cell. The space between the outer membrane and the plasma membrane, the periplasmic space (PPS), is evident. ×116 050

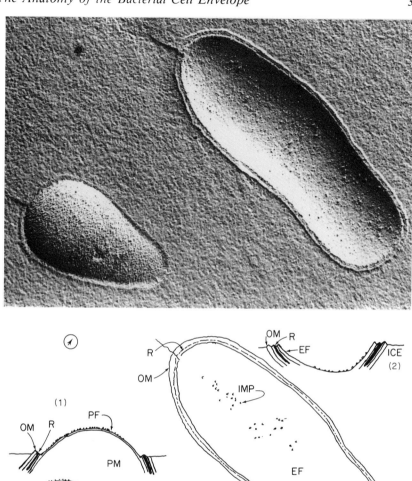

Figure 15. Freeze-fractured cells of *E. coli* showing the fracture faces of the two halves of the plasma membrane with the outer membrane and rigid layer in cross fracture. The fracture planes in the two cells, which tend to follow the interior of bilayer membranes, are illustrated in profile in the line drawings which show the appearance of (1) the PF face (the outer surface of the inner half of the plasma membrane bilayer) which is richly endowed with intramembrane protein particles (IMP), and (2) the EF face (the inner surface of the outer half of the plasma membrane bilayer) which characteristically has fewer intramembrane particles associated with it. The slightly enlarged periplasmic space at the poles of the cells is a common feature of gram-negative organisms. The encircled arrow shows the direction of shadowing. ×41 800

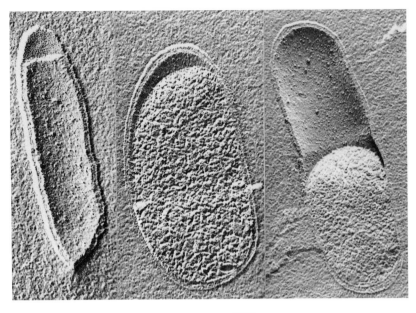

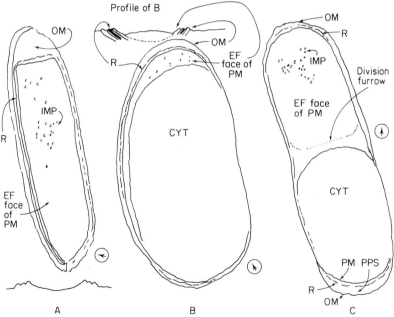

Figure 16. Three views of freeze-fractured cells of *E. coli* showing details of the layers in the cell envelope. In A, a rare fracture plane through the outer membrane (OM) is seen at the top of the fragment of the cell envelope; lying immediately above this is the rigid layer (R) and outer half of the plasma membrane (EF face). In B, a cross fracture showing cytoplasm (CYT) and an EF fracture face of the plasma membrane, with the distinct R layer and outer membrane most clearly revealed at the poles of the cell. In C, the envelope layers are revealed in tangential fracture at the top of the picture and in true cross fracture at the bottom, with the cell showing an early stage in division.
A, ×45 925; B, ×45 485; C, ×31 350

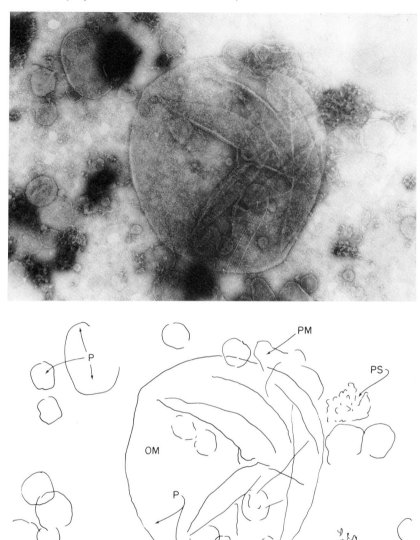

Figure 17. Negatively stained preparation of a total envelope fraction of *E. coli* after disruption with glass beads, showing large fragments of outer membrane (OM) with many porin complexes (P), just resolved as fine doughnut structures, forming a regular lattice. Some plasma membrane fragments (PM) are also visible, these tending to be much more irregular in shape. Cytoplasmic polysomes (PS) are also visible in the background.
× 39 930

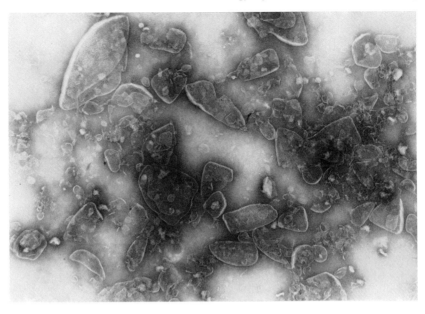

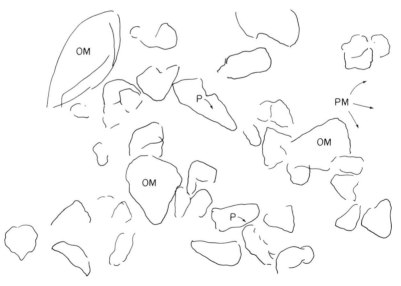

Figure 18. A similar negatively stained total envelope fraction from *Pseudomonas aeruginosa*, showing fragments of outer membrane (OM) carrying porin complexes, along with more irregularly shaped plasma membrane fragments (PM). × 30 580

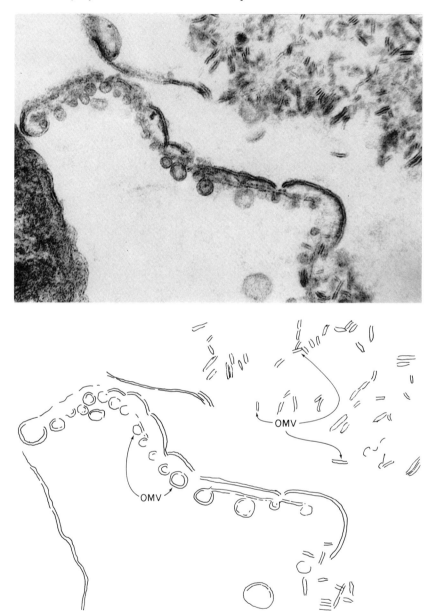

Figure 19. A thin-section of an autolysed cell of *Pseudomonas aeruginosa* showing fragmentation of the outer membrane into small flattened vesicles rich in LPS (OMV). Many of these are seen in cross-section and appear as triple-tracked (dark–light–dark) structures. These small vesicles are frequently shed from gram-negative bacteria without loss of viability. ×116 050

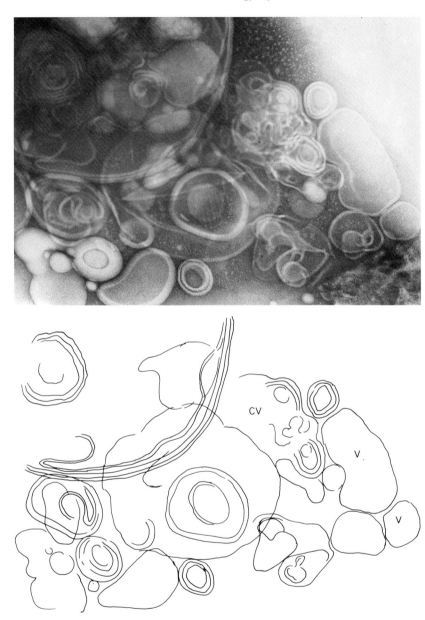

Figure 20.

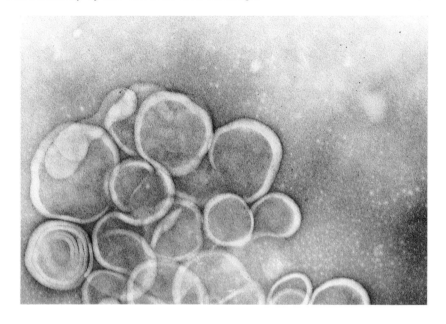

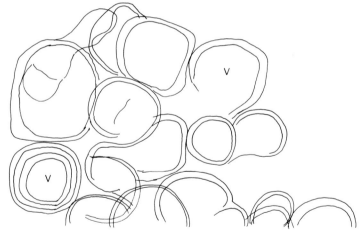

Figure 21.

Figures 20 and 21. Lipopolysaccharide extracted from *E. coli* envelope fractions by the aqueous phenol method. Many single and multilamellar vesicles (V) are seen along with more complex convoluted structures (CV) composed of multiple layers of lipopolysaccharide. Figure 20, × 104 500; Figure 21, × 143 000

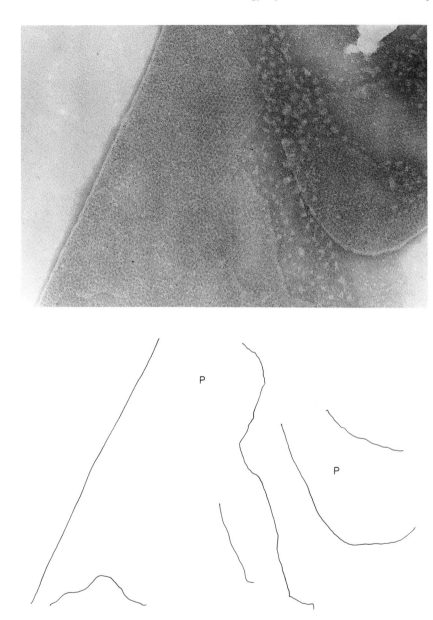

Figure 22. Total envelope fraction of *E. coli* after extensive washing in hot sodium dodecyl sulphate, negatively stained to reveal the rigid layer and associated proteins (P) arranged as hexagonally packed complexes. × 104 500

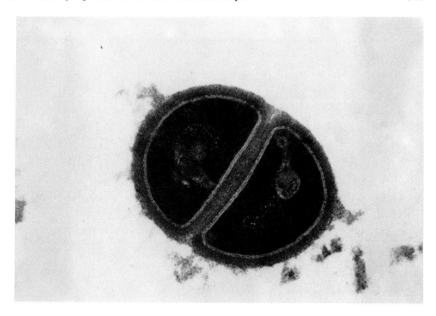

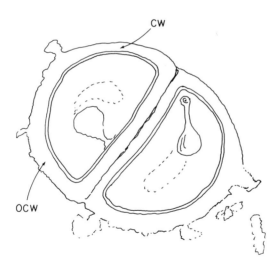

Figure 23. A thin section of a dividing cell of *Micrococcus luteus* showing a relatively thick amorphous cell wall (CW). The septum shows the beginning of the central splitting which will eventually spread across the cell to release two daughter cells. The region of older wall (OCW) is recognizable by its surface irregularity, caused by wall fragments being sloughed off into the medium. ×48 675

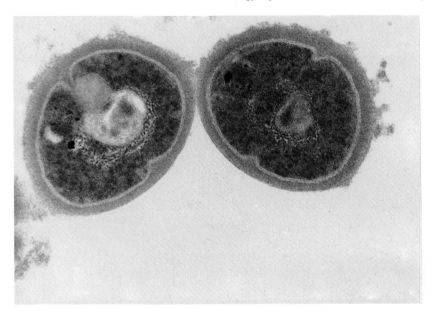

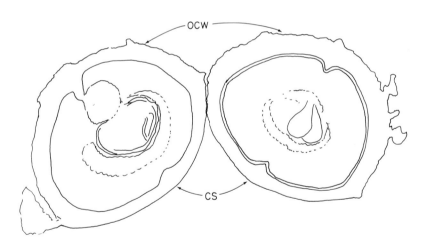

Figure 24. Thin-section of *Micrococcus luteus* after division, with the two daughter cells about to separate. The newly cleaved septum (CS) has a very sharply defined surface whereas the older cell wall (OCW) is much more uneven, with fragments being continuously released. ×48 675

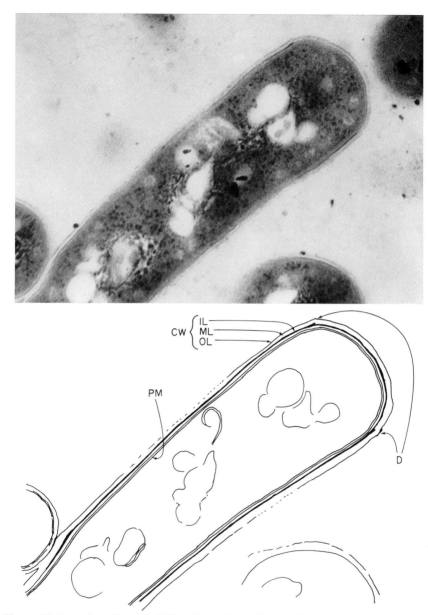

Figure 25. A section of a cell of *Mycobacterium phlei* showing the cell wall (CW) with layers of material which stain differentially. An outer dense layer (OL) overlies an unstained layer (ML), which in turn has a densely staining layer (IL) on its inner surface. Beneath the cell wall layers the triple track of the plasma membrane (PM) can be seen. The lugs (D) on the cell wall which remain after cleavage following the previous cell division are evident on all three wall layers. Walls in this group, in common with other acid-fast bacteria, are rich in complex lipid. × 53 900

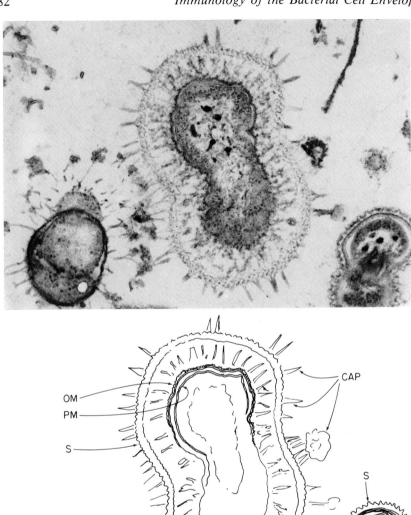

Figure 26. An unidentified bacterium from the rumen, seen in thin section. It shows an elaborate structured layer (S) which appears beneath condensed capsular material (CAP). Underlying the structured layer is a large compartment filled with unidentified stained material. Beneath this, the cell wall layers are characteristic of a gram-negative bacterium with outer (OM) and plasma (PM) membranes clearly defined. Part of a second cell is evident in the same micrograph, which also shows a well-defined structured layer (S). ×44 275

as opposed to the more usual diameter of 12–20 nm. In the spirochaetes, the flagellar filaments (axial filaments) are not exposed as surface antigens but lie beneath the outer layer of the cell envelope.

Many of the features discussed briefly above are illustrated in the following electron micrographs. Salient features are noted by lettering the appropriate areas in the line drawings which accompany each micrograph.

ACKNOWLEDGEMENTS

I wish to thank Dr. Julian Beesley for providing Figure 6, Dr. Alan Williams for providing Figure 26 and the material shown in Figures 12 and 13, and Ian McKie for the photographs of Figures 1 and 2. Figure 2 was developed from a drawing originally published by Dr. B. Lugtenberg (see further reading) although the responsibility for the version shown is mine.

FURTHER READING

Lugtenberg, B., and van Alphen, L. (1983). Molecular architecture and functioning of the outer membrane of *Escherichia coli* and other Gram-negative bacteria. *Biochim. Biophys. Acta*, **737**, 51–115.

Shockman, G. D., and Barrett, J. F. (1983). Structure, function and assembly of cell walls of Gram-positive bacteria. *Annu. Rev. Microbiol.*, **37**, 501–518.

Sleytr, U. B., and Messner, P. (1983). Crystalline surface layers on bacteria. *Annu. Rev. Microbiol.*, **37**, 311–340.

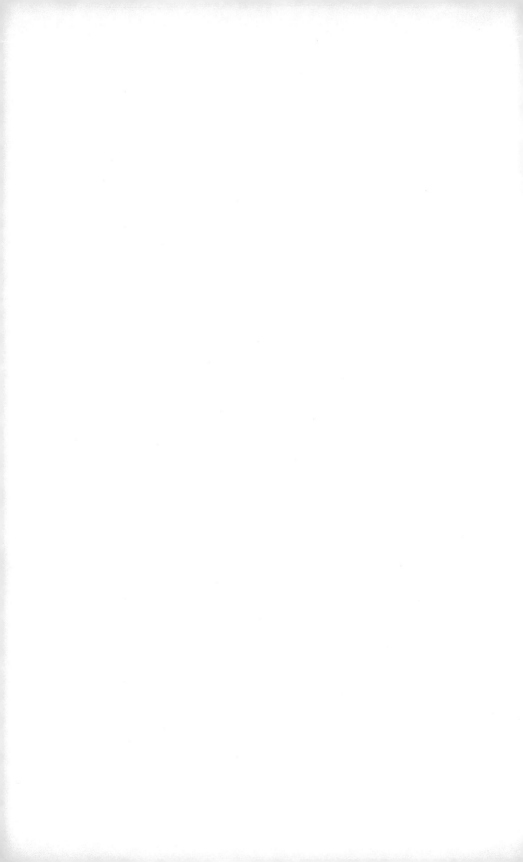

Index